Updates on Renal Replacement Therapy

Edited by Henry H.L. Wu

Published in London, United Kingdom

Updates on Renal Replacement Therapy
http://dx.doi.org/10.5772/intechopen.107663
Edited by Henry H.L. Wu

Contributors
Mathew George Kunthara, Maiko Alejandro Tavera Díaz, Susan Atieno Onyango, Grace Nyawira Njuguna, Božidar Vujičić, Koraljka Benko, Ana Petretić, Nenad Nemarnik, Matko Spicijarić, Dean Markić, Matej Bura, Fabio Kadum, Sanjin Racki, Alen Ružić, Mansour Ghafourifard, Dhaval Patel, Gurleen Kaur, Hussain Majeed, Megan Joseph, Randah Dahlan, Ali Alkatheeri, Tomoyuki Takura, Naotsugu Ichimaru, Atushi Aikawa, Haseeba Shouket, Eman Abdelmohsen Sanad, Djamila-Djahida Batouche, Djilali Batouche, Kamel Elhalimi

First published in London, United Kingdom, 2024 by IntechOpen
IntechOpen is the global imprint of INTECHOPEN LIMITED, registered in England and Wales, registration number: 11086078, 5 Princes Gate Court, London, SW7 2QJ, United Kingdom

British Library Cataloguing-in-Publication Data
A catalogue record for this book is available from the British Library

Additional hard and PDF copies can be obtained from orders@intechopen.com

Updates on Renal Replacement Therapy
Edited by Henry H.L. Wu
p. cm.
Print ISBN 978-1-83769-174-6
Online ISBN 978-1-83769-175-3
eBook (PDF) ISBN 978-1-83769-176-0

For EU product safety concerns:
IN TECH d.o.o., Prolaz Marije Krucifikse Kozulić 3, 51000 Rijeka, Croatia,
info@intechopen.com or visit our website at intechopen.com.

Meet the editor

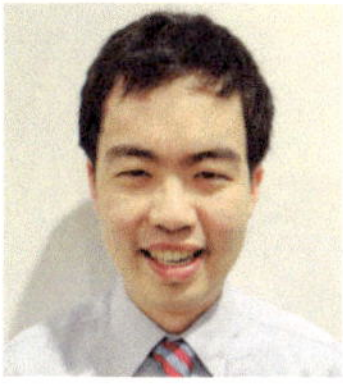

Dr. Henry H.L. Wu is currently a Ph.D. candidate in medicine and health at the Kolling Institute of Medical Research, University of Sydney, Australia, and a visiting researcher at the University of New South Wales, Australia. Dr. Wu was a National Institute of Health Research (NIHR) academic clinical fellow in nephrology at the University of Manchester, England from 2019 to 2021, where his research focused on older people and complex health needs. He has research experience in chronic kidney disease (CKD) epidemiology, geriatric nephrology, glomerulonephritis, and COVID-19 clinical nephrology. Dr. Wu has published widely in key journals and presented at major international nephrology conferences. He has been invited as a peer reviewer for various journals. He is an associate editor of Nutrition and Health, a review editor of the nephrology section of Frontiers in Medicine, and an editorial board member of BMC Nephrology and PloS One. Dr. Wu was a co-organizer of the Royal Society of Medicine Geriatric Nephrology Symposium in late 2021 and was selected as the mentee for the International Society of Nephrology Mentorship Program for the Geriatric-Palliative Nephrology Section. He is also currently an early/mid-career researcher and a member of the International Society of Nephrology CardioRenal Toolkit Workgroup. Dr. Wu was elected for full membership to Sigma Xi, The Scientific Honor Research Society, in May 2023.

Contents

Preface

There is an increased incidence of chronic kidney disease (CKD) progressing to renal failure, as our aging population continues to expand across the globe. Hence, the number of people indicated for renal replacement therapy in the form of dialysis (hemodialysis and peritoneal dialysis) and renal transplantation is also increasing. National and international registry data have highlighted the growing incidence and prevalence of renal replacement therapy. Renal replacement therapy is not an appropriate option for all adults. Older patients living with advanced frailty status and a high number of comorbidities may prefer supportive care without renal replacement therapy to achieve a better quality of life in the short time they have left considering their poor overall prognosis. For those who are deemed suitable candidates for renal replacement therapy, there are many facets of care to consider in aiming for the successful delivery of renal replacement therapy – from guiding patient choice and educating patients regarding their preferred modality of renal replacement therapy to optimizing treatment adequacy and managing treatment-related complications, to ensuring there are appropriate levels of caregiver and financial support, and to integrating advances in innovation and technology in maximizing renal replacement therapy outcomes.

Renal failure may also occur as a result of acute kidney injury (AKI), which could be due to CKD and/or other causes. Renal replacement therapy in the form of continuous renal replacement therapy or other dialysis modalities may be indicated within an intensive care setting. For individuals in these circumstances, there are challenging decisions to make on whether to initiate renal replacement therapy, selection of renal replacement therapy modality, prescription and optimization of renal replacement therapy in intensive care, and at what point it may be in the patient's best interest to withdraw renal replacement therapy and consider palliative treatment.

This book provides a comprehensive global update on the delivery of renal replacement therapy, featuring extensive discussion on recent advances within various aspects of this topical area.

Dr. Henry H.L. Wu
Renal Research,
Kolling Institute of Medical Research,
The University of Sydney and Royal North Shore Hospital,
Sydney, Australia

Chapter 1

Renal Replacement Therapy in Intensive Care Unit

Dhaval Patel, Hussain Majeed, Megan Joseph and Gurleen Kaur

Abstract

This chapter presents a comprehensive overview of the latest advancements in renal replacement therapy (RRT) including Continuous Renal Replacement Therapy (CRRT), focusing on key topics such as acute kidney injury (AKI), renal replacement techniques, patient selection, vascular access, dialyzer membranes, anticoagulation strategies, optimal RRT prescription, drug dosing, laboratory monitoring, and complications of RRT. The incidence of AKI in intensive care unit (ICU) is estimated to be from 5% to 50%. It carries substantial morbidity and mortality. In this chapter, we aim to emphasize the significance of AKI in ICU and indications that necessitate effective RRT. The chapter explores various renal replacement techniques with emphasis on CRRT, including continuous venovenous hemodialysis, hemodiafiltration, and hemofiltration. The clinical indications and contraindications for CRRT are discussed. Vascular access options, dialyzer membrane characteristics, and anticoagulation strategies are examined, providing insights into their impact on treatment outcomes and patient safety. Additionally, highlighted points include the importance of optimal RRT prescription, drug dosing adjustments, and laboratory monitoring in CRRT. It addresses potential complications associated with CRRT and offers strategies for their prevention and management. Overall, this book chapter aims to serve as a valuable guide for healthcare professionals, providing them with updated information to optimize patient care and improve outcomes in individuals with AKI undergoing RRT in ICU.

Keywords: renal failure, acute kidney injury, continuous renal replacement therapy (CRRT), hemofiltration, hemodialysis, peritoneal dialysis

1. Introduction

1.1 Acute kidney injury

Acute kidney injury (AKI) is a widespread problem. It is often used interchangeably with acute renal failure. The incidence of AKI in intensive care unit (ICU) is wide ranging from 5% to 50% and specific to the type of ICU. AKI can have quite a profound impact on the patient and is associated with severe morbidity and mortality. Mortality can range from 40% to >60%. There are consensus definitions of AKI, and they are broken down into three types.

1.2 KDIGO criteria

An AKI can be defined or diagnosed by various criteria. The most used criteria are the KDIGO (Kidney Disease Improving Global Outcomes) criteria. Others include RIFLE (Risk, Injury, Failure, Loss of kidney function and End-stage kidney disease) and AKIN (Acute Kidney Injury Network) criteria. KDIGO defines AKI as:

- Increase in serum creatinine by greater than or equal to 0.3 mg/dl within 48 hours

- Increase in serum creatinine greater than equal to 1.5 times baseline which is known or presumed to have occurred within the past 7 days or

- Urine volume less than 0.5 ml/kg/h for 6 hours.

1.3 Types of AKI: pre-renal vs. intrinsic vs. post-renal

AKI can be broken up into pre-renal, intrinsic, post-renal causes. Pre-renal is caused when the kidney has ischemia due to decreased generalized perfusion or specifically to the kidney. This can occur through many processes such as hypovolemia, hypotension, hemorrhage, acute heart failure exacerbation, ACE inhibitor use etc.

Intrinsic renal disease can be caused by many varied factors. Renal vascular disease can affect small and large vessels within the kidney. These can be caused by vasculitis, microangiopathic and hemolytic anemias, malignant hypertension, etc. Intrinsic disease can also be glomerular disease that can be primary or secondary to systemic disease. This can cause nephritic or nephrotic pattern of disease. Tubular or interstitial can cause intrinsic disease that causes AKI, also known as ATN, these are caused by ischemic or nephrotoxic exposure, such as medications or contrast dye.

Lastly, post-renal disease is obstructive and can be anywhere in the urinary tract. This can be due to prostatic disease, nephrolithiasis, cancer, etc.

1.4 KDIGO criteria - AKI severity staging

KDIGO guidelines [1] split severity into three groups based on specific creatinine levels and urine output (**Table 1**).

Other guidelines such as RIFLE use reduction in GFR as well. Though both serum creatinine and urine output can be used to diagnose, serum creatinine tends to be a stronger predictor of ICU mortality whereas urine output does not independently predict mortality. Some studies suggest that when both criteria were met, elevated

Stage	Serum creatinine	Urine output
Stage 1	• Increase in sCr to 1.5–1.9 times baseline • Increase sCr by ≥0.3 mg/dl	• UOP <0.5 ml/kg/h for 6–12 hours
Stage 2	• Increase in sCr to 2.0–2.9 times baseline	• UOP < 0.5 ml/kg/h for ≥12 hours
Stage 3	• Increase in sCr to 3 times baseline • Increase in sCr to ≥4.0 mg/dl	• Improved hemodynamic stability compared to standard IHD • Anuria for ≥12 hours

Table 1.
KDIGO AKI stages [1].

serum creatinine and reduced urine output, the risk of death or use of RRT was more strongly correlated. Urine output is also dependent on fluid intake, if the patient has limited fluid intake even a healthy individual cannot meet this criterion. Because of this many experts do not agree on diagnosing of an AKI based solely on urine output.

2. What are the types of renal replacement techniques?

2.1 What is renal replacement therapy?

Renal replacement therapy (RRT) is for patients with severe kidney injury. Hemodialysis is a method that uses a dialysis machine to filter the patient's blood and remove waste products and any volume surplus. The machine uses catheters that fit into the venous system, arteriovenous fistula (AVF) or arteriovenous grafts (AVGs) that will drain the blood and replace it after it is cycled through.

Blood flows through the hemofilter and comes to a semipermeable membrane, using the process of diffusion to separate waste and volume from the patient's blood. The smaller contents such as water and electrolytes can be filtered through and larger molecules such as cells and proteins are maintained in the blood. The semipermeable membrane has different pore sizes that can determine what is able to move through, 10–100 angstroms that will allow smaller molecules <5000 Da.

For diffusion to occur a change in concentration must pull certain toxins and water from the blood out of the circulation. A dialysate fluid is used around the semipermeable membrane to provide the concentration difference. Dialysate fluid usually uses bicarbonate as a buffer such that bicarbonate can be added to the blood; it can have low levels of potassium so that potassium from the blood can be pulled out. Dialysate runs countercurrent to the plasma to maximize the solute difference on both sides.

Multiple modalities of RRT are available, categorized as intermittent hemodialysis (IHD) and continuous renal replacement therapy (CRRT). IHD can be used in patients who are more hemodynamically stable. It can also be used for patients on lower dosing and stable requirement of pressors in ICU at the discretion of nephrologist and critical care physician. They get HD at different intervals depending on need and renal function. CRRT or continuous dialysis is usually 24 hours a day and is used in an ICU setting. There are also hybrid therapies such as sustained low efficiency dialysis (SLED) and extended duration dialysis (EDD). Hybrid therapies are used infrequently, though, this tends to be ICU and institution specific.

CRRT machines can do hemodialysis as described above with diffusive clearance. They can also use hemofiltration which is a convective clearance. The fluids are removed with hydrostatic pressure so that all the toxins and electrolyte abnormalities are removed from the plasma. This can remove small, medium, or large solutes. The greater the fluid movement the more "solute drag" is had, where solutes are moved out of the plasma because of the force of fluid movement. Replacement fluid is then added back to the plasma. The fluid is physiological and contains electrolytes and proteins that are closer to what the body needs or should have. The replacement fluid will have normal concentrations of potassium, bicarbonate, etc. The replacement fluid can be added before the filtration which would dilute the plasma and cause less solute clearance. However, it can prevent clotting and preserve the filter. When added after filtration it is called post-dilution. This can allow for more solute clearance but a higher chance of clotting. A mix of both will allow for balancing the negative consequences. This added fluid will be pulled out through ultrafiltration.

Ultrafiltration works by having fluid cross a semi-permeable membrane. This is done in response to a pressure gradient that can be osmotic, oncotic, or hydrostatic. There can be positive pressure in the plasma pushing fluid out or negative pressure in the dialysate drawing fluid from the plasma. This creates a transmembrane pressure that can control how much fluid is being drawn from the blood.

There are multiple types of CRRT modalities depending on the needs of the patient. These include continuous venovenous hemofiltration (CVVH), continuous venovenous hemodialysis (CVVHD), and continuous venovenous hemodiafiltration (CVVHDF).

CVVH uses hydrostatic pressure with the concept of convection that removes solutes and dialysate fluid is not used. The fluid pulled from the plasma is high, about 20–25 ml/kg/h so there is significant volume depletion. This must be replaced according to the goal that is desired for maintaining even fluid balance or a net negative balance. The addition of fluid dilutes the elevated concentrations of solutes such as urea or creatinine. Predilution also allows urea to be moved out of RBCs into the plasma so once it goes through the filter it can be removed easier.

CVVHD removes solute by diffusion, in which dialysate is used. This is how hemodialysis is done generally and the dialysate fluid runs countercurrent at a rate of 1–2 l/h. The ultrafiltration in this setting is based on desired fluid removal that is desired; no IV fluid replacement is needed.

CVVHDF combines these two modalities. It uses replacement of fluid and dialysate to pull solutes as well as dilute the plasma. The ultrafiltration volume is variable and replacement fluid is used to maintain volume status.

SLED, or **sustained low-efficiency daily dialysis**, is a term to describe prolonged intermittent kidney replacement therapy (PIRKT). The indication is AKI requiring dialysis and they are patients who are too hemodynamically unstable to tolerate standard IHD. SLED is an alternative to CRRT. CRRT, blood pressures are more stable compared to standard intermittent RRT, because the rate of solute and fluid is slower. Mortality rates are comparable with other forms of RRT, including CRRT. PIKRT should be performed at least three times per week to provide adequate dialysis dose. The time per session ranges from 6 to 18 hours. But typically, is about 8 hours per session. Truly, the length of the session depends on the need of the patient and the hemodynamic stability. A systemic review by Aldahbi et al. published in 2021 [2] found no advantage of using CRRT over SLED in hemodynamically unstable AKI patients.

SCUF (slow continuous ultrafiltration) is a RRT technique that removes excess fluid and solutes from the blood in a gradual and continuous manner. This method operates at a slower rate, minimizing abrupt shifts in fluid and electrolyte balance and reducing the risk of hemodynamic instability in critically ill patients. Unlike CRRT, SCUF primarily focuses on fluid removal rather than solute clearance, making it a suitable choice for patients with fluid overload but stable solute levels. However, it may not be as effective in managing severe electrolyte imbalances or uremic toxins as other dialysis modalities.

Peritoneal dialysis (PD) is another modality that can be used. This involves using the patient's peritoneal membrane, the thin membrane that lines the abdominal cavity, as a filter to remove waste products and excess fluid from the body. A catheter with two tubes is placed surgically into the patient's abdomen; one tube is used for inserting the fluid and the other is used for draining the used solution. The solution contains a specific concentration of electrolytes and dextrose that pulls waste products and excess fluids. It remains in the cavity for a certain amount of time, known as the dwell time. This allows the peritoneal membrane to act as a semi-permeable

RRT type	Description	Advantages	Disadvantages
Continuous venovenous hemofiltration	• Uses hydrostatic pressure and convection to remove solutes through a filter. • Dialysate fluid is not used. • High fluid removal rate of 20–25 ml/kg/h, requiring replacement fluids to maintain fluid balance. • Predilution dilutes elevated concentrations of solutes and aids in their removal.	• Effective removal of solutes and fluid through convection	• Requires significant volume replacement
Continuous venovenous hemodialysis	• Removes solutes by diffusion using dialysate fluid. • Dialysate runs by counter-current at a rate of 1 to 2 l/h. • No IV fluid replacement is needed, and ultrafiltration is based on desired fluid removal.	• Well-established technique similar to standard hemodialysis	• Limited solute clearance compared to other modalities
Continuous venovenous hemodiafiltration	• Combines hemofiltration and hemodialysis. • Uses both replacement fluid and dialysate to remove solutes and dilute plasma. • Variable ultrafiltration volume and replacement fluid are used to maintain volume status.	• Enhanced solute clearance compared to CVVH and CVVHD	• Increased complexity and requirement for replacement fluid
Sustained low-efficiency daily dialysis	• PIRKT for hemodynamically unstable patients. • An alternative to CRRT. • Solute and fluid removal rate is slower, providing more stable blood pressures compared to standard IHD. • Typically performed at least three times per week with session durations ranging from 6 to 18 hours, often around 8 hours.	• Improved hemodynamic stability compared to standard IHD	• Longer session durations may limit patient mobility and comfort
Slow continuous ultrafiltration	• Gradual and continuous removal of excess fluid and solutes. • Focuses on fluid removal rather than solute clearance. • Slower rate minimizes abrupt shifts in fluid and electrolyte balance, reducing the risk of hemodynamic instability. • Suitable for patients with fluid overload but relatively stable solute levels.	• Minimizes hemodynamic instability and electrolyte shifts	• Limited solute clearance compared to other modalities

RRT type	Description	Advantages	Disadvantages
Peritoneal dialysis	• Uses the peritoneal membrane in the abdomen as a filter. • Dialysis solution is introduced into the peritoneal cavity, allowing waste products and excess fluid to diffuse across the peritoneum. • Multiple exchanges are performed throughout the day or overnight. • No anticoagulation required. • Not suitable for emergencies or patients with abdominal scarring. • Requires time for catheter insertion and is not ideal for life-threatening hyperkalemia or pulmonary edema.	• Convenient and can be performed at home	• Limited solute clearance compared to other modalities • May not be suitable for patients with high solute loads

Table 2.
RRT types along with their respective advantages and disadvantages [2, 3].

membrane. After the dwell time, the dialysis solution that now has waste products and excess fluid is drained out by gravity using the cycler machine. This process of fluid going in, dwelling, and draining is repeated multiple times during the day or overnight depending on the patient's requirements. PD has certain advantages, namely: it does not require anticoagulation, it is better tolerated and is cheaper than using an expensive dialysis machine and dialysis nurse or tech. However, it's not always feasible to emergently place a PD catheter when emergency dialysis is required. It's preferred that at least 2 weeks be allowed before using the PD catheter after it is inserted. Because the solute and volume clearance are slow, it is not a desirable choice for life-threatening hyperkalemia or pulmonary edema. Patients who have had abdominal surgery or peritoneal scarring cannot use the peritoneum as a dialytic membrane (**Table 2**).

3. Clinical indications and contraindications

CRRT is indicated in severe AKI in hemodynamically unstable patients. Many patients in the hospital have a mild AKI in the setting of acute tubular necrosis, drug induced nephropathy, or pre-renal hypoperfusion, these will require IV fluids and time and, the kidneys will recover. ICU patients tend to have more severe cases of AKI with significant tubular necrosis where fluid resuscitation may not improve the kidney function.

Indications for CRRT [4]:

1. Fluid overload: CRRT can help to remove excess fluid from the body in patients with fluid overload, which can occur because of heart failure, liver failure, or other medical conditions.

2. Electrolyte imbalances: CRRT can be used to correct electrolyte imbalances in the blood, such as hyperkalemia, hypernatremia, and metabolic acidosis.

3. Toxin removal: CRRT can be used to remove toxins from the blood, such as those that result from drug overdoses, poisonings, or metabolic disorders as well as in uremia.

Relative contraindications for CRRT:

1. Bleeding disorders: Patients with bleeding disorders or who are at elevated risk of bleeding may not be good candidates for CRRT, since the anticoagulants used in CRRT can increase the risk of bleeding.

2. Hemodynamic instability: Patients with severe hemodynamic instability, such as those with severe hypotension, may not be able to tolerate the fluid and electrolyte shifts that can occur during CRRT.

3. Active infection: Patients with active infections or who are at elevated risk of infection may not be good candidates for CRRT, since the use of a catheter to connect the patient to the CRRT machine can increase the risk of infection.

4. Coagulopathy: Patients with coagulopathy, or who are at elevated risk of developing blood clots, may not be good candidates for CRRT, since the hemofilter used in CRRT can promote clot formation.

4. Types of vascular access

Vascular access involves the insertion of a catheter into a large vein to provide access for the CRRT machine. There are several types of vascular access options available for CRRT for placement of central venous catheters (CVCs). Either subclavian vein, internal jugular vein or femoral vein can be used for CVC placement. CRRT capable catheters need to be able to handle blood flow of 200–250 ml/min. Internal jugular vein is the preferred site.

Given that vascular access is required for CRRT, the introduction of a vascular catheter into a vein always poses a risk of infection. The femoral site has been commonly known to carry a higher risk of infection as compared to other potential sites of vascular access such as jugular or subclavian veins. Typical risk factors for infection include improper catheter care, prolonged catheterization, immunocompromised status, and underlying comorbidities.

Interestingly, a large trial in JAMA in 2008 (by Parienti et al.) [5] found that, in terms of infections and its complications, jugular and femoral sites were equivalent. However, internal jugular vein insertion may be preferable in obese patients.

According to a systematic review and meta-analysis published in the Journal of Critical Care in 2019 (by Clark et al.) [6], the overall rate of catheter-related bloodstream infection (CRBSI) in CRRT was approximately 7.4 per 1000 catheter-days. However, the specific infection rates associated with femoral vascular access were not explicitly mentioned in the study.

The right internal jugular vein is the preferred site for a temporary catheter in CRRT due to its direct route to the superior vena cava. The catheter tip should be positioned at the junction of the SVC and the right atrium. The left jugular vein has a more indirect path to the right atrium, potentially causing inadequate blood flows and filter issues. The femoral veins are a secondary option due to their accessibility. Subclavian veins are used as a last resort due to concerns about stenosis, especially if the patient may require an AVF or AVG in the same arm in the future.

Subclavian vein stenosis in CRRT is a potential complication, though its exact incidence varies. Prolonged catheter use, catheter-related factors, and individual patient characteristics contribute to its development. Rates range from 1% to 10%. Careful catheter insertion techniques, appropriate catheter size selection, and regular monitoring are important for mitigating the risk. Prompt evaluation and intervention, such as percutaneous transluminal angioplasty (PTA), may be necessary if subclavian vein stenosis occurs to maintain effective CRRT.

A recent study by Xu et al. [7] evaluated the safety and efficacy of a newly developed PTA technique for maintaining vascular access in patients undergoing CRRT. The study found that the PTA technique was safe and effective in maintaining vascular access in patients with central venous stenosis, and it significantly reduced the incidence of catheter-related infections and thrombosis. The study recommended the use of the PTA technique for the maintenance of vascular access in patients with central venous stenosis undergoing CRRT.

Transhepatic and trans lumbar approaches are alternative methods for dialysis access when traditional options are not possible. The transhepatic approach involves inserting a catheter through the liver, while the trans lumbar approach involves accessing the lumbar vein through the lower back. These methods require expertise in interventional radiology and carry risks such as infection and catheter dysfunction. They are temporary solutions until more permanent access can be established.

In summary, vascular access is a critical aspect of CRRT, and the choice of access site should be individualized to each patient's clinical condition.

5. Dialyzer membrane

In both IHD and CRRT, standard dialyzers are used. Semipermeable hollow fiber dialyzers are the current standard of care. KDIGO suggests using a biocompatible membrane for both IHD and CRRT (2C) [1].

There are many distinct types of membranes available. Modified cellulose and synthetic membranes such as ones made from Poly sulfone are thought to be compatible membranes. All dialyzers activate the complement system. The dialyzer membrane that activates the complement system such that it leads to fever, hypotension, vasodilation, leucopenia, and hypoxia are "bioincompatible". It should be noted that a Cochrane meta-analysis in 2008 [8] did not show any difference between bioincompatible and biocompatible membranes.

The other property to be considered is flux. Flux is the permeability of dialyzer membrane. Clearance of beta-2 microglobulin defines low (<10 cc/min), medium (10–20 cc/min) and high (>20 cc/min) flux, respectively. It has been a matter of debate whether high flux membranes would be more beneficial as it can clear larger solutes. To this point, there is some evidence from a couple meta-analyses that showed potential benefit for high flux dialyzer membrane in hemodialysis patients [9].
A well-designed RCT is needed to further study this.

6. Anticoagulation

CRRT requires anticoagulation to prevent clotting of the extracorporeal circuit, which can lead to circuit failure, decreased filter life, and an increased bleeding risk. There are several different methods of anticoagulation for CRRT [10], including:

- Unfractionated heparin (UFH)
- Low molecular weight heparin (LMWH)
- Regional citrate anticoagulation (RCA)
- Prostacyclin

The choice of anticoagulant is based on a variety of factors, including the patient's underlying medical conditions, bleeding risk, and the preference and experience of the treating physician.

6.1 Unfractionated heparin

UFH is a commonly used anticoagulant for CRRT. It works by binding to anti-thrombin III, which subsequently inhibits thrombin and other coagulation factors. Dosing is typically titrated to achieve a target activated partial thromboplastin time (aPTT) or activated clotting time (ACT). Typical ranges for aPTT are between 45–60 seconds and 180–220 seconds for ACT. UFH carries the often-cumbersome need for careful monitoring of the patient's clotting function and frequent dosing adjustments to maintain the target aPTT or ACT.

6.2 Low molecular weight heparin

LMWH is another type of heparin occasionally used for CRRT. It has a similar mechanism of action to UFH, but comparatively holds a lower affinity to anti-thrombin III. As a result, they have a more predictable anticoagulant effect. As such, LMWH does not require monitoring of clotting function, and dosing is usually based on the patient's weight.

6.3 Regional citrate anticoagulation

RCA is a method of anticoagulation involving the infusion of citrate into the extra-corporeal circuit. Citrate's mechanism of action is binding to ionized calcium, which is necessary for the activation of coagulation factors. By chelating ionized calcium, citrate inhibits coagulation within the circuit. RCA also requires careful monitoring of the patient's acid–base and electrolyte status, as citrate metabolism can lead to metabolic alkalosis, hypocalcemia, and hypernatremia. However, these effects can be diminished by infusing calcium into the circuit and using a low bicarbonate dialysate or chloride based intravenous fluids. Using a higher chloride citrate solution can also blunt the alkalotic effect. Hypernatremia can be prevented by using lower sodium dialysate or appropriate replacement fluids.

A recent meta-analysis published in 2022 compared the efficacy of citrate vs. heparin anticoagulation in critically ill patients on undergoing CRRT [10]. The study

Anticoagulation method	Mechanism	Advantages	Disadvantages
Unfractionated heparin	Binds to antithrombin III, inhibits thrombin and factor Xa	Widely available, reversible, familiar dosing	Increased bleeding risk, requires monitoring, heparin-induced thrombocytopenia
Low molecular weight heparin	Binds to antithrombin III, inhibits factor Xa more than thrombin	Longer half-life, predictable dosing	Risk of bleeding, accumulation in renal dysfunction, expensive
Regional citrate anticoagulation	Citrate infused pre-filter, calcium replacement post-filter	Reduced bleeding risk, no systemic anticoagulation required	Need for calcium monitoring, risk of metabolic derangements

Table 3.
Comparing major types of anticoagulation in CRRT [10].

noted no significant difference in mortality, metabolic alkalosis, and circuit loss between the two groups. It did note that the citrate group had the advantage of an overall longer filter life and significantly lower risk of bleeding and heparin-induced thrombocytopenia. As such, RCA was deemed to have priority for CRRT in critically ill patients (**Table 3**).

6.4 Monitoring clotting function and dosing

It is essential to monitor the clotting function of the blood during CRRT and adjust the anticoagulant dosing accordingly.

During CRRT, the clotting function of the blood is monitored using either the aPTT or the ACT. The aPTT measures the time it takes for clotting to occur in a blood sample after the addition of an activator, while the ACT measures the time it takes for clotting to occur in a blood sample after the addition of an activator and a contact activator. Both tests are used to monitor the effectiveness of UFH anticoagulation.

The dose of UFH for CRRT is typically titrated to achieve a target aPTT or ACT. The initial dose is usually 500–1000 units per hour, with adjustments made every 4–6 hours based on the patient's clotting function. LMWH dosing is based on the patient's weight, with dalteparin typically given as a subcutaneous injection at a dose of 5000 units every 12 hours. There is insufficient data to currently recommend for the use of LMWH in CRRT circuit.

RCA dosing is based on the infusion rate of citrate, which is typically started at a rate of 4–6 mmol/min and adjusted based on the patient's ionized calcium levels (iCa). Goal is to maintain iCa between 1 and 1.4 mg/dl (0.25–0.35 mmol/l).

6.5 Complications

Despite appropriate anticoagulant dosing and monitoring, complications can still occur during CRRT. One of the main complications of CRRT is circuit clotting, which can lead to decreased filter life and increased risk of bleeding. Other complications include bleeding from anticoagulation, metabolic derangements from RCA, and hypotension from the fluid removal during CRRT.

6.6 Conclusion

The choice of anticoagulant for CRRT is a complex one that should be made on a case-by-case basis. There is no single "best" anticoagulant, and the best choice will vary depending on the patient's individual circumstances.

7. Optimal RRT prescription, initiation timing, drug dosing, and lab monitoring, complications of RRT

7.1 Optimal RRT modality

The choice of RRT depends on the institution, resources available, nurses training and patient's clinical status. Either IHD, PD, PIKRT such as SLED or CRRT can be used in ICU. CRRT tends to be the preferred modality in most ICUs. Given, CRRT does not require blood flow rates as high as IHD, CRRT tends to be the preferred modality for hemodynamically unstable patients. However, there is not any evidence that supports one modality over another.

A systematic review and meta-analysis published in 2021 (by Ye et al.) [11] compared different modalities of RRT through 31 randomized controlled trials. The review concluded that there was no overall difference in mortality between CRRT and IHD. However, CRRT was noted to increase renal recovery compared to IHD. Slow-efficiency extended dialysis with hemofiltration may be the most effective intervention at reducing mortality, but more research is needed. PD is associated with good efficacy and the least number of complications but may not be practical in all settings. ICU clinicians should feel comfortable that the differences between CRRT, IHD, slow efficiency extended dialysis, and PD are small, and any of these modalities is a reasonable option to employ in critically ill patients.

SLED can be useful if the patient requires multiple procedures that would interrupt CRRT, Since CRRT needs to be operating with as few interruptions as possible over 24 hours. Some institutions use SLED to transition patients from CRRT to standard IHD as hemodynamic stability improves.

One meta-analysis found no statistically significant difference between SLED and CRRT regarding patient-centered outcomes such as mortality, kidney function, recovery, dialysis dependence, length of stay in ICU, and fluid rate. SLED is also generally less expensive to administer and has similar safety for patients as CRRT.

Timing of onset: Multiple trials have compared the timing of RRT initiation in critically ill patients with AKI. Early RRT initiation (within 12 hours of identification) was not associated with improved outcomes and may be associated with increased risk of adverse events. Delayed RRT initiation (until indications develop) is preferred [12], but there are likely to be limits to how long RRT can be safely delayed. The optimal timing of RRT initiation is still unknown.

- The STARRT-AKI trial [13] found no difference in mortality at 90 days between patients who received early RRT and those who received delayed RRT. However, patients who received early KRT were more likely to remain RRT-dependent at 90 days and to require rehospitalization.

- A meta-analysis of nine studies [14] found no difference in mortality at 28, 60, or 90 days between patients who received early RRT and those who received delayed RRT.

- The AKIKI-2 trial [15] found that mortality was higher in patients who had RRT deferred until an urgent indication developed or the BUN exceeded 140 mg/dL, but the difference was not statistically significant.

Based on the available evidence, delayed RRT initiation is preferred in critically ill patients with AKI. However, the optimal timing of RRT initiation is still unknown and may vary depending on individual patient characteristics.

Session length: Session length depends on the modality of dialysis and patients' ability to tolerate it. IHD is about 3–4 hours 2–3 times a week. PIKRT is 3 times a week but for 8–16 hours a day. CRRT is optimally applied for 24 hours a day.

Dialysate flow rate: The flow rate ranges from 100 to 400 ml/min. The dialysate flow rate is adjusted for the anticipated duration of the session. There is a finite amount of dialysate volume per session, based on how much the machine can accommodate. If the session is needed to last more than 8 hours for example, a lower flow rate may be needed. The dialysis flow rates for CRRT and PIKRT are lower than IHD 100–200 ml/min compared to IHD 300-400 ml/min.

CRRT dialysate dosing: The 'Randomized Evaluation of Normal versus Augmented Level of RRT' (RENAL) trial [16] and the 'Acute Renal Failure Trial Network' (ATN) [17] trials were two large clinical trials that evaluated the higher intensity (40 or 35 cc/kg/h) vs. lower intensity (25 or 20 cc/kg/h) dosing of CRRT. There was no difference found between lower intensity vs. higher intensity groups. Lower intensity dosing is currently recommended.

Ultrafiltration rate: The rate is determined by hemodynamic stability and urgency to remove excess fluid. With hemodynamically unstable patients, UF of 50 ml/h is a good starting place and can increase over time, However, if a patient is severely volume overloaded and can tolerate higher volume removal, a much higher ultra filtration rate can be targeted. For IHD, multiple liters of fluid negativity per session can be targeted based on hemodynamic stability.

Blood flow: The highest blood flow that the catheter will allow is used. It is usually initiated at100mL/min for CRRT and gradually increased to 200 cc/min. The higher the blood flow, the less likely a clot forms in the extracorporeal circuit. IHD can be initiated at 300–400 ml/min.

Drug Dosing: Volume of distribution, Vd and protein binding determine the effectiveness of a drug for a patient on CRRT 24 hours a day. Ideally, an ICU pharmacist should help dose medications for patients on CRRT 24 hours a day. If a drug is less than 2000 Da in weight, it might be readily removed on CRRT. Such drugs may need a higher dosing than usual dosing. The higher the protein bound content, the lesser the likelihood the drug will be cleared during CRRT. If a patient is volume overloaded, the higher Vd should be accounted for compared to ideal body weight and drug should be dosed accordingly. When possible and where available, follow plasma concentrations of drugs to achieve therapeutic levels. If a patient is on intermittent dialysis, it may be possible to dose a drug whose clearance may be affected by dialysis outside the dialytic time.

Complications: The major complications Include hypotension and abnormalities in electrolytes, albumin, calcium, and phosphate. As far as hypotension, PIKRT or SLED is well tolerated. Like CRRT, the slow blood flow rates and low UF allows hemodynamically unstable patients to tolerate it well. Hypophosphatemia only occurs with prolonged or frequent PIKRT and requires phosphate supplementation.

It is typically recommended that electrolytes and acid–base status be monitored every 6–12 hours initially for CRRT. Should the patient remain stable with minimal electrolyte changes after 24–48 hours, lab monitoring frequency can be further spaced to every 12–24 hours.

In recent years, there have been some updates in CRRT monitoring technology, aimed at improving the accuracy and efficiency of the process. For example, newer CRRT machines now incorporate advanced sensors and algorithms that can detect changes in blood flow and pressure, helping to prevent clotting and other complications.

Another recent development is the use of electronic medical records (EMRs) and data analytics tools to track patient outcomes and identify potential areas for improvement. This approach has been shown to reduce errors and improve overall quality of care in CRRT patients.

Author details

Dhaval Patel[1]*, Hussain Majeed[2], Megan Joseph[2] and Gurleen Kaur[1]

1 Core Faculty of Northeast Georgia Medical Center, Internal Medicine Residency, Gainesville, GA, USA

2 Northeast Georgia Medical Center, Internal Medicine Residency Program, USA

*Address all correspondence to: dhavalpatel05@gmail.com

References

[1] Kidney Disease: Improving Global Outcomes (KDIGO) Acute Kidney Injury Work Group. KDIGO Clinical Practice Guideline for Acute Kidney Injury. Kidney International Supplements. 2012;**2**(1-138):19-36

[2] Dalbhi SA, Alorf R, Alotaibi M, Altheaby A, Alghamdi Y, Ghazal H, et al. Sustained low efficiency dialysis is non-inferior to continuous renal replacement therapy in critically ill patients with acute kidney injury: A comparative meta-analysis. Medicine (Baltimore). 2021;**100**(51):e28118. DOI: 10.1097/MD.0000000000028118. PMID: 34941056; PMCID: PMC8702221

[3] Macedo E, Mehta RL. Continuous Dialysis Therapies: Core Curriculum 2016. American Journal of Kidney Diseases. 2016;**68**(4):645-657. DOI: 10.1053/j.ajkd.2016.03.427

[4] Golper TA. Indications, technical considerations, and strategies for renal replacement therapy in the intensive care unit. Journal of Intensive Care Medicine. 1992;**7**(6):310-317. DOI: 10.1177/088506669200700604. PMID: 10147940

[5] Parienti J, Thirion M, Mégarbane B, et al. Femoral vs jugular venous catheterization and risk of nosocomial events in adults requiring acute renal replacement therapy: a randomized controlled trial. Journal of the American Medical Association. 2008;**299**(20):2413-2422. DOI: 10.1001/jama.299.20.2413

[6] Ramritu P, Halton K, Cook D, Whitby M, Graves N. Catheter-related bloodstream infections in intensive care units: a systematic review with meta-analysis. Journal of Advanced Nursing. 2008;**62**(1):3-21. DOI: 10.1111/j.1365-2648.2007.04564.x. PMID: 18352960

[7] Xu R, Wang T, Dmytriw AA, Wang X, Li L, Yang K, et al. Percutaneous transluminal angioplasty and stenting for vertebral artery stenosis. Cochrane Database of Systematic Reviews. 2020;**2020**(7):14-15:CD013692. DOI: 10.1002/14651858.CD013692. PMCID: PMC7389776

[8] Alonso A, Lau J, Jaber BL. Biocompatible hemodialysis membranes for acute renal failure. Cochrane Database of Systematic Reviews. 2008. Issue 1. Art. No.: CD005283. DOI: 10.1002/14651858.CD005283.pub2

[9] Palmer SC, Rabindranath KS, Craig JC, Roderick PJ, Locatelli F, Strippoli GFM. High-flux versus low-flux membranes for end-stage kidney disease. Cochrane Database of Systematic Reviews. 2012. Issue 9. Art. No.: CD005016. DOI: 10.1002/14651858.CD005016.pub2

[10] Li R, Gao X, Zhou T, Li Y, Wang J, Zhang P. Regional citrate versus heparin anticoagulation for continuous renal replacement therapy in critically ill patients: A meta-analysis of randomized controlled trials. Therapeutic Apheresis and Dialysis. 2022;**26**(6):1086-1097. DOI: 10.1111/1744-9987.13850. Epub 2022 Apr 20. PMID: 35385216

[11] Ye Z, Wang Y, Ge L, Guyatt GH, Collister D, Alhazzani W, et al. Comparing renal replacement therapy modalities in critically ill patients with acute kidney injury: a systematic review and network meta-analysis. Critical Care Explorations. 2021;**3**(5):e0399. DOI: 10.1097/CCE.0000000000000399. PMID: 34079944; PMCID: PMC8162503

[12] Gaudry S, Hajage D, Benichou N, Chaïbi K, Barbar S, Zarbock A, et al. Delayed versus early initiation of renal replacement therapy for severe acute kidney injury: a systematic review and individual patient data meta-analysis of randomised clinical trials. Lancet. 2020;**395**(10235):1506-1515. DOI: 10.1016/S0140-6736(20)30531-6. Epub 2020 Apr 23. PMID: 32334654

[13] STARRT-AKI Investigators; Canadian Critical Care Trials Group; Australian and New Zealand Intensive Care Society Clinical Trials Group; United Kingdom Critical Care Research Group; Canadian Nephrology Trials Network; Irish Critical Care Trials Group, Bagshaw SM, Wald R, NKJ A, Bellomo R, da Costa BR, et al. Timing of initiation of renal-replacement therapy in acute kidney injury. The New England Journal of Medicine. 2020;**383**(3):240-251. DOI: 10.1056/NEJMoa2000741. Erratum in: N Engl J Med. 2020 Jul 15. PMID: 32668114

[14] Lai TS, Shiao CC, Wang JJ, Huang CT, Wu PC, Chueh E, et al. Earlier versus later initiation of renal replacement therapy among critically ill patients with acute kidney injury: a systematic review and meta-analysis of randomized controlled trials. Annals of Intensive Care. 2017;**7**(1):38. DOI: 10.1186/s13613-017-0265-6. Epub 2017 Apr 5. PMID: 28382597; PMCID: PMC5382114

[15] Gaudry S, Hajage D, Martin-Lefevre L, Lebbah S, Louis G, Moschietto S, et al. Comparison of two delayed strategies for renal replacement therapy initiation for severe acute kidney injury (AKIKI 2): a multicentre, open-label, randomised, controlled trial. Lancet. 2021;**397**(10281):1293-1300. DOI: 10.1016/S0140-6736(21)00350-0. PMID: 33812488

[16] Finfer S, Cass A, Gallagher M, Lee J, Su S, Bellomo R; RENAL Study Investigators. The RENAL (Randomised Evaluation of Normal vs. Augmented Level of Replacement Therapy) study: statistical analysis plan. Critical Care and Resuscitation. 2009;11(1):58-66. PMID: 19281446

[17] Palevsky PM, O'Connor T, Zhang JH, Star RA, Smith MW. Design of the VA/NIH Acute Renal Failure Trial Network (ATN) Study: Intensive versus conventional renal support in acute renal failure. Clinical Trials. 2005;**2**(5):423-435. DOI: 10.1191/1740774505cn116oa. PMID: 16317811; PMCID: PMC1351394

Chapter 2

Dialytic Treatment of Acute Renal Failure in Children

Djamila-Djahida Batouche, Djilali Batouche and Kamel Elhalimi

Abstract

Renal replacement therapy (RRT) ensures the removal of water and solutes that are not or no longer sufficiently ensured by the kidneys: Acute renal failure (AKI) remains the oldest indication, regardless of the patient's age. All the methods of extracorporeal purification (peritoneal dialysis, conventional hemodialysis, and continuous extracorporeal purification) have been developed in children to compensate for renal function when it becomes totally or partially inadequate, and primarily or secondarily the RRT must be initiated without delay in life-threatening situations (hyperkalemia, metabolic acidosis, lysis syndrome, pulmonary edema refractory to medical treatment...). There are insufficient data to define the optimal time for initiation of RRT outside of life-threatening situations. Despite the lack of specific studies, the benefit of ERA in life-threatening situations seems reasonable, which is why most experts recommend its use in these situations. The CRRT has proven its effectiveness in pediatrics. The continuous and progressive nature of CRRT, particularly hemofiltration, makes it the therapy of choice for unstable ICU patients. The choice of the RRT method in a given center is therefore based on the type of patient to be treated, but also on technical availability, experience, and local skills.

Keywords: child, neonate, peritoneal dialysis, salt and water depletion, hemodiafiltration, continuous extrarenal therapy

1. Introduction

Kidney failure, currently called acute kidney injury in children and adults alike, is growing daily and can be life threatening if associated with organ failure. The substitutive treatment of this renal failure is the renal replacement therapy (RRT). This ensures the removal of water and fluids that are not or are no longer sufficiently supplied by the kidneys: Acute renal failure (ARF) remains the oldest indication, regardless of the age of the patients [1]. Our objective will provide a synthesis in the area of RRT in children through a few literature reviews. The incidence of the use of RRT varies in the published series from 0.7 to 2.4% of admissions, that is, a maximum of 20 cases per year for the largest units [1–5] and its occurrence worsens the life-threatening. Overall fluid overload is a factor associated with mortality [1–6].

IntechOpen

2. Principles modalities of renal replacement therapy

Prior to the late 1980s, RRT was limited to peritoneal dialysis (PD) and hemodialysis (HD). In intensive care, all the renal therapy methods (peritoneal dialysis, conventional hemodialysis, and continuous extracorporeal purification, such as hemofiltration (HF) and hemodiafiltration (HDF)) have been developed in children to supplement renal function when it becomes insufficient in all or part, whether in primary or secondary way. These methods became quickly very popular, especially in Europe, and gradually gained prominence in intensive care units. HD is based essentially on diffusion, hemofiltration on convection, and hemodiafiltration on the diffusion/convection combination.

The advent of hemofiltration (HF) methods has provided resuscitators with therapies that they have been able to appropriate more easily while reducing hemodynamic complications but at the cost of reduced efficacy (clearance), thus justifying their continued use [7].

For the convective modality, the exchanges take place through a semipermeable membrane according to a hydrostatic pressure gradient. An ultrafiltrate is then removed from the patient's blood, composed of plasma water and molecules of a molecular weight less than the diameter of the pores of the membrane. A large quantity of plasma water is thus withdrawn from the patient, requiring replacement with a replacement liquid, either upstream of the filter (predilution) or downstream (post-dilution).

The DP, therefore, does not require an extracorporeal blood circuit, the peritoneum acts as a semi-permeable membrane, and the exchanges between the blood and the dialysis solution (infused into the peritoneal cavity by a catheter placed by the resuscitator in the peritoneal cavity) take place through the walls of the rich vascular network of the peritoneal membrane, according to the concentration gradients. Water extraction is possible by adding glucose polymers to the dialysate, creating an oncotic pressure gradient that generates water transfer from the vascular sector to the dialysate.

PD is the most commonly initiated technique in infants and newborns because of the hemodynamic stability it provides, and the age and weight of the child.

The advantages and disadvantages of each method are summarized in **Table 1**.

Variable	CRRT	PD	IHD
Continuous therapy	Yes	Yes	No
Hemodynamic stability	Yes	Yes	No
Fluid balance achieved	Yes, pump controlled	Yes/no, variable	Yes, intermittent
Easy to perform	No	Yes	No
Metabolic control	Yes	Yes	Yes, intermittent
Optimal nutrition	Yes	No	No
Continuous toxin removal	Yes	No/yes, depends on the nature of the toxin—larger molecules not well cleared	No
Anticoagulation	Yes, requires continuous anticoagulation	No	Yes/no, intermittent anticoagulation

Variable	CRRT	PD	IHD
Rapid poison removal	Yes/no, depending on patient size and dose	No	Yes
Stable intracranial pressure	Yes	Yes/no, less predictable than CRRT	Yes/no, less predictable than CRRT
ICU nursing support	Yes, high level of support	Yes/no, moderate level of support (if frequent, manual cycling can be labor intensive)	No, low level of support
Dialysis nursing support	Yes/no, institution dependent	Yes/no, institution dependent	Yes
Patient mobility	No	Yes, if IPD used	No
Cost	High	Moderate. Increases with increased dialysis fluid used	High/moderate
Vascular access required	Yes	No	Ye
Recent abdominal surgery[a]	Yes	No	Yes
VP shunt	Yes	Yes/no, relative contraindication	Yes
Prune belly syndrome	Yes	Yes/no, relative contraindication	Yes
Ultrafiltration control,	Yes	Yes/no variable	Yes, intermittent
PD catheter leakage	No	Yes	No
Infection potential	Yes	Yes	Yes
Use in AKI-associated inborn errors of metabolism	Yes	No	Yes
Use in AKI-associated ingestions	Yes	No	Yes

[a]Omphalocele, gastroschisis, frequent or extensive abdominal surgery.
IPD intermittent peritoneal dialysis, VP ventriculoperitoneal, ICU intensive care unit.

Table 1.
Comparison of the advantages and disadvantages of continuous renal replacement therapies (CRRT) and peritoneal dialysis (PD) and intermittent hemodialysis (IHD).

3. Indications for initiating acute dialysis in children

The decision to initiate acute dialysis depends first on fluid balance, degree of azotemia, electrolyte disturbances, and acid-base metabolism.

In addition to renal causes (e.g., hemolytic uremic syndrome) or hemodynamic causes (after cardiac intervention for congenital heart disease), in rare cases indications for acute dialysis are also intoxication (ethylene glycol, barbiturates) or a metabolic disorder (urea cycle deficits and hyperammonemia).

For HD, HF, and HDF a central venous access with a large light is placed by the resuscitator. The size of the central catheter depends on the weight of the child (**Table 2**).

In low-weight newborns with problems getting blood to them, using two single-lumen catheters in two different veins is an efficient alternative [8].

Weight	Catheter size
3–5 kg	6,50 F (frequent surgical denudation)
5–20 kg	8 F
20–30 kg	10 F
> 30 kg	11–13 F

Table 2.
Choice of bilumeric dialysis catheter size by child's weight.

4. Peritoneal dialysis

It is a relatively simple technique, which can be used regardless of the age or weight of the child, including the newborn or the premature because of the difficulties of vascular access, the risk of bleeding, and hypotension in an extracorporeal circulation [9].

In case of respiratory distress, the child should be intubated and ventilated.

Access to the peritoneum may be possible by placing a rigid catheter near the resuscitator at the patient's bedside or by placing a Tenckhoff catheter that is surgically introduced with subcutaneous tunneling and positioning control, under cover of antibiotic prophylaxis (2nd-generation IV cephalosporin, 20 mg/kg); it is heparinized at 500 IU/L.

The initial cycles last approximately 1 hour, with a volume of 10 mL/kg (at the beginning to avoid leakage), with a 30-minute break to reach in 2 to 3 days an optimal volume of recruitment of the peritoneal exchange surface, of the order of 30 to 50 mL/kg/cycle and according to the clinical needs and the patient's tolerance. Industrial solutions of neutral pH (bicarbonate buffer) are preferred, with iso-osmolarity at first, and then use the intermediate osmolarity solution if necessary. A glucose concentration of 3.8 to 4.2% is required in the case of a high water overload. Risks of PD: leakage around the catheter, migration, catheter dysfunction, and peritonitis. Hemodynamic tolerance is generally correct; occasionally there is pain with abdominal filling.

5. Continuous hemofiltration (HF, HDF, continuous HD)

These techniques are preferred in respiratory and/or hemodynamic failure situations; they require the placement of a dialysis catheter), an HF machine, and a biocompatible filter. The preferred ultrasound insertion site is the right internal jugular vein in terms of purification quality [10, 11].

The femoral site is a perfectly acceptable alternative in the context of extreme urgency and remains the most used in the English literature [12].

Machinery pumps (blood, dialysate, restitution) guarantee the accuracy of the water balance. Pediatric filters with areas ranging from 0.2 to 1.2 m^2 are available in all commercial markets depending on the brand of dialysis generator used (**Figure 1**).

A wide range of pediatric and neonatal Hemofilters, made of MediSulfone® proprietary membrane, has been developed to create the best treatment for low-body-weight patients.

Frequently, the circuit must be de-coagulated with heparin therapy (10 to 20 IU/kg/hour to achieve an activated cephalin time between 50 and 65 seconds) or with regional citrate anticoagulation (ionized calcium monitoring).

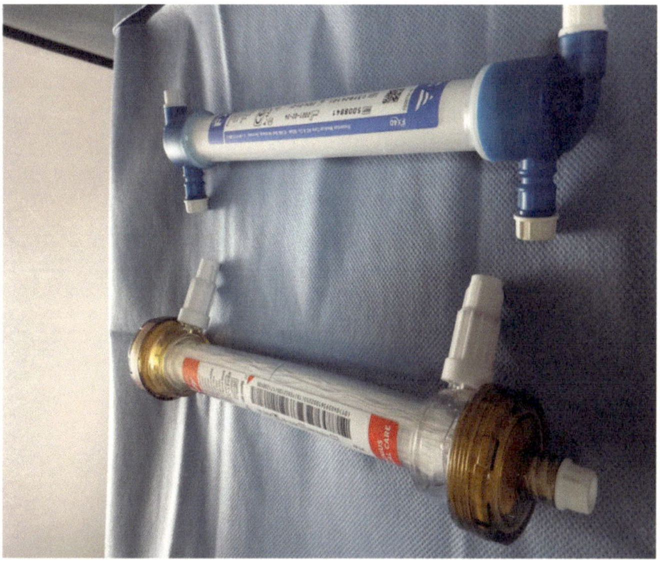

Figure 1.
Diagram of a pediatric hemofilter.

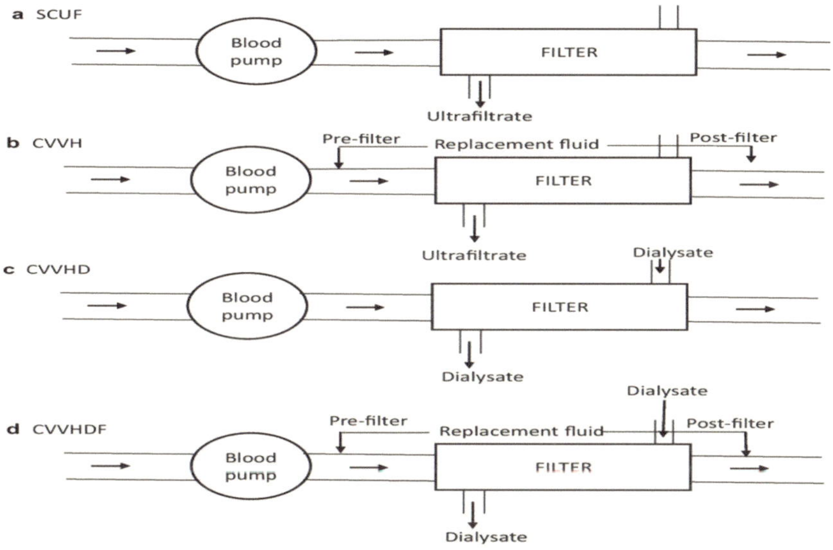

Figure 2.
Circuit diagrams for the various modes of continuous kidney replacement therapy (CKRT) by ref. [14] in Indian J Pediatr. Blood flows from left to right from the patient to the blood pump and then to the filter, from which it is returned to the patient. (a) Slow continuous ultrafiltration (SCUF): In this modality, there is no diffusive clearance and only ultrafiltrate (UF) is generated across the filter; this method is preferred for isolated UF removal when kidney function is normal, (b) Continuousvenovenous hemofiltration (CVVH): Replacement fluid is run eitherpre- or post-filter in a volume to replace the effluent; excess effluent is removed to ensure the UF desired for negative fluid balance; clearance is convective rather than diffusive. (c) Continuous venovenous hemodialysis (CVVHD): Blood flows across the filter in a countercurrent fashion with the dialysate fluid, and the effluent predominantly consists of dialysate fluid with minimal, if any, UF, as in intermittent hemodialysis. (d) Continuous venovenous hemodiafiltration (CVVHDF): This modality combines CVVH with CVVHD, such that the blood and dialysis fluid run in counter-current directions, the replacement fluid is either pre- or post-filter, and the effluent comprises the dialysate and replacement fluids.

Blood flow (BF) ranges from 3 to 10 mL/kg/minute. The blood pump flow rate should be at least 50 mL/min to maintain a filtration fraction <20%, which is easily achieved with a functioning 8 Fr catheter and HF of 0.3 m^2 [13].

This corresponds approximately to 2000 mL/h for 1.73 m^2 (in HDF, it is necessary to take into account the dialysate flow rate, or QD: total dose = QUF + QD).

In all cases, a filtration fraction (FF = QUF/[1 - Ht] x QS) of less than 15–20% should be maintained to avoid coagulation of the filter.

In pure continuous hemofiltration (CVVH, CAVH) and in the course of the derived methods which are the techniques without restitution (SCUF), the clearance is ensured by convection (**Figure 2**).

The following table describes the advantages and disadvantages of each treatment modality.

6. The choice of the therapeutic modality

6.1 Intermittent hemodialysis

Like HF, it requires a dialysis catheter, dialysis machine, and filter as well as a water treatment system. It may be preferred for hemodynamically stable patients with acute poisoning or acute decompensation of CKD to avoid costly and time-consuming continuous use.

In children with intermittent hemodialysis lasting <6 hours, blood flow should start at 3 ml/kg per minute and reach 5 ml/kg per minute in subsequent sessions, and dialysate flow should be at least 300 ml/min up to twice the blood flow in ml/min [15].

Another method, sustained low-efficiency dialysis (SLED), is a form of prolonged intermittent renal replacement therapy (PIRRT), combines the advantages of intermittent hemodialysis and CKRT, although the literature on the use of PIRRT in children is limited [16].

6.2 When to start a dialysis session?

EER should be initiated without delay in life-threatening situations (hyperkalemia, metabolic acidosis, lysis syndrome, pulmonary edema refractory to medical therapy [17]).

In children, water and sodium overload of more than 10% and most likely more than 20% should be considered as a criterion for initiating an ERA.

Several series published in the literature have shown that water overload before RRT is a risk factor for mortality [12, 17–22].

However, despite the absence of specific studies, the benefit of ERA in acute prognostic situations seems reasonable, which explains why most experts recommend using RRT in these situations [15, 23, 24].

The best time to start an RRT remains an unresolved question. Very few studies have assessed the potential benefits of an early start to RRT.

The study of Gettings [25] in polytrauma patients treated with continuous techniques shows greater survival when ERA was started before urea reached 20 mmol/l.

The beneficial impact of the dialysis dose on prognosis would be to start very early. However, a start after relative hemodynamic stability has been achieved might be more reasonable. Whatever the situation, the only certainty is that it is not necessary to wait for the complications of nitrogen retention before starting the purification [26].

A prospective randomized study by Bouman [27] compared an early onset of hemofiltration within 12 h of diagnosis of AKI to a later onset (urea greater than 40 mmol l^{-1}, serum potassium greater than 6.5 mmol l^{-1}, presence of pulmonary edema).

Time from diagnosis of ARF to onset of hemofiltration averaged 6 h in the early group and 42 h in the late group. Survival between the two groups was identical.

A meta-analysis of 12 studies with 4880 participants of all ages found no significant difference between early or late-onset dialysis in terms of survival but in terms of cost [28].

7. Impact of choice of dialysis modality

The choice of continuous therapy varies widely in the pediatric literature [29].

HDI has the obvious advantage of rapid ultrafiltration or solute removal over the DP or RRTC.

In hemodynamically stable patients, no RRT modality is better suited than HDI for rapid removal of an offending solute. This method of treatment is particularly important in the following cases: cases of ingestion of drug toxicity, tumor lysis syndrome, and hyperammonemia observed in the pediatric population [30–32].

For the ability to adjust the composition of the dialysate to treat various electrolytes (i.e., hyperkalemia, hypernatremia) HD is a major advantage over DP or RRTC [33].

In some literature series, most hypernatremic dehydration in children was treated with PD [34, 35].

Bunchman et al. [36] reviewed survival outcomes in 226 pediatric patients receiving various forms of RRT, including PD, IHD, and CRRT, over 7 years. Patients were treated with CRRT (n = 106), IHD (n = 61), or PD (n = 59).

The survival rate is 54% of the overall population studied: 40% survival in the group treated with hemofiltration, 49% in the group treated with peritoneal dialysis, and 81% survival in the group treated with intermittent hemodialysis. ($P < 0.01$ HD vs. HF or PD).

In a series of 62 children with organ dysfunction syndrome (22-fold related to septic shock), continuous hemodiafiltration was more effective in controlling fluid overload than peritoneal dialysis (Lowrie) [37].

The hemodynamic tolerance of intermittent hemodialysis has been studied in adults [38, 39] but not in children, but in the Maghreb countries personal experience has led us to take into consideration what the literature has offered us by taking specific measures (with respect to volume, reduction of the temperature of the dialysis baths and sodium enrichment of the dialysis bath in particular, and daily dialysis session [40]).

A new machine can perform KRT in neonates and young infants using low extracorporeal blood volume and a slow blood flow rate while permitting precise calibration of ultrafiltration (CARPEDIEM) NIDUS developed in French and countries developed and confirming their safety and feasibility in infants with AKI [41, 42].

These machines are not marketed in india [43] and in the a Maghreb and in our country we use Prismaflex ®, to deliver CKRT to infants.

8. Conclusion

The data for RRT modality choice in the treatment of pediatric AKI are limited. At the present time, there have been no randomized clinical trials comparing PD vs.

IHD vs. CRRT for the treatment of children with AKI and no prospective studies have evaluated the effect of dialysis modality on the outcomes of children with AKI in the ICU setting.

The decision about dialysis modality should therefore be based on local expertise, resources available, and the patient's clinical status.

Author details

Djamila-Djahida Batouche[1,2,3*], Djilali Batouche[4] and Kamel Elhalimi[1,2]

1 Department of Pediatric-neonatal Anesthesia, ICU EHU Oran, Oran, Algeria

2 Faculty of Medicine Oran 1, Oran, Algeria

3 Research Laboratory LERMER, University Oran 1, Oran, Algeria

4 Clinical Research Multihealth and Pharmacovigilance, Company Freelance, Paris, France

*Address all correspondence to: batouchedjamiladjahida@gmail.com

References

[1] Flynn. Joseph T. Choice of dialysis modality for management of pediatric acute renal failure. Pediatric Nephrology. 2002;**17**:61-69

[2] Bailey D, Gauvin F, Phan V, et al. Risk factors for acute renal failure in critically ill children: A prospective descriptive epidemiologic study. Pediatric Critical Care Medicine. 2007;**8**(1):29-35

[3] Schneider J, Khemani R, Grushkin C, Bart R. Serum creatinine as stratified in the RIFLE score for acute kidney injury is associated with mortality and length of stay for children in the pediatric intensive care unit. Critical Care Medicine. 2010;**38**:933-939

[4] Macher MA. Insuffisance rénale aigue chez l'enfant. In: EMC, Néphrologie. Paris: Elsevier Masson SAS; 2007 18-064-10

[5] Hackbarth R, Maxvold N, Bunchman T. Acute renal failure and end-stage renal disease. In: Nichols DG, editor. Rogers Textbook of Pediatric Intensive Care. 4th ed. Philadelphia: Lippincott, Williams & Wilkins; 2008. pp. 1661-1676

[6] Askenazi DJ, Goldstein SL, Koralkar R, Fortenberry J, Baum M, Hackbarth R, et al. Continuous renal replacement therapy for children < 10 kg: A report from the prospective Pediatric continuous renal replacement therapy registry. The Journal of Pediatrics. 2013;**162**:587-592

[7] Walters S, Porter C, Brophy PD. Dialysis and pediatric acute kidney injury: Choice of renal support modality. Pediatric Nephrology. 2009;**24**:37-48

[8] El Masri K, Jackson K, Borasino S, Law M, Askenazi D, Alten J. Successful continuous renal replacement therapy using two single-lumen catheters in neonates and infants with cardiac disease. Pediatric Nephrology. 2013;**28**(12):2383-2387

[9] Coulthard MG, Vernon B. Managing acute renal failure in very low birthweight infants. Archives of Disease in Childhood. 1995;**73**:F187-F192

[10] Little MA, Conlon PJ, Walshe JJ. Access recirculation in temporary hemodialysis catheters as measured by the saline dilution technique. American Journal of Kidney Diseases. 2000;**36**:1135-1139

[11] Sutherland SM, Alexander SR. Continuous renal replacement therapy in children. Pediatric Nephrology. 2012;**27**(11):2007-2016

[12] Symons JM, Chua AN, Somers MJ, Baum MA, Bunchman TE, Benfield MR, et al. Demographic characteristics of pediatric continuous renal replacement therapy: A report of the prospective pediatric continuous renal replacement therapy registry. Clinical Journal of the American Society of Nephrology. 2007;**2**:732-738

[13] Maclaren G, Butt W. Controversies in paediatric continuous renal replacement therapy. Intensive Care Medicine. 2009;**35**:596-602

[14] Krishnasamy S, Sinha A, Bagga A. Management of acute kidney injury in critically ill children. Indian Journal of Pediatrics. 2023;**90**(5):481-491. DOI: 10.1007/s12098-023-04483-2

[15] Renal Replacement Therapy in Adult and Pediatric Intensive Care. Recommendations by an expert panel from the French Intensive Care Society

(SRLF) with the French Society of Anesthesia Intensive Care (SFAR) French Group for Pediatric Intensive Care Emergencies (GFRUP) the French dialysis society (SFD). Annals of Intensive Care. 2015;**5**(1):58

[16] Sethi SK, Mittal A, Nair N, et al. Pediatric continuous renal replacement therapy (PCRRT) expert committee recommendation on prescribing prolonged intermittent renal replacement therapy (PIRRT) in critically ill children. Hemodialysis International. 2020;**24**:237-251

[17] Gillespie RS, Seidel K, Symons JM. Effect of fluid overload and dose of replacement fluid on survival in hemofiltration. Pediatric Nephrology. 2004;**19**:1394-1399

[18] Foland JA, Fortenberry JD, Warshaw BL, et al. Fluid overload before continuous hemofiltration and survival in critically ill children: A retrospective analysis. Critical Care Medicine. 2004;**32**:1771-1776

[19] Goldstein SL, Somers MJ, Baum MA, et al. Pediatric patients with multi-organ dysfunction syndrome receiving continuous renal replacement therapy. Kidney International. 2005;**67**:653-658

[20] Hayes LW, Oster RA, Tofil NM, Tolwani AJ. Outcomes of critically ill children requiring continuous renal replacement therapy. Journal of Critical Care. 2009;**24**:394-400

[21] Sutherland SM, Zappitelli M, Alexander SR, et al. Fluid overload and mortality in children receiving continuous renal replacement therapy: The prospective pediatric continuous renal replacement therapy registry. American Journal of Kidney Diseases. 2010;**55**:316-325

[22] Batouche D, Elhalimi K, Kerboua K, Sadaoui L, Benatta NF, Negadi M. Statut volémique chez l'enfant en insuffisance rénale aiguë admis aux soins intensifs: approche étiologique. Néphrologie & Thérapeutique. 2015;**11**(5):298

[23] Lameire N, van Biesen W, Vanholder R. Acute renal failure. Lancet. 2005;**365**:417-430

[24] Bagshaw SM, Cruz DN, Gibney RT, Ronco C. A proposed algorithm for initiation of renal replacement therapy in adult critically ill patients. Critical Care. 2009;**13**:317

[25] Gettings LG, Renolds HN. Outcome in post-traumatic acute renal failure when continuous renal replacement therapy is applied early vs. late. Intensive Care Medicine. 1999;**8**:805-813

[26] Klahr S. Obstructive nephropathy. Internal Medicine. 2000;**39**:355-361

[27] Bouman C, Oudemans-Van Straaten HM, Tijssen Jan GP. Effects of early high-volume continuous venovenous hemofiltration on survival and recovery of renal function in intensive care patients with acute renal failure: A prospective, randomized trial. Critical Care Medicine. 2002;**30**:2205-2211

[28] Isabel FA, Buamscha DG, Ciappon AI. Timing of kidney replacement therapy initiation for acute kidney injury. Cochrane Database of Systematic Reviews. 2022;**11**(11):CD010612

[29] Parakininkas D, Greenbaum LA. Comparison of solute clearance in three modes of continuous renal replacement therapy. Pediatric Critical Care Medicine. 2004;**5**:269-274

[30] Cortina G, McRae R, Hoq M, et al. Mortality of critically ill children requiring continuous renal replacement therapy:

Effect of fluid overload, underlying disease, and timing of initiation. Pediatric Critical Care Medicine. 2019;**20**:314-322

[31] McBryde KD, Kershaw DB, Bunchman TE, Maxvold NJ, Mottes TA, Kudelka TL, et al. Renal replacement therapy in the treatment of confirmed or suspected inborn errors of metabolism. The Journal of Pediatrics. 2006;**148**:770-778

[32] Brophy PD, Flynn JT, Kershaw DB, Smoyer WE, Mottes T, Maxvold NJ, et al. Pediatric overdose: Effective treatment with high-efficiency hemodialysis (abstract). Journal of the American Society of Nephrology. 1999;**10**:137A

[33] Pazmino PA, Pazmino BP. Treatment of acute hypernatremia with hemodialysis. American Journal of Nephrology. 1993;**13**:260-262

[34] Yildiz N, Erguven M, Yildiz M, Ozdogan T, Turhan P. Acute peritoneal dialysis in neonates with acute kidney injury and hypernatremic dehydration. Peritoneal Dialysis International. 2013;**33**(3):290-296

[35] Moritz ML, del Rio M, Crooke GA, Singer LP. Acute peritoneal dialysis as both cause and treatment of hypernatremia in an infant. Pediatric Nephrology. 2001;**16**:697-700

[36] Bunchman TE, Mcbryde KD, Mottes TE, Gardner JJ, Maxvold NJ, Brophy PD. Pediatric acute renal failure: Outcome by modality and disease. Pediatric Nephrology. 2001;**16**:1067-1071

[37] Lowrie LH. Renal remplacment therapys in pediatric multiorgane dysfunction syndrome. Pediatric Nephrology. 2000;**14**:6-12

[38] Schortgen F. Tolérance et efficacité des séances d'épuration extrarénale. Réanimation. 2003;**12**:318-326

[39] Shiffl H, Lang SM, Fischer R. Daily hemodialysis and the out-comes of acute renal failure. The New England Journal of Medicine. 2002;**346**:305-310

[40] Batouche DD, Benouaz S, Okbani R, Benatta NF, Berrachdi W, Lahmer M. Hémodialyse quotidienne pour un bon contrôle de la pression artérielle chez l'enfant en insuffisance rénale aiguë. Néphrologie & Thérapeutique. 2017;**13**(5):399

[41] Goldstein SL, Vidal E, Ricci Z, et al. Survival of infants treated with CKRT: Comparing adapted adult platforms with the Carpediem™. Pediatric Nephrology. 2022;**37**:667-675

[42] Menon S, Broderick J, Munshi R, et al. Kidney support in children using an ultrafiltration device: A multicenter, retrospective study. Clinical Journal of the American Society of Nephrology. 2019;**14**:1432-1440

[43] Coulthard MG, Crosier GC, Smith J, Drinnan M, Whitaker M, Beckwith R, et al. Haemodialysing babies weighing <8 kg with the Newcastle infant dialysis and ultrafiltration system (Nidus): Comparison with peritoneal and conventional haemodialysis. Pediatric Nephrology. 2014;**29**(10):1873-1881

Chapter 3

Preservation of Peritoneal Membrane Structure and Function in Peritoneal Dialysis

Mathew George Kunthara

Abstract

Peritoneal dialysis (PD) is a type of renal replacement therapy which is based on the use of peritoneum, which acts as a semipermeable membrane with diffusion and convection. Long term use can produce structural and functional changes of the membrane by the activation of the resident fibroblasts and infiltrating inflammatory cells, mesothelial to mesenchymal transition, further leading to fibrosis, angiogenesis and ultrafiltration failure. This is due to use of bioincompatible fluids, frequent peritoneal inflammation, uremic milieu and other multiple factors. The peritoneal fibrosis has two parts: fibrosis and inflammation, which induces each other via TGF/SMAD pathway and IL-6 signaling, respectively. The advent of newer biocompatible fluids along with additives has significantly reduced the production of glucose degradation products (GDPs). In addition, the identification of the biomarkers in peritoneal effluent is necessary, which, after being correlated with peritoneal biopsy, may help us to guide future studies and assessment of the efficacy of therapeutic interventions. Various interventions are being tried based on experimental studies from animal models, pharmacology and gene therapy with promising results, with new insights in near future. This article reviews the main aspects associated with the functional and structural alterations related to PD and discusses interventions whereby we may prevent them to preserve the peritoneal membrane.

Keywords: peritoneal dialysis, ultrafiltration, encapsulating peritoneal sclerosis, mesothelial to mesenchymal transition (MMT), VEGF (vascular endothelial growth factors), GDP (glucose degradation products)

1. Introduction

Peritoneal dialysis (PD) is a life-sustaining therapy used by >100,000 patients with ESRD worldwide, accounting for approximately 10 to 15% of the dialysis population [1]. Despite these benefits, only a small number of dialysis patients receive PD, in Europe about 13% and in the USA about 10% and 6% in India [2, 3]. The major obstacles for a successful long-term PD are infections and the deleterious functional alterations in the peritoneal membrane following prolonged exposure to dialysis fluids; which is responsible for increased morbidity and mortality. These alterations, such as progressive fibrosis and vasculogenesis, leading to increased solute transport and ultrafiltration (UF) failure, are seen in more than 50% of patients on PD.

Rippe proposed the existence of three pores of different sizes in peritoneal membrane: a large pore of 100–200 Å corresponding to interendothelial cell clefts allowing transport of large molecular weight solutes; a small pore of 40–60 Å, which allows for transport of water and low molecular weight (LMW)solutes and an ultrasmall pore of 4–6 Å that allows for the passage of only water.

2. The normal peritoneal transport barrier

2.1 Distributed concept of ultrafiltration barrier

The three potential barriers to both solute and water are (1) anatomic peritoneum (2) cellular-interstitial matrix surrounding the blood vessels (3) capillary endothelium. Blood vessels are the main source of UF and the water flow from the capillaries to the interstitium depends on the difference between the capillary luminal pressures and the effective pressure on the interstitial side. The concentration profile occurs due to diffusion of the small solutes via the tissue interstitium along with simultaneous uptake into the capillaries. The largest gradients of osmotic pressure will therefore be across blood vessels closest to the peritoneum.

Figure 1A describes the distributed concept of UF barrier and **Figure 1B** shows changes in membrane [4].

The distributed model proposes that "the influence of a specific capillary on PD transport is the function of that capillary's proximity to mesothelial to the dialysate interface". The proliferation of vessels near the interface increases the "effective" peritoneal surface area; especially during peritonitis and following exposure to high glucose containing fluids.

2.2 Pore matrix concept of endothelial barrier

Flessner [4] has postulated a new concept which says that the large and small pores will be represented as a single entity with the difference in transport characteristics;

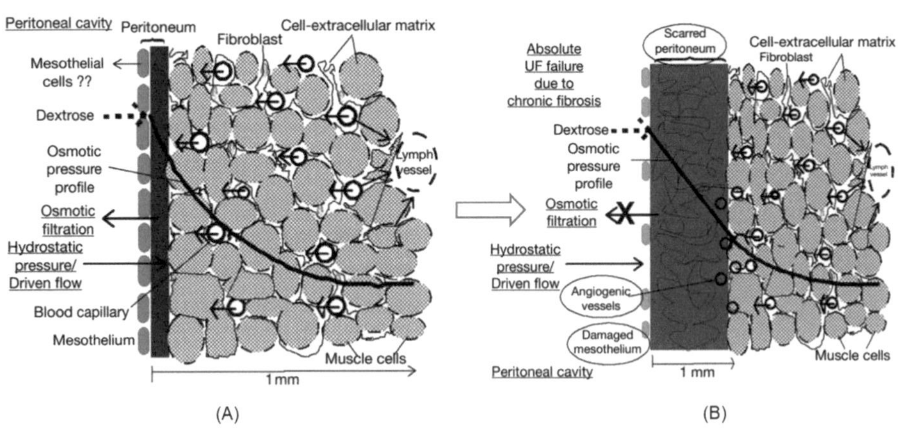

Figure 1.
(A and B) Distributed concept of normal ultrafiltration barrier. Dextrose diffuses from dialysate into tissue and sets up an osmotic pressure profile (thick curved line).

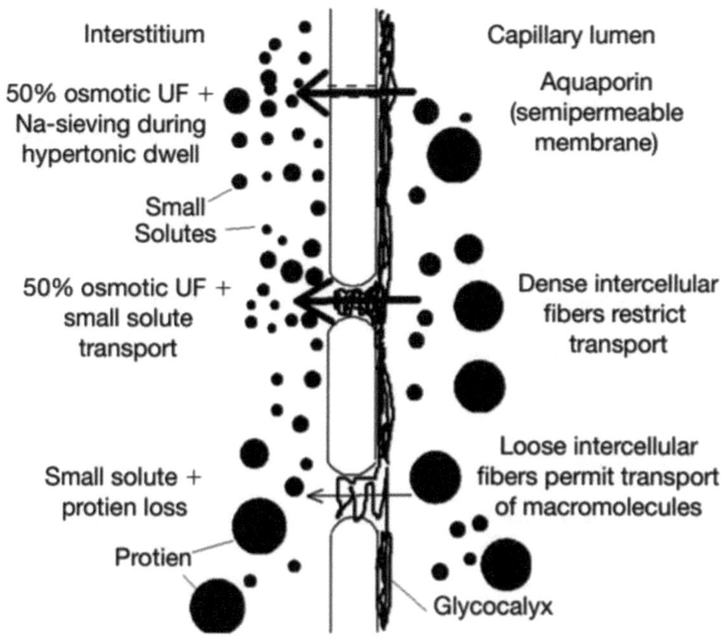

Figure 2.
Pore-matrix concept of endothelial barrier incorporating the luminal glycocalyx [4].

being a function of the density of intercellular glycoprotein matrix; as in **Figure 2**. This additional layer of glycocalyx alters the microenvironment near the true, size-selective boundary.

Moreover, albumin concentration below the glycocalyx but above the tight junction is likely much lower than that in the interstitium. This is because the albumin is unable to diffuse against the ultrafiltrate flow through the gap in the glycocalyx. The glycocalyx density is decreased by perfusion of oxidized LDL, adenosine, ischemia reperfusion injury and TNF-α.

3. Natural history of peritoneal membrane in CAPD

The peritoneal fibrosis has two parts; fibrosis process itself and the inflammation which is promoted by the non-physiologic content of solutions and infections. In the fibrotic process, there is loss of mesothelial cells with fibroblastoid changes leading to mesothelial-to-mesenchymal transition mediated by TGF-ß (Transforming growth factor) and VEGF (Vascular endothelial growth factor) signaling pathways. The inflammation pathway is mediated by the IL-6 (Interleukin-6) and other chemokines. Both the pathways are interlinked to each other and will be potentiating each other.

4. Regulation of peritoneal inflammation and leukocyte trafficking

During acute episodes of peritonitis, there is early activation of proinflammatory cytokines (TNF-, IL-1, and IFN-) and rapid recruitment of neutrophils with subsequent replacement by monocytes. This initial influx of neutrophils is due to the expression of CXC chemokine, MIP-1/KC, and the release of sIL-6R which facilitates the formation of sIL-6R/IL-6 complexes. These trans-signaling complexes suppress the release of other CXC chemokines, ensuring clearance of neutrophils, and simultaneously promoting the secretion of the CC chemokines, such as monocyte chemoattractant protein 1 (MCP-1) and RANTES, triggering the recruitment of mononuclear leukocytes and regulate the process of apoptosis. The IL-6/sIL-6R signaling also selectively promotes T cell recruitment into the peritoneal membrane through a gp130-dependent, STAT1/3-dependent activation pathway (as shown in **Figure 3**).

The most consistent change observed in peritoneal tissues of a patient on PD is an increase in the sub-mesothelial thickness associated with peritoneal fibrosis.

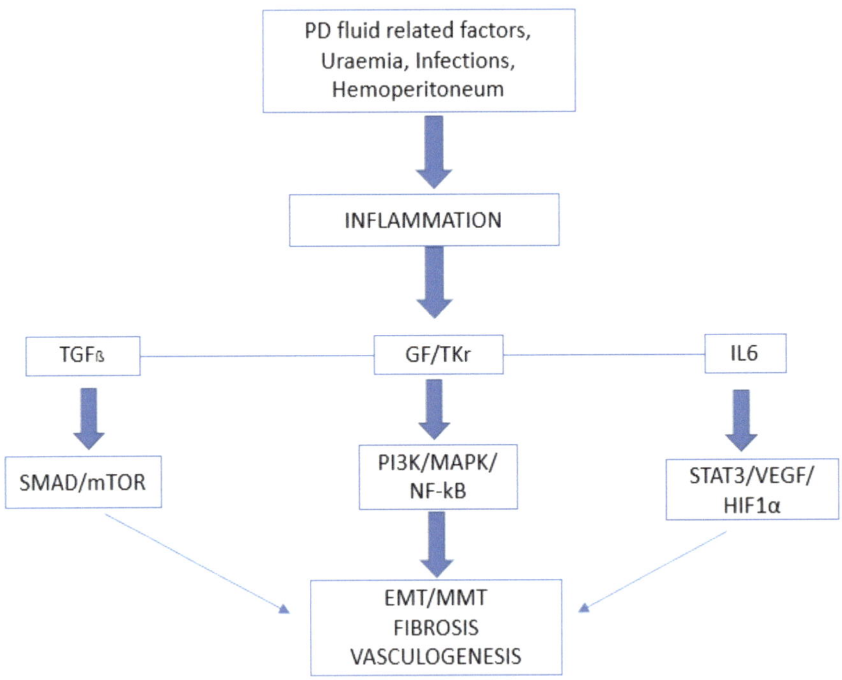

Figure 3.
Molecular network that regulate EMT [5]. Courtesy: Gonzalez 2016. Abbreviations: TGF ß—Transforming growth factor ß; GF—growth factor; TKr—Tyrosine kinase receptor; IL-6—interleukin 6; and EMT/MMT—Epithelial/Mesothelial to mesenchymal transition.

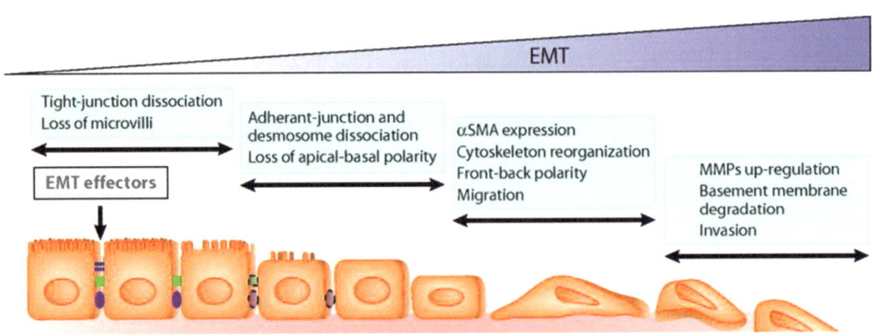

Figure 4.
Key events during EMT (Courtesy: [6]).

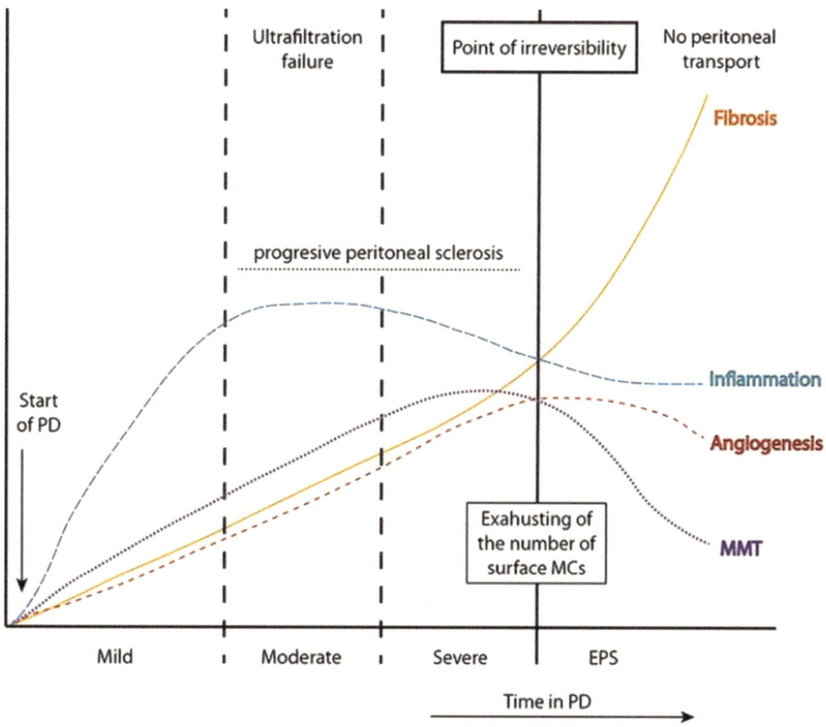

Figure 5.
Natural history of peritoneal membrane changes (Courtesy: [5]).

The use of non-physiologic PD solutions along with uremic milieu, has led to the production of advanced glycation end products (AGEs) in peritoneal tissues which induces vasculogenesis and fibrosis. The interaction between fibrosis and angiogenesis may occur at the level of inducing cytokines; TGF-ß leading to SMAD pathway and inflammatory cytokines induce VEGF and angiogenesis; this is how EMT (epithelial to mesenchymal transition)/MMT (mesothelial to mesenchymal transition) occurs (shown in **Figure 4**).

There are two pathologic types of PD related fibrosis. Most common type is simple peritoneal sclerosis which is seen in almost all patients. The other one is Encapsulating peritoneal fibrosis (EPS) that evolves rapidly with intense fibrosis and inflammation leading to life threatening visceral encapsulation (as shown in **Figure 5**).

5. Consequences of peritoneal fibrosis

The peritoneum is an acellular, avascular layer of tissue. Significant scarring of the peritoneum is often present after 6 or more years of CAPD. Solute transport is rapid across this avascular, acellular layer and uptake into abnormal blood capillaries is rapid. However, with the loss of the interstitial cell matrix and the increase in the distance of the blood capillaries from the peritoneum, the water transport to peritoneal cavity will be nearly zero [4]. Immunolocalization of collagen 1α-1 revealed that this protein was predominantly expressed in the sub-mesothelial compact zone of EPS peritoneal samples, whereas non-EPS patients exhibited diffuse and homogeneous Col1a-1 staining.

For more advanced peritoneal conditions with potential EPS development, EPS-prone states [7] is defined by (i) PD duration >3 years (ii) history of recurrent ± severe peritonitis (iii) presence of acquired UF failure or high-fast membrane transport (iv) high exposure to high GDP PD fluids, (v) repeated hemoperitoneum.

6. Risk factors for peritoneal membrane damage

A. Diabetes: In diabetes there will be upregulation of vascular endothelial growth factor (VEGF), driven by local hypoxia induced by vasculopathy of the micro-vasculature and also due to increased GDPs. They also have lower lumen-to-vessel diameter ratios and higher postcapillary venule diameters.

B. Uraemia: There will be increased expression of several proteoglycan components (versican, matrix metalloproteinase-2 [MMP-2] and hyaluronan) in patients with uraemia along with upregulation of AGE receptors (RAGE). It has been shown that presence of the C allele of RAGE protects against peritoneal fibrosis.

C. Dietary salt intake: There will be upregulation of TGF-β1 and IL-6 expression in the peritoneal membrane, resulting in an enhanced EMT; in addition, to an increase in peritoneal small solute transport leading to UF failure.

7. Genetic factors

A. IL-6 POLYMORPHISM: There can be G and C allele variant IL-6 polymorphism. IL-6 level is linked to peritoneal small solute transport and to albumin leakage. Those with GC or CC genotype had much higher IL-6 levels in their serum and in the drained dialysate than did patients with a GG genotype, along with upregulation of IL-6mRNA in the membrane [8].

B. eNOS: eNOS genotype aa or ab (versus bb) was an independent predictor of reduced peritoneal membrane transport rate [9].

C. Receptor for AGE: Numata et al. observed that a polymorphism of RAGE, the presence of the C allele in RAGE –429 T/C, were not present in patients with EPS [10]. Anti-RAGE antibodies also prevented the AGE associated upregulation of TGF-β1.

D. Il-1β: polymorphism has shown increased infection rate (lower with T/T vs. C/T & T/T) [11].

E. IL-1RN: polymorphism was an independent predictor of technique survival.

F. CCL18: Increased expression of CCL18 was associated with functional deficiency, increased fibrosis and atherosclerosis.

The risk factors for the peritoneal membrane damage are summarized in **Figure 6**.

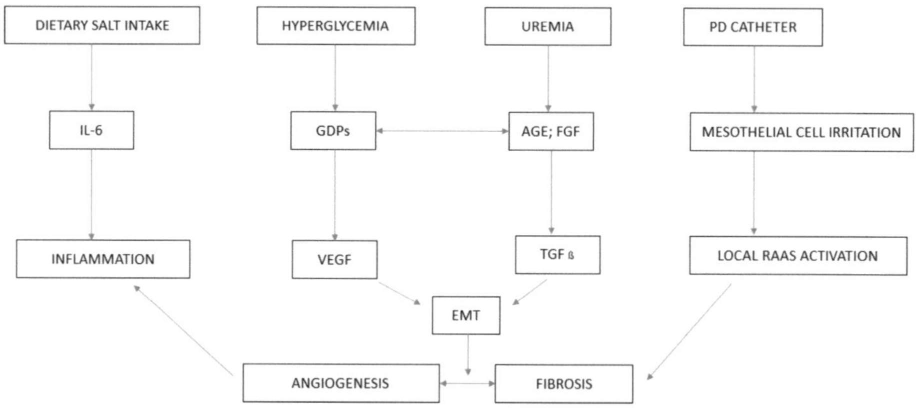

Figure 6.
Factors affecting peritoneal membrane degradation. Abbreviations: IL-6—Interleukin-6; VEGF—vascular endothelial growth factor; TGF—Transforming growth factor; and RAAS—renin angiotensin aldosterone system. Courtesy: Pletinck et al. [12].

8. Diagnosis of peritoneal fibrosis

A. Effluent biomarkers: Nowadays, early detection of membrane damage can be done with biomarkers. Some of them are CA-125, IL-6 and PAI-1. A low effluent level of CA 125 has recently been found as a prognosis factor for the membrane damage [13]. Cases of plasminogen activator inhibitor and CCL18, in peritoneal effluent are also associated with the prognosis of the membrane [14]. Other biomarkers are VEGF, MMP-2, TGF-ß, CTGF, TNF-α.

B. Histopathology: is the gold standard. The biopsy findings if using bioincompatible fluids were mesothelial layer disappearance, thickening of the sub-mesothelial compact zone, hyalinizing vasculopathy, angiogenesis, along with co-expression of α-smooth muscle actin and cytokeratin. The biopsy findings in those who used biocompatible fluids were associated with more well-preserved MC layer (56% vs. 26%), mild thickening with less dense sub-mesothelial compact zone (47% vs. 69%) and an absence of hyalinizing vasculopathy (4% vs. 30%) [15].

9. Conventional PD fluids

First generation Fluids: contain 35–40 mM lactate buffer with an acidic pH of 5.5. The low pH will be aggravating the detrimental effects of the high lactate on peritoneal mesothelium. During heat sterilization and storage, more of (GDPs) (e.g., formaldehyde, acetaldehyde, glyoxal, methylglyoxal, 5-hydroxymethylfurfural (5-HMF), 3-Deoxyglucosone (3-DG) and 3,4-dideoxyglucosone3-ene (3,4-DGE)) are formed, leading to membrane damage (shown in **Figure** 7).

Second generation Fluids: The buffers (such as lactate ± bicarbonate) are in separate chamber and are kept in very low pH to prevent formation of GDPs. Prior to use, they are mixed to a pH of 7–7.5 and are administered. They are detailed below.

Icodextrin: is an osmotic agent (Mol.wt-16,800 Da) derived from the starch, used in long night dwell with very low GDP, since they are absorbed into the

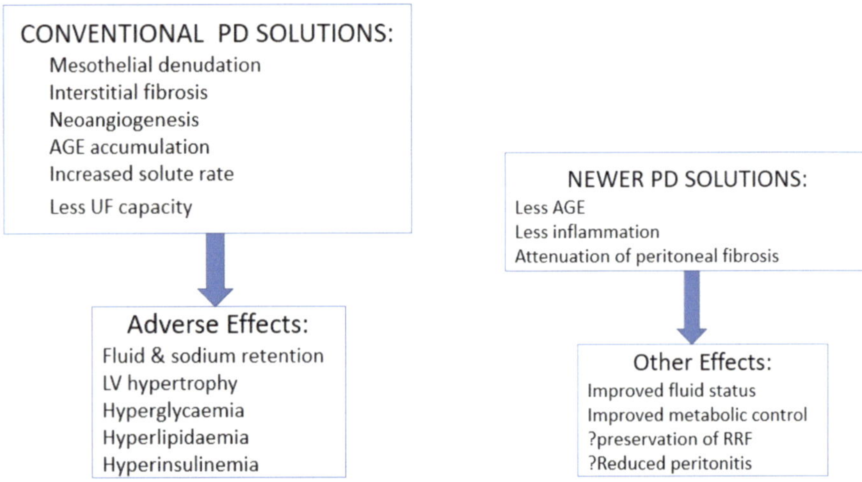

Figure 7.
Potential beneficial effects of newer peritoneal dialysis solutions [16]. (Courtesy: Garcia nature reviews 2012). Abbreviations: RRF—residual renal function; LV—left ventricle; and AGE—advanced glycosylated end products).

circulation, with no sodium sieving. It has an UF capacity comparable to 4.25% dextrose fluid. Despite this, acidic PD fluid has been associated with increased local and systemic inflammation with increased permeability and IL-6. Even though this reaction is reaction, long term exposure may irreversibly change peritoneal morphology. The ISPD guidelines recommends use of icodextrin in high transporters for better volume control.

Amino acid solutions: A bag of 1.1% 21 amino acid PD fluid used in one exchange a day provide 22gm of amino acids (2/3rd essential & 1/3rd nonessential) which is 25% of daily requirement and generate an UF equal to 2 L 1.5% dextrose. It has an acidic pH of 6.6 with very low GDPs and low VEGF. For optimized nutrition of malnourished patients and to prevent increased serum nitrogen levels and metabolic acidosis, they should be applied at a ratio of 1:4 with glucose-containing PD fluids [17]. Nutrineal in one exchange with icodextrin (Extraneal) and Physioneal (Baxter) for other exchange as a regimen (NEPP regimen) has shown to preserve mesothelial integrity but with increased VEGF.

10. Newer PD fluids

1. Trio gambrosol- tri compartment with two small chambers with 50% glucose and last chamber with calcium, magnesium, chloride & lactate.

2. Physioneal- two chamber with chamber A containing glucose in 1.5%, 2.5%, 4.5% at a pH of 2.1 along with calcium & magnesium salts and chamber B with buffer lactate & bicarbonate at a pH 9.0. Volume of chambers in 3:1 ratio and solutions in both chamber mixed prior infusion, at least 1.6 L instilled during each infusion (to avoid accidental infusion of buffer only chamber and alkalosis).

3. Balance- double chamber with glucose & electrolyte and other with buffer in equal volumes.

Fluid	pH	Buffer	GDP (μmol/L)	Osmotic agent
Icodextrin	5.8	Lactate	45	7.5% polyglucose
Amino acid	6.6	Lactate		1.1% amino acid
Trio Gambro	6.3	Lactate	65	Dextrose
Physioneal	7.4	Bicarbonate+lactate	253	Dextrose
Balance	7.0	Lactate	42	Dextrose
Bicavera	7.4	Bicarbonate	42	Dextrose
Delflex NpH	7.0	Lactate+bicarbonate	70	Dextrose

Table 1.
Newer PD fluids and constituents.

4. Bicavera-double chamber which has used bicarbonate as buffer used along with glucose containing calcium& magnesium chloride. This is the only PD fluid which used bicarbonate alone as buffer.

5. Delflex Neutral pH- Only FDA approved neutral pH PD fluid. GDP levels are 55, 70, 95 μmol/L depending on 1.5%, 2.5%, 4.5% glucose content (**Table 1**).

The Euro-Balance trial, demonstrated improved residual renal function together with decreased peritoneal UF with the pH neutral, low GDP fluid, as compared to the first generation, acidic high GDP solution [18]. The BalANZ trial has shown a lower risk of anuria and lower ultrafiltration and higher solute clearance rates with the use of low GDP fluid during the first 9 months of PD. Peritonitis incidence and severity were reduced in the BalANZ trial [19]. The TRIO trial comparing biocompatible solution (Gambrosol Trio) to standard PD fluid (Dianeal) showed contrasting results with slower rated of GFR decline but with higher peritonitis rate.

11. Novel PD fluid protoypes

The introduction of novel osmotic agents, is a promising way to improve the biocompatibility (**Figure 8**).

1. The addition of 3.5% taurine-based PD fluid achieved equivalent ultrafiltration as glucose-based PD fluid and induced less mesothelial and fibroblast cell proliferation(rat model) [20].

2. Hyperbranched polyglycerol containing PD fluid achieved similar solute and water transport and induced less peritoneal membrane damage (rat model)but data on metabolism are lacking [21].

3. By the addition of dipeptide alanyl-glutamine to first- and second-generation PD fluid improved mesothelial cell stress response and cell survival with reduced peritoneal fibrosis [22]. A phase 3 trial is needed.

4. Addition of L-carnitine to acidic, glucose PD fluids resulted in superior ultrafiltration and improved insulin sensitivity [23].

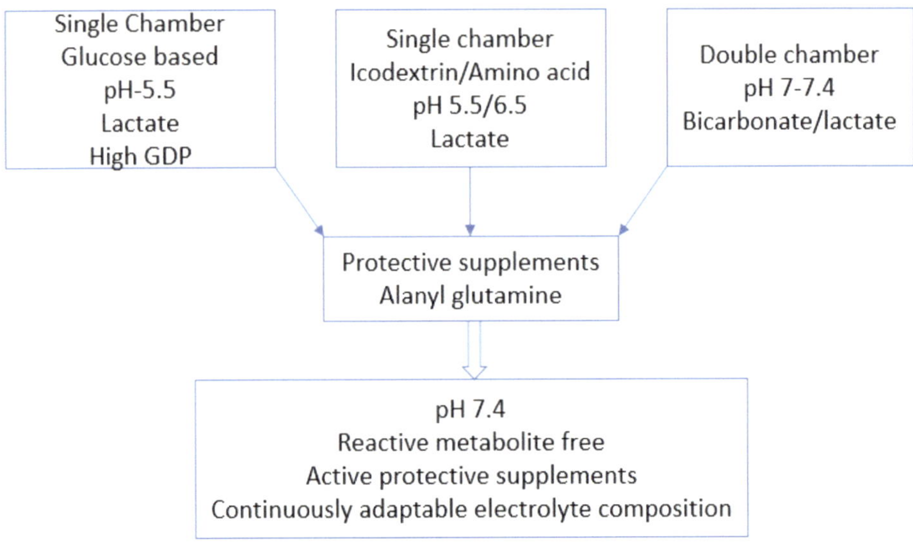

Figure 8.
Novel PD fluid prototypes.

Other preventive strategies:

Peritoneal resting: especially for high solute transport with Type 1 UF failure because this partially reverses some of the functional alterations of peritoneal transport. De souse et al. [24] found decreased D/P creatinine with increased UF capacity, after 4 weeks of peritoneal resting.

12. Newer agents to ameliorate membrane damage

1. Inhibitors of the RAAS system: The mesenchymal cells can locally activate RAAS; in autocrine and paracrine fashion. The administration of RAAS inhibitors results in blockage of the TGF-β, fibronectin and VEGF. Koleysnk et al. [21] and Jing et al. [25], found that ACE inhibitors appeared to have a slower rate of decline in ultrafiltration and residual function, effectively protect against peritoneal fibrosis in long-term peritoneal dialysis.

2. Hyaluronic acid: Preservation of hyaluronan concentration in PD effluent is deemed to be a marker of preservation of peritoneal integrity. It has protective role against abrasion and infection, through the initiation of increased synthesis of growth factors.

3. I.P. Tinzaparin & Bemiparin: Del peso et al. [26] showed an improvement in UF capacity.

4. Paricalcitol: VDR activator reduced IL-17 and increased Tregs leading to antifibrotic and anti-inflammatory effects.

5. Rapamycin: mTOR inhibitors diminish IL-17 and decreases fibrosis with anti-MMT action but delayed healing, limiting its use in specific situations. It also decreases synthesis of VEGF.

6. Tamoxifen: Estrogen receptor modulator, which inhibit MMT, reduces membrane thickness, invasion of the compact zone by mesenchymal mesothelial cells leading to reduced peritoneal MC migration and improved fibrinolytic capacity. A Dutch study showed a decreased mortality among patients with EPS after treatment with Tamoxifen.

7. Nebivolol & Heparin (IP): increases fibrinolytic capacity associated with increased tPA levels. Apart from anticoagulation, heparin also has anti-inflammatory, immunomodulatory, antiangiogenic, antiproliferative, antifibrotic properties. Low-molecular-weight heparins can also inhibit VEGF and fibroblast growth factor activity.

8. Benfotiamine: A derivative of thiamine, has been associated with decreased AGE and decreased oxidation by increasing transketolase [27].

9. Pyridoxamine: beneficial role against UF failure; by reduction in accumulation of AGEs and the expression of angiogenic cytokines leading to decreased transport rates for small solutes and reduced blood vessel density [28].

10. NSAIDs: In a rat model, oral administration of celecoxib drastically reduced prostaglandin E2, angiogenesis and lymph angiogenesis [29] and preserved ultrafiltration. Liu et al. observed that selective COX inhibition resulted in blunting of TGF-β production by mesothelial cells when exposed to high glucose concentrations and resulted in reduction of fibrosis and blunted ultrafiltration failure. No data on oral administration.

11. Sulodexide: consists of 80% LMW heparin and 20% heparan sulphate. Apart from anticoagulation, it has immunomodulating, anti-inflammatory and antiproliferative, and anti-angiogenic properties. Oral sulodexide inhibits either VEGF directly by binding to it or by inhibiting its interaction with receptor.

12. PPAR Y agonist: Rosiglitazone, decreases AGE and fibrosis but the adverse effects have limited its use. The anti-inflammatory properties were mediated by an increase in peritoneal levels of IL-10 along with recruitment of CD4+ CD25+ FoxP3+ cellsD3+ lymphocytes.

13. Tranilast: proposed to have some effects on peritoneal MCs, being the therapeutic potential for the treatment of peritoneal fibrosis [30].

The potential MMT modulators untested in PD are depicted in **Table 2**:

A study in a rat model, by using the stem cells demonstrated that the xenografts of human umbilical mesenchymal stem cells prevented the PD-induced membrane alterations [31].

By the advent of the proteomics and functional genomics analysis of the MC and the EMT, these fine biomarkers can be used for the accurate follow-up of the progressive peritoneal membrane deterioration. They also will identify the master molecules which governs the mesenchymal transition of MC. These molecular profiles of the EMT process in future might become an excellent tool to test the biocompatibility of newer PD fluids. Although further studies are needed, it is expected that increasing knowledge will provide a novel approach for therapeutic benefits in the treatment of peritoneal fibrosis, thus maintaining the peritoneal membrane for an extended period in PD patients.

Antifibrotic agents	Mechanism of action
1) Tetrapeptide	TGF ß inhibition
2) Dipyridamole	TGF ß inhibition
3) Pentoxyfylline	Inhibition of ECM production
4) Emodin	Inhibition of ECM production
5) Simvastatin	Increases fibrinolytic activity
Antiangiogenic	
1) Anecortave acetate	Inhibits VEGF production
2) Pegaptanib	Inhibits VEGF-VEGFR binding
3) Anti-VEGFRII	Blocks receptor VEGFRII
4) TNP 470	Decreases VEGF expression
Inhibition of EMT	
1) Rho-ROCK inhibitor (Y27632)	TGF-β/Smads inhibitors
2) Anti-oxidant agent	NF-κB inhibition
3) Notch inhibitors	Inhibit the induction of snail and repression of VE-cadherin
4) JNK inhibitors (PS600125)	Inhibition of both ZEB and Rho pathway
5) CBR1 antagonists	TGF-β/Smads inhibitors

Courtesy: Gonzalez 2016.

Table 2.
Potential MMT modulators untested IN PD.

Conflicts of interest

None.

Disclosures

None.

Source of funding

Nil.

Abbreviations

AGE	advanced glycation end products
EMT	epithelial to mesenchymal transition
EPS	encapsulating peritoneal sclerosis
GDP	glucose degradation product
IL-6	interleukin 6
LMW	low molecular weight

DOI: http://dx.doi.org/10.5772/intechopen.111586

MC	mesothelial cells
MMT	mesothelial to mesenchymal transition
PD	peritoneal dialysis
RAGE	receptor for AGE
RANTES	regulated on activation, normal T cell expressed and secreted
RRF	residual renal function
STAT	signal transducer and activator of transcription
TGF	transforming growth factor
UF	ultrafiltration
VEGF	vascular endothelial growth factor

Author details

Mathew George Kunthara
Osmania Medical College, India

*Address all correspondence to: mathewgeorgekunthara@gmail.com

References

[1] ESRD Patients in 2004: Global Overview of Patient Numbers, Treatment Modalities and Associated Trends. Available from: https://pubmed.ncbi.nlm.nih.gov/16204281/ [Accessed: January 14, 2021]

[2] Mehrotra R, Devuyst O, Davies SJ, Johnson DW. The current state of peritoneal dialysis. Journal of American Society Nephrology. 2016;**27**(11):3238-3252

[3] Kramer A, Pippias M, Noordzij M, Stel VS, Afentakis N, Ambühl PM, et al. The European Renal Association – European Dialysis and Transplant Association (ERA-EDTA) registry annual report 2015: A summary. Clinical Kidney Journal. 2018;**11**(1):108-122

[4] Flessner MF. Peritoneal ultrafiltration: Physiology and failure. Peritoneal Dialysis – From Basic Concepts to Clinical Excellence. 2009;**163**:7-14

[5] Gónzalez-Mateo G, Gallardo JM, AntonioSánchez-Tomero J, Majano P, Flores-Maldonado E, Paniagua R, et al. Pharmacological Preservation of Peritoneal Membrane in Peritoneal Dialysis. Some Special Problems in Peritoneal Dialysis. 2016. Available from: https://www.intechopen.com/books/some-special-problems-in-peritoneal-dialysis/pharmacological-preservation-of-peritoneal-membrane-in-peritoneal-dialysis [Accessed: January 14, 2021]

[6] Aroeira LS, Aguilera A, Sánchez-Tomero JA, Bajo MA, del Peso G, Jiménez-Heffernan JA, et al. Epithelial to mesenchymal transition and peritoneal membrane failure in peritoneal dialysis patients: Pathologic significance and potential therapeutic interventions. Journal of the American Society of Nephrology. 2007;**18**(7):2004-2013

[7] de Sousa-Amorim E, del Peso G, Bajo MA, Alvarez L, Ossorio M, Gil F, et al. Can EPS development be avoided with early interventions? The potential role of tamoxifen—A Single-Center Study. Peritoneal Dialysis International. 2014;**34**(6):582-593

[8] Pecoits-Filho R, Carvalho MJ, Stenvinkel P, Lindholm B, Heimbürger O. Systemic and intraperitoneal interleukin-6 system during the first year of peritoneal dialysis. Peritoneal Dialysis International. 2006;**26**(1):53-63

[9] Wong TY-H, Szeto C-C, Szeto CY-K, Lai K-B, Chow K-M, Li PK-T. Association of ENOS polymorphism with basal peritoneal membrane function in uremic patients. American Journal of Kidney Diseases. 2003;**42**(4):781-786

[10] Numata M, Nakayama M, Hosoya T, Hoff CM, Holmes CJ, Schalling M, et al. Possible pathologic involvement of receptor for advanced glycation end products (RAGE) for development of encapsulating peritoneal sclerosis in Japanese CAPD patients. Clinical Nephrology. 2004;**62**(6):455-460

[11] Shu K-H, Chuang Y-W, Huang S-T, Cheng C-H, Wu M-J, Chen C-H, et al. Association of interleukin-1β gene polymorphism and peritonitis in uremic patients undergoing peritoneal dialysis. Blood Purification. 2011;**32**(3):156-160

[12] Pletinck A, Vanholder R, Veys N, Van Biesen W. Protecting the peritoneal membrane: Factors beyond peritoneal dialysis solutions. Nature Reviews Nephrology. 2012;**8**(9):542-550

[13] Barreto DL, Hoekstra T, Halbesma N, Leegte M, Boeschoten EW,

Dekker FW, et al. The association of effluent Ca125 with peritoneal dialysis technique failure. Peritoneal Dialysis International. 2015;**35**(7):683-690

[14] Ahmad S, North BV, Qureshi A, Malik A, Bhangal G, Tarzi RM, et al. CCL18 in peritoneal dialysis patients and encapsulating peritoneal sclerosis. European Journal of Clinical Investigation. 2010;**40**(12):1067-1073

[15] del Peso G, Jiménez-Heffernan JA, Selgas R, Remón C, Ossorio M, Fernández-Perpén A, et al. Biocompatible dialysis solutions preserve peritoneal mesothelial cell and Vessel Wall integrity. A case-control study on human biopsies. Peritoneal Dialysis International. 2016;**36**(2):129-134

[16] García-López E, Lindholm B, Davies S. An update on peritoneal dialysis solutions. Nature Reviews Nephrology. 2012;**8**(4):224-233

[17] Dombros NV, Prutis K, Tong M, Anderson GH, Harrison J, Sombolos K, et al. Six-month overnight intraperitoneal amino-acid infusion in continuous ambulatory peritoneal dialysis (CAPD) patients--no effect on nutritional status. Peritoneal Dialysis International. 1990;**10**(1):79-84

[18] Williams JD, Topley N, Craig KJ, Mackenzie RK, Pischetsrieder M, Lage C, et al. The Euro-Balance Trial: The effect of a new biocompatible peritoneal dialysis fluid (balance) on the peritoneal membrane. Kidney International. 2004;**66**(1):408-418

[19] Johnson DW, Brown FG, Clarke M, Boudville N, Elias TJ, Foo MWY, et al. Effects of biocompatible versus standard fluid on peritoneal dialysis outcomes. JASN. 2012;**23**(6):1097-1107

[20] Nishimura H, Ikehara O, Naito T, Higuchi C, Sanaka T. Evaluation of taurine as an osmotic agent for Peritoneal Dialysis Solution. 2009. DOI: 10.1177/089686080902900216

[21] Du C, Mendelson AA, Guan Q, Dairi G, Chafeeva I, da Roza G, et al. Hyperbranched polyglycerol is superior to glucose for long-term preservation of peritoneal membrane in a rat model of chronic peritoneal dialysis. Journal of Translational Medicine. 2016;**14**(1):338

[22] Kratochwill K, Boehm M, Herzog R, Lichtenauer AM, Salzer E, Lechner M, et al. Alanyl–glutamine dipeptide restores the cytoprotective stress proteome of mesothelial cells exposed to peritoneal dialysis fluids. Nephrology Dialysis Transplantation. 2012;**27**(3):937-946

[23] Bonomini M, Liberato LD, Rosso GD, Stingone A, Marinangeli G, Consoli A, et al. Effect of an l-carnitine-containing peritoneal dialysate on insulin sensitivity in patients treated with CAPD: A 4-month, prospective, multicenter randomized trial. American Journal of Kidney Diseases: The Official Journal of the National Kidney Foundation. 2013;**62**(5):929-938

[24] Sousa ED, Peso GD, Alvarez L, Ros S, Mateus A, Aguilar A, et al. Peritoneal resting with heparinized lavage reverses peritoneal type I membrane failure. A Comparative Study of the Resting Effects on Normal Membranes: Peritoneal Dialysis International. 2014. DOI: 10.3747/pdi.2013.00286

[25] Effect of renin–angiotensin system inhibitors on prevention of peritoneal fibrosis in peritoneal dialysis patients - JING - 2010 - Nephrology - Wiley Online Library. DOI: 10.1111/j.1440-1797.2009.01162.x

[26] Effect of Self-administered Intraperitoneal Bemiparin on Peritoneal Transport and Ultrafiltration Capacity

in Peritoneal Dialysis Patients with Membrane Dysfunction. A Randomized, Multi-centre Open Clinical Trial | Nephrology Dialysis Transplantation | Oxford Academic. Available from: https://academic.oup.com/ndt/article/27/5/2051/1838368 [Accessed: January 28, 2021]

[27] Kihm LP, Müller-Krebs S, Klein J, Ehrlich G, Mertes L, Gross M-L, et al. Benfotiamine protects against peritoneal and kidney damage in peritoneal dialysis. Journal of American Society Nephrology. 2011;**22**(5):914-926

[28] Kakuta T, Tanaka R, Satoh Y, Izuhara Y, Inagi R, Nangaku M, et al. Pyridoxamine improves functional, structural, and biochemical alterations of peritoneal membranes in uremic peritoneal dialysis rats. Kidney International. 2005;**68**(3):1326-1336

[29] Cyclooxygenase-2 Mediates Dialysate-Induced Alterations of the Peritoneal Membrane | American Society of Nephrology. Available from: https://jasn.asnjournals.org/content/20/3/582 [Accessed: January 27, 2021]

[30] Fukuyama J, Ichikawa K, Hamano S, Shibata N. Tranilast suppresses the vascular intimal hyperplasia after balloon injury in rabbits fed on a high-cholesterol diet. European Journal of Pharmacology. 1996;**318**(2):327-332

[31] The Therapeutic Potential of Human Umbilical Mesenchymal Stem Cells from Wharton's Jelly in the Treatment of Rat Peritoneal Dialysis-Induced Fibrosis - Fan - 2016 - STEM CELLS Translational Medicine - Wiley Online Library. DOI: 10.5966/sctm.2015-0001

Chapter 4

Timing of Initiation of Kidney Replacement Therapy in Acute Kidney Injury in the Critically Ill Patient

Maiko Alejandro Tavera Diaz

Abstract

Acute kidney injury (AKI) represents one of the most frequent complications in critically ill patients. In recent years, mortality rates have exceeded 50%, and 10% of them require kidney replacement therapy (KRT). Since the 60's, the question of when to start KRT has been raised, classically the time of temporality when life-threatening (hyperkalemia, metabolic acidosis, uremia, and fluid overload); in the last decade, the possibility of early initiation was raised as a strategy to achieve better outcomes. Current evidence shows that the timing of late onset has the same results as the strategy of early onset. We will also review the considerations in relation to renal capacity and demand generated by the acute pathology in a critically ill patient and the set of variables to make better decisions.

Keywords: acute kidney injury, critically ill patients, kidney replacement therapy, uremic toxins, indications for hemodialysis

1. Introduction

Classically, acute kidney injury (AKI) is defined as a decrease in the glomerular filtration rate (eGFR) in a period of less than 3 months accompanied by the retention of nitrogenous products and changes in the internal environment, and anuria or oliguria may or may not be present [1].

In 2004, the Acute Dialysis Quality Initiative (ADQI) group considered that staging the damage is important in the diagnosis of AKI because small increases in creatinine or decreased diuresis are associated with greater morbidity and mortality and longer hospital stay [2].

In the Acute Kidney Injury Network (AKIN) Classification System, the value of increased serum creatinine (sCr) greater than 0.3 mg/dl is added with greater diagnostic sensitivity and eliminates the Loss and ESRD stages [3]. The Kidney Disease Improving Global Outcomes (KDIGO) workgroup in 2012 [4] encompasses an elevation of sCr greater than 0.3 mg/dl or an increase greater than 50% above the baseline value in a period of 7 days; in each of the three stages, a range is placed in relation to the fold increase in creatinine in relation to the basal range, and the other parameter that is taken into account is urine production [4]. Comparison of the KDIGO criteria, creatinine has greater predictive ability than urinary volume.

After reaching consensus on the definition of AKI by the Acute Disease Quality Initiative (ADQI) group, the AKI incidence in the general ward has been 20% [5], with rates increasing by approximately 10% per year [6]. The incidence of AKI in the intensive care unit (ICU) has been 30 to 50%, and 10% require kidney replacement therapy (KRT) [7, 8]. The hospital mortality of AKI has been 27.5% in those who did not require KRT and from 33 to 53% [9] in those who required KRT. This incidence has not changed over time probably due to more serious pathologies and increasingly long-living patients.

The development of AKI in the ICU is considered a predictor of mortality with a specificity of 71% and a sensitivity of 93% similar to the APACHE II score with a specificity of 75% and a sensitivity of 93% and where the relationship between AKI and mortality in the ICU is significant (odds ratio 3.99; 95% CI 2.125–7.481) [10].

2. Classification and biomarkers

The KDIGO guidelines classify the severity of ARF into three stages according to functional 2os2rome (sCr and diuresis), one of which is the elevation of creatinine with respect to baseline, and if the baseline value is not known, the corresponding creatinine values are taken into account, depending on sex, age and race; another variable is the reduction in urinary 2os2rom as a function of time. It is known that creatinine is not the best marker of renal function, in addition to being a late marker, and can be interpreted in different clinical situations such as states of fluid overload (FO), and the creatinine value should be corrected by the FO. There are also drugs that affect the tubular secretion of creatinine (trimethoprim-sulfamethoxazole, cimetidine, and ranitidine) and changes in the rate of sCr production (muscle hypercatabolism, the elderly).

It is important to identify predisposing and susceptibility factors that may develop AKI, such as heart failure, diabetes mellitus, liver disease, chronic kidney disease (CKD), sepsis, emergency surgery, cardiac surgery, and the use of nephrotoxic drugs. The use of biomarkers in populations at clinical risk will allow the detection of subclinical AKI in those at risk of renal complications after exposure to a noxa and allow opportunities for preventive intervention strategies to improve clinical outcomes and reduce the need for KRT [11]. The ADQI consensus conference (**Table 1**) recommends a combination of damage and functional biomarkers (**Table 2**) to improve the diagnostic accuracy of AKI and has made it possible to modify the KDIGO classification in stage 1 AKI with three subcategories (1S, 1A, and 1B) and AKI stage 2 and 3 with subcategories (2 A biomarker negative, 2B biomarker positive) (recommendation grade B) [12, 13].

3. Considerations at the start of kidney replacement therapy

The question of when to start KRT dates back 60 years, where Parsons F. et al. described a retrospective cohort of 17 patients with sepsis of surgical origin with AKI and who underwent intermittent hemodialysis with BUN values >180 mg/dl and had an 88% mortality. One year later, the same work group reported another cohort of 17

	Structural injury	
	No damage	**Damage**
Stable GFR	**Not here** No loss of function no cellular damage	**Subclinical AKI** Cellular damage Without loss of function Conserved creatinine Positive damage response biomarkers Positive cell regulation biomarkers
Decreased GFR	**Functional here** Loss of function Without cellular damage Elevated creatinine Negative tubular function biomarkers	**Established here** Cellular damage With loss of function Elevated creatinine Positive damage response biomarkers Positive cell regulation biomarkers

The ADQI consensus conference recommends a combination of damage and functional biomarkers to improve the diagnostic accuracy of AKI and have allowed modification of the KDIGO classification in stage 1 AKI with three subcategories (1S, 1A, and 1B) and stages 2 and 3 from AKI with subcategories (2A biomarker negative and 2B biomarker positive) [12].

Table 1.
AKI classification.

Biomarkers glomerular filtration	**Tubular function biomarkers**	**Tubular damage biomarkers**	**Damage response biomarkers**	**Cellular regulation biomarkers**
Creatinine Cystatin	FEU, FENA Furosemide stress test	Urinary sediment. Albuminuria	MCP1, IL6, IL10, IL18, KIM-1, LFABP	NGAL TIMP2-IGFBP7

Biomarkers are classified into glomerular filtration, tubular function, tubular damage, injury response, and cell regulation [12].
Urinary insulin-like growth factor-binding protein (IGFBP-7) and tissue inhibitor of metalloproteinase (TIMP-2), neutrophil gelatinase-associated lipocalin (NGAL), interleukin-6, interleukin-10, interleukin-18, Kidney Injury Molecule-1 (KIM-1), liver-type fatty acid-binding protein (L-FABP), Fractional Excretion of Sodium (FENa), and Fractional Excretion of Urea (FEUrea).

Table 2.
Biomarker IN AKI.

patients with AKI due to sepsis with daily BUN increases of 30 mg/dl in which early intervention in dialysis treatment decreased mortality to 25% [14].

The KDIDO-2012 guideline recommends the Initiate KRT emergently when life-threatening changes in fluid, electrolyte, and acid-base balance exist (Not Graded). The clinical context should be considered, and trends from laboratory tests should be evaluated, rather than single nitrogen values (Not Graded). These appraisals are far from being practical and we hope that, with the updated evidence of recent years and the forthcoming recommendations from the KDIGO, they will provide a clearer guideline [15].

The decision to start KRT should not only be based on kidney function or KDIGO stage, but many aspects mentioned below should also be evaluated (**Figure 1**).

The kidneys have a finite capacity; when the demands exceed the renal capacity in the context of AKI, an imbalance with non-renal organ dysfunction is generated. Renal demands and capacity should be assessed taking the following considerations:

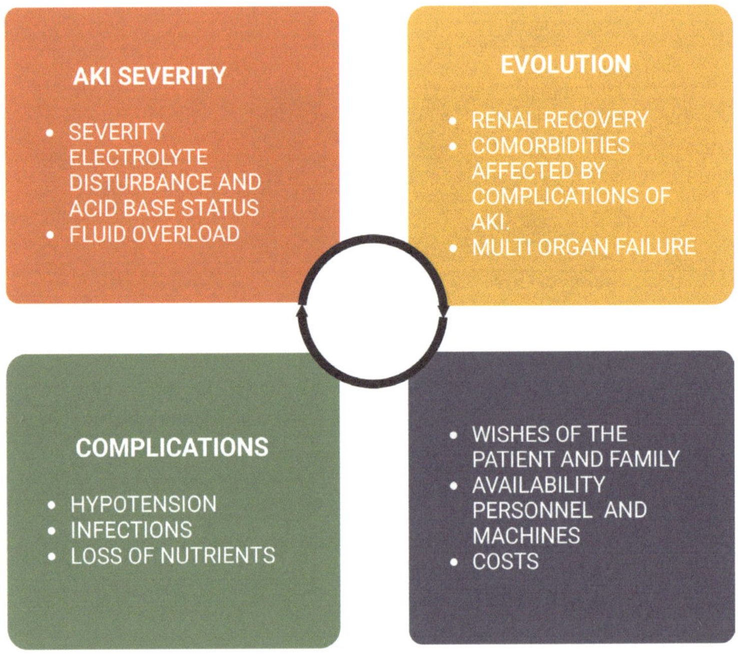

Figure 1.
Considerations at the start of kidney replacement therapy. To consider the initiation of KRT, patient comorbidities, severity of acute illness, severity of AKI, and the expressed will of the patient, family, human resources, and available machines and costs are taken into account [16].

1. Chronic diseases: Chronic heart disease, chronic lung disease, CKD and chronic liver disease present loss of functional reserve and have lower tolerance to fluid overload, solute overload and inflammatory response leading to clinical worsening.

2. Severity of acute disease: elevated vasoactive inotropic score (VIS), SOFA, APACHE and SAPS III scores, refractory hemodynamic instability, macromicrovascular alterations, mitochondrial damage, oxidative stress, inflammatory response, capillary leak syndrome and vasoactive dependence express the degree of severity of acute pathology and in these clinical conditions, loss of renal functional capacity is likely not tolerated.

3. The degree of fluid and solute overload (acids, K, urea myoglobin, and other unmeasurable uremic toxins) generates organ dysfunction in other organs with less functional reserve.

4. The sCr and diuresis are used as markers of renal function; they are not specific and have many limitations in their interpretation, besides being late markers. In the evaluation of renal capacity, the trend of elevated nitrogen levels is important. The use of biomarkers (NGAL, TIMP-IGFB 7) and other tools such as the furosemide stress test (FST) allow the assessment of renal capacity, but they are still far from perfect as markers of damage (**Figure 2**).

5. The initiation of KRT should also consider the risks inherent to the treatment, such as: catheter-associated infections, worsening hemodynamic instability, and nutrient elimination associated with dialytic therapy.

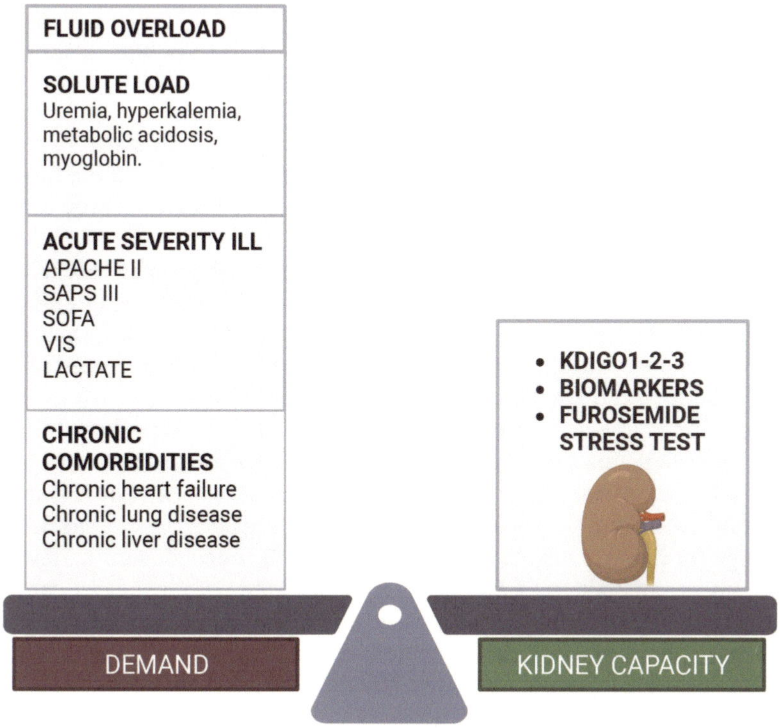

Figure 2.
Kidney capacity and demand. The relationship of renal capacity and demands refers to the state of functional reserve of the kidneys. They are not able to withstand the severity of acute illness, fluid overload, and metabolic overload, where previous comorbid conditions may be a factor in a lower tolerance to the development of AKI [16].

6. It is important to know the wishes of the patient and family, to evaluate with the medical team whether dialysis is part of a therapeutic plan of the multidisciplinary team and that it does not represent a futile measure, and to consider the availability of nursing staff, machines, and costs [16].

4. Management of complications of acute kidney injury and classic indications for kidney replacement therapy

4.1 Hyperkalemia

In AKI, the incidence of hyperkalemia is 13 to 24% and hypokalemia 11 to 17%; dyskalemia values (<3.5 to >5.5 mmol/L) are associated with longer hospital stay and mortality [17, 18]. The prevalence of hyperkalemia increases linearly with the fall in glomerular filtration rate and with the severity of AKI, 3.4% occurring without AKI, 8.8% in AKI stage 1, 17% in AKI stage 2, and 32.2% in AKI stage 3 [19]. It may also be secondary to intracellular potassium release (rhabdomyolysis, tissue injury, and hemolysis) and altered transfer to the intracellular space (metabolic acidosis, insulin deficit) [18].

Independent of AKI, there are factors that contribute to the development of concomitant hyperkalemia in AKI, such as the use of nonsteroidal anti-inflammatory drugs, renin-angiotensin-aldosterone inhibitors (RAASI), and potassium-sparing diuretics; diabetes mellitus (DM); heart failure (HF); chronic kidney disease (CKD); severe tissue breakdown; and potassium intake in crystalloid solutions or oral potassium supplements [20].

The KDIGO Conference on Potassium Controversies recommended cardiac monitoring and 12-lead electrocardiogram (ECG) for potassium levels >6.0 mmol/L. There is evidence to support that severe hyperkalemia levels do not necessarily exhibit ECG changes, as will be described later [21].

Mortality increases in a linear relationship with increasing potassium, K = 4.5–5.0 mmol/L with odds ratio (OR) 1.25; K = 5.0–5.5 mmol/L with OR 1.42; K = 5.5–6.0 mmol/L with OR 1.67; K = 6.0–6.5 mmol/L with OR 1.63; K > 6.5 mmol/L with OR 1.72 where the risk of mortality is higher. Hyperkalemia, if not decreased by >1.0 mEq/L within 48 h after measurement, predicts death [22].

There is important evidence in a meta-analysis [23] with more than 1 million patients with dyskalemia that was associated with all-cause, cardiovascular mortality and shows a U-shaped curve for hypokalemia (3.0 mmol/L) with HR 1.49 and in hyperkalemia (>5. 5 mmol/L) with HR 1.22. Likewise, values considered within the normal range for healthy subjects do not seem to be as innocuous for patients with AKI, since potassium values ≥4.8 mmol/L are associated with higher all-cause mortality with an adjusted HR of 1.12. Decreased eGFR was a strong risk factor for hyperkalemia (>5.5 mmol/L); also, the interaction of hyponatremia with hyperkalemia was associated with higher 30-day (HR 1.15) and 90-day (HR 1.16) mortality. Values of "normokalemia" seem to have an impact on mortality in patients with AKI, but these findings need to be confirmed in prospective studies [24]. Li et al., in a retrospective observational study in adjusted multivariate analysis, shows the risk of all-cause mortality for K values 4.1–4.79 mmol/L with HR 1.45; K 4.8–5.49 mmol/L with HR 2.15 and for K > 5.5 mmol/L with HR 2.34 [25].

Mortality is related to not only the severity of hyperkalemia but also the prolonged duration of hyperkalemia and lack of correction of the disorder, rapid increases in serum potassium, massive cell turnover, and underlying heart disease. In a study of 408 patients excluding patients with end-stage renal disease (ESRD) and on hemodialysis (HD), hyperkalemia of prolonged duration was associated with concomitant AKI (OR = 3.88; $p = 0.03$), metabolic acidosis (OR = 4.84; $p < 0.01$), tissue necrosis (OR = 4.55; $p < 0.01$), and potassium supplements (OR = 5.46; $p < 0.01$), and all of them are associated with higher hospital mortality [26].

Mortality is attributed to changes in heart rhythm and its consequences such as hemodynamic instability, myocardial ischemia, and sudden cardiac death [27]. Under normokalemia conditions, the cardiomyocyte cell membrane is polarized (resting potential at −90 mV). In moderate hyperkalemia, the cell membrane partially depolarizes, bringing the resting potential closer to the threshold potential for action potential initiation, where fast sodium channels are activated, increasing excitability and conduction velocity, and it electrocardiographically manifests as a T-wave spike. In severe hyperkalemia (K ≥ 6.5 mmol/L), voltage-dependent inactivation of sodium channels and activation of internal rectifying potassium channels lead to reductions in conduction velocity, and cells enter a state refractory to excitation and is expressed electrocardiographically with widening of complexes and blockades driving [28, 29].

ECG findings do not have a relationship with hyperkalemia levels in patients with 9 AKI and ESRD [30]; ECG is an insensitive tool for the diagnosis of hyperkalemia even with K values between 6 and 7.2 mmol/L and with K values >7.3 mmol/L the predictive value is minimal; non-traditional electrocardiographic changes are also described [31].

In a prospective study [32] of 77 patients that included both AKI and CKD, 94% associated with a fall in eGFR and 70.9% had metabolic acidosis, 10.4% developed mild hyperkalemia (5.5–5.9 mmol/L), moderate 40.3% (6–6.4 mmol/L), and severe 49.3% (>6.5 mmol/L); electrocardiographic changes occurred in 74.6% of patients, the most frequent findings being atrial fibrillation (13.4%), peaked T wave (11.9%), widened QRS, and prolonged PR (10.5%); none of these electrocardiographic findings were more significant with greater severity. The sensitivity in the electrocardiographic detection of hyperkalemia was 0.28 for the emergency physician and 0.36 for the cardiologist. The diagnosis improved with K values >6.5 mmol/L and in another study with values >7.8 mmol/L. The lack of sensitivity in the electrocardiographic diagnosis in these study groups may be biased by the slow increases in K in ESRD and the use of hemodialysis. The electrocardiographic findings may be masked by the effect of fluid overload and other electrolyte disorders such as concomitant hypocalcemia. In this sense, hypocalcemia can induce QT prolongation and widening of T waves and may mask the changes in T wave morphology caused by hyperkalemia [33, 34].

There is no conclusive evidence that the electrocardiogram can guide the treatment of 3iperkalemia and electrolyte monitoring is necessary.

In a prospective cohort of patients with AKI, it was identified that 60.8% developed dyskalemia, and 8 evolution groups were identified according to the kalemia characteristics. Group 7 was characterized by K values that were normal on hospital admission and increased to hyperkalemia; group 8 were those that never returned to a normal kalemia value and corresponded to uncorrected hyperkalemia. In both groups, the increase in mortality was identified, 37% for group 7 and 63% for group 8, and the latter group had a higher risk (40%) of requiring KRT [35].

When hyperkalemia is associated with arrhythmias and/or hemodynamic instability despite medical treatment, the initiation of intermittent hemodialysis or sustained low-efficiency dialysis (SLED) or continuous kidney replacement therapy (CKRT) is indicated. In situations where rapid and prolonged K generation is generated, such as in rhabdomyolysis, tissue lysis syndrome and tissue ischemia, where hyperkalemia values are persistent and the K load exceeds the elimination capacity by CKRT, intermittent hemodialysis is recommended [36].

It is important to consider that the longer the duration of hyperkalemia and without the ability to correct itself, the higher the mortality and we see that mortality is associated with extreme values of dyskalemia.

4.1.1 Management of acute hyperkalemia

There is limited evidence, and the existing one is based on the recommendation of experts or studies with a small number of patients for the analysis of the treatment of acute hyperkalemia in AKI, and many of the studies of this disorder come from patients with CKD (**Table 3**).

4.1.1.1 Membrane stabilizers

Calcium gluconate and calcium chloride

The recommendation for the use of calcium gluconate is based on expert opinion; there are no randomized studies.

	Mechanism	Onset (min)	Duration (hours)	Effect on potassium plasma level	Dose	Side effects
Calcium gluconate 10%	Membrane stabilization	1–3 min	1–2	None	10–20 ml iv within 5 min	Hypercalcemia Digoxin toxicity
Calcium chloride 10%	Membrane stabilization	5 min	1–2	None	10–20 mL iv within 5 min	Tissue necrosis
Hypertonic sodium 20%	Membrane stabilization	5– 10 minutes	2	None	10–20 mL IV within 5 min	Hypernatremia Volume overload
Regular insulin/ dextrose	Shift K in to the cells	10– 20 minutes	4–6	-0.7 ± 0.6 mEq/L at 60 min	Regular insulin 5 or 10 U + Glucose level > 200 mg/dl, none dextrose. Glucose 100–200 mg/dl, supplemental 25 gr dextrose 50% (50 ml). Glucose level < 200 mg/dl, supplemental 50 gr dextrose 50% (100 ml) at 60 min	Hypoglycemia Hyperglycemia
Sodium Bicarbonate	Shift K in to the cells	90 min	2–4	-0.47 ± 0.31 mmol/L at 30 min	100 mL of 8.4% iv at 30 min. either 125–250 ml of 4.2% iv at 30 min.	Hypernatremia Volume overload Hypocalcemia
B2 – Agonist	Shift K in to the cells	30 min	2–6	-0.5 ± 0.1 mmol/L at 60 min	0.5 mg IV either 10 mg nebulization over 15 min	Tachycardia, tremors
Patiromer	K removal	180-420 min	12–24	0.75 mmol/L at 48 hours	8.4–25.2 g per day	Gastrointestinal intolerance and hypomagnesemia
Zyrconium	K removal	120 min	24–48	-0.67 mEq/L at 48 hours	10 g one to three times a day	Gastrointestinal side effects and edema
Furosemide	K removal	15 min	2–3 hours	-0.3 mmol/L at 3–6 hours	40–80 mg IV	Volume depletion
Hemodialysis	K removal	immediately	3 hours	-1 mmol/L at 60 min	3–4 hours on modality intermittent hemodialysis	Arrhythmias

Table 3.
Drugs for the management of hyperkalemia [37, 38].

Calcium gluconate increases intracellular calcium entry and binds to calcium-dependent calmodulin and protein kinase II (CaMKII), which allows sodium channel activation, leading to intracellular sodium entry, thus restoring action potential in phase 0 dV/dt. Also, hypertonic physiological solution increases extracellular sodium and allows greater intracellular displacement of sodium, managing to increase the speed of the action potential; it is an option as a membrane stabilizer [18, 39].

Membrane stabilizers should be started early, after identification of hyperkalemia >6.5 mmol/L or when some ECG change is evident in the context of hyperkalemia. The recommended dose is from 10 ml (2.3 mmol of Ca^{2+}) to 20 ml of 10% undiluted calcium gluconate, administered over 3 to 5 minutes; if ECG changes persist, it can be administered again later 5 min; the effect lasts between 30 to 60 minutes [40]. Another option as a membrane stabilizer is calcium chloride, which has three times the concentration of Ca^{2+} (6.8 mmol of Ca^{2+}) than calcium gluconate, but tissue damage secondary to skin extravasation has been described. There are no randomized studies available showing a clear benefit of hypertonic saline.

In an observational and prospective study of 111 patients with a mean $K > 7.1$ mmol/L, 243 pathological ECGs were found, of which in 79 cases, they were identified as major rhythm disorders (AV block, sinus bradycardia, right and left bundle block, escape beats, atrial fibrillation, ventricular tachycardia), and of these only 9 cases improved with calcium gluconate in a dose of 10 ml at 10% and was repeated up to three times. Calcium gluconate may only be effective in major rhythm disorders with limited evidence and did not cause statistically significant improvement in non-rhythmic ECG disorders [41].

4.1.1.2 Intracellular redistribution of potassium

Insulin-dextrose

The insulin binds to glucose transporter type 4 receptor on skeletal muscles and allows the translocation of intracellular Na^+-K^+ ATPase to the cell membrane and induces the transfer of potassium from the extracellular space to the intracellular space. Insulin stimulates the phosphorylation of FXYD1 (phospholigen) by atypical protein kinase C, increasing the Na-K ATPase Vmax for potassium transfer into the intercellular space [42].

Regular insulin allows a reduction of K in a range of 0.5 to 0.9 mEq/L and dextrose alone in a range of 0.2 to 0.6 mEq/L; current evidence recommends both treatments as first line of treatment [18].

In a randomized crossover study in 10 patients per group on chronic hemodialysis, in the 4lucosa infusion alone group (100 ml of 50% 4lucosa) versus the 4lucosa + insulin group (100 ml of 50% 4lucosa + 10 IU of regular insulin), K Values were measured at 60 minutes and there was a significant decrease in K 0.83 ± 0.53 mmol/l ($p < 0.001$) in the combined treatment compared to the glucose alone group (0.50 ± 0.31 mmol/l) [43].

In a retrospective cohort study of 174 critically ill patients with concomitant hyperkalemia in ARF or CKD, two groups were evaluated, those receiving 5 IU of regular insulin and those receiving 10 IU of regular insulin. Both groups received 25 g of dextrose along with intravenous insulin and 1 hour after receiving insulin a second dose of 25 g of dextrose was administered and a third dose of 25 g of dextrose if blood glucose was less than 70 mg/dl and hourly blood glucose was measured and K control were performed after 2 or 3 hours of insulin administration. The rate of hypoglycemia at the sixth hour was higher in the 10-unit insulin group 19.5% and 9.2% in the 5-unit group (p = 0.052); in severe hypoglycemia, there was no difference between the groups. K reduction was similar (−0.8 ± 0.7 mEq/L in the 5-unit group vs. −0.7 ± 0.6 mEq/L in the 10-unit group (p = 0.430)) [17]. (p = 0.052); in severe hypoglycemia, there were no differences between groups. The reduction of K was similar (−0.8 ± 0. 7 mEq/L in the 5-unit group vs. −0.7 ± 0.6 mEq/L in the 10-unit group (p = 0.430)) [17]. Regular insulin doses of 5 units reduce K levels without difference with higher doses and with fewer hypoglycemic events.

In a systematic review of 11 studies, different doses of insulin are described. In eight studies, 10 units of regular insulin were administered and of these, in 5 studies the method of administration was a bolus and in two studies as an infusion over 15 to 30 minutes, and in another three studies regular insulin was administered 5 IU/Kg equivalent to 20 units in 60 minutes. Regarding the glucose dose, it was 25 g in six studies, 30 g in one study, 40 g in two studies, 50 g in one study, and 60 g in another study. The incidence of hypoglycemia was 30% in the group that used 25 g of glucose; when 60 g of glucose was administered, no hypoglycemia was reported. When a bolus dose of 10 units of regular insulin was used, the serum potassium decrease at 60 minutes was 0.78 ± 0.25 mmol/L, and with the administration of insulin infusion of 20 units over 60 minutes, the decrease in serum potassium was 0.79 ± 0.25 mmol/L, with no significant difference between both groups (P = 0.98) [44].

A meta-analysis of 10 retrospective cohort studies (n = 3437) with low or moderate risk of bias evaluated standard doses (10 IU regular insulin) vs. alternative doses (5 IU regular insulin or 0.1 IU/kg). K reduction was similar in the two groups (mean difference − 0.02 mmol/L, 95% CI −0.11–0.07, I2 = 53%), with no difference in hospital mortality (OR 1.03, 95% CI 0.58–1.81, I2 = 0%); in the alternative dose group there was a lower risk of hypoglycemia (OR 0.55, 95% CI 0.43–0.69, I2 = 8%); and severe hypoglycemia (OR 0.41, 95% 0.27–0.64) [37].

The use of dextrose and insulin constitutes the first line of treatment for intracellular K redistribution; when comparing 5 units vs. 10 units of regular insulin, the K decrease values are similar, and with fewer hypoglycemia events in the first group, the recommended dose of 50 ml dextrose 50% (25 g) is a safe regimen to avoid hypoglycemia [18].

In case of severe hyperkalemia, a dose of 20 units of regular insulin with 60 g of glucose (200 ml 30% dextrose) for 60 minutes is recommended, and an alternative in non-severe hyperkalemia is a dose of 10 units of regular insulin, and 25 g (50 mL 50% dextrose) to glucose is a safe regimen to avoid hypoglycemia.

Sodium bicarbonate

Evidence for the use of sodium bicarbonate is limited and heterogeneous including patients with ESRD, AKI, and various therapeutic interventions for the management of hyperkalemia.

Sodium bicarbonate allows intracellular entry of sodium through the Na + /H + (NHE) exchanger; higher intracellular sodium activates sodium-potassium adenosine triphosphatase (NaK + ATPase) and allows transfer of potassium from the extracellular space to the intracellular space [18].

Studies on sodium bicarbonate show that it is not able to rapidly reduce serum potassium levels with optimal efficacy, and the onset of its action can take several hours; therefore, it is not recommended as first-line treatment [18].

There is controversy regarding its usefulness, due to the small decrease in K values <1 mmol/L and slow onset. Some predictors of a better response to the use of bicarbonate are mentioned, such as the presence of hyperkalemia >6 mmol/L, metabolic acidosis with pH < 7.35 or bicarbonate <17 mmol/L, AKI and the use of bicarbonate doses >120 mEq [36]. There are clinical situations where its use should be avoided, such as in organic acid acidosis (diabetic ketoacidosis, lactoacidosis) and hypervolemia [45].

In a retrospective study of 106 patients, of which 38 patients correspond to the sodium bicarbonate group (regular insulin and bicarbonate) and 68 patients to the control group (regular insulin without bicarbonate), the primary objective was to compare the absolute reduction in serum potassium between initial concentrations and at 2-hour intervals, up to 8 hours. Median initial potassium concentration was higher in the bicarbonate group (6.6 vs. 6.1 mmol/L (P = 0.009)); the lowest potassium concentration was reached within the first 8-h period, with no difference between both groups (bicarbonate group 5.35 mmol/L) vs. (control group 5.15 mmol/L (P = 0.255)). We saw that adding bicarbonate did not improve the absolute reduction of K. It must be clarified that this study has several limitations and randomized controlled trials are required to confirm the efficacy of bicarbonate [46].

The different concentrations of 1.4% or 8.4% sodium bicarbonate have the same capacity to reduce potassium values, even a transient increase of K in patients with CKD is mentioned, the lack of evidence should be considered due to a small number of patients in the studies [47].

Potassium homeostasis and management of dyskalemia in kidney diseases: conclusions from a Kidney Disease: Improving Global Outcomes (KDIGO) Controversies Conference recommends a bicarbonate dose of 1 amp of 50 ml of 8.4% over 15 minutes. The European Resuscitation Council Guidelines recommend sodium bicarbonate 1 mmol/kg IV in case of a metabolic acidosis (pH < 7.2) and/or in cardiac arrest [21, 48].

In the BICAR-ICU study [49], 4.2% sodium bicarbonate in patients with severe metabolic acidosis (pH < 7.2) reported lower K values and less hemodialysis requirement when compared with the control group. The use of hypertonic sodium bicarbonate (100–250 mL of 8.4% sodium bicarbonate over 20 min) is also recommended in patients with severe metabolic acidosis and AKI, who have a contraindication to the use of calcium gluconate. It is important to mention that sodium bicarbonate has side effects, such as fluid overload and hypocalcemia; the aforementioned electrolyte disorder is crucial for cardiac contractility, for which its monitoring and replacement are important.

Beta-agonists

Beta-adrenergic agonists activate pancreatic β receptors, causing increased insulin secretion, which activates Na-K-ATPase and stimulates K movement into cells [18, 50].

The standard doses are 10 and 20 mg for the inhaled forms and between 0.5 and 2.5 mg intravenously; the effect begins between 15 and 30 minutes regardless of the formulation used. K decreases were 0.3 mmol/L with 10 mg and 0.6 mmol/L with 20 mg, with a duration of effect of 2 hours [51].

In a randomized, double-blind, placebo-controlled trial of few patients (n 17) with ERSD, there was an increase in K by 0.1 mmol/L in the first minute after inhalation; when compared to placebo (p < 0.001), the increase in K was transient without generating arrhythmias and was attributed to the β 1-activity of these drugs. Also, the values of glycemia, insulin, and heart rate increase after 5 minutes of salbutamol inhalation [51].

The paradoxical elevation of K by beta-agonists is slight and transient; it is not known if they have a clinical effect in critically ill patients and raises doubts about the use of these drugs.

4.1.1.3 Elimination of potassium

Diuretics

Loop diuretics act by inhibiting the NKCC2 channel on the apical surface of the thick cells of the ascending limb of the loop of Henle, generating natriuresis and kaliuretic effect. The use of furosemide in AKI is useful for the management of fluid overload and as a stress test to assess the progression of sustained AKI and to determine the need for hemodialysis; the use of diuretics in non-responders should not delay the use of other types of therapies for the management of hyperkalemia [18, 52].

New resins

Patiromer is a non-absorbable and sodium-free potassium-chelating polymer. It is not ideal for the management of severe acute hyperkalemia, since the decrease in serum K is 0.21 ± 0.07 mmol/L in 7 hours and 0.75 mmol/ L in 48 hours; its use is focused on patients with CKD and ESRD [18, 38].

Sodium zirconium cyclosilicate (zs-9)

ZS-9 is a crystal that is selective for potassium and ammonium ions, and they exchange sodium for potassium. A systematic review and meta-analysis of data from phases II and III clinical trials found that ZS-9 produced a decrease in K of −0.17 mEq/L 1 hour after dosing, and − 0.67 mEq/L at 48 hours; at this time, it is not recommended for severe acute hyperkalemia [18, 53].

In a review of seven randomized controlled trials, it shows that the use of IV insulin + dextrose and salbutamol in any of the pharmacological presentations are the most effective in lowering serum potassium. Evidence on the benefits of IV sodium bicarbonate is limited [54].

In severe hyperkalemia and refractory to medical treatment, KRT is indicated; the details of the indication and timing of KRT will be discussed later.

Kidney replacement therapy.

In a large retrospective study of AKI complications in critically ill patients in the multivariate logistic regression model adjusted for AKI-related complications, KRT was found to be associated with increased hospital survival (OR 0.75; 95% CI, 0.58 to 0.96), and KRT decreased mortality by 45% in patients with hyperkalemia [19].

The causes of death in AKI attributed to hyperkalemia, metabolic acidosis, volume overload and uremia with the onset KRT allowed correction of these alterations, was associated with improved hospital survival (OR, 0.75; 95 % CI, 0.58 to 0.96) [19].

In RCTs such as ELAIN and STARRT, late onset of CKRT was associated with K values >6 mmol/l and/or ECG abnormalities; in the AKIKI study, the value was K > 6 mmol/L (or > 5.5 mmol/L without improvement despite medical treatment); in the IDEAL-ICU, the K values were higher (> 6.5 mmol/L), and 4% had a K of 7 mmol/L for the start of dialysis treatment in a delayed strategy or there were no significant differences between the groups in other adverse events, nor in mortality. Medical treatment for hyperkalemia could prevent or delay the initiation of KRT in patients with AKI and avoid complications of dialysis therapy and additional costs [55–58].

4.2 Metabolic acidosis

Acidemia is the accumulation of protons in the plasma, whose expression is a low blood pH. Severe acidemia is defined when the pH is <7.20, but it is not a universally accepted term. Metabolic acidosis is classified based on time, as acute (hours to days) and chronic (weeks to months), and based on the presence of an anion gap (AGMA) and no anion gap (NAGMA). In AKI, metabolic acidosis is caused by decreased renal synthesis of bicarbonate and decreased excretion of nonvolatile acids in the urine [59].

Metabolic acidosis has an impact on several systems. At the cardiac level, Ca 2+ transport decreases through the SR Ca 2+ -ATPase (SERCA) channels, the ryanodine receptor (RyR) and the Na + /Ca 2+ (NCX) exchanger, having a negative inotropic effect, due to less coupling and decreased sensitivity of troponin C regulatory sites to Ca2+. Also, in acidosis, it conditions a delayed β-adrenergic response and decreases the affinity of β-adrenergic receptors for vasoactive (norepinephrine, epinephrine) and inotropic agents, decreasing the responsiveness to catecholamines [60].

The impact of the drop in pH generates a lower affinity of hemoglobin for oxygen at the tissue level (Bohr effect), shifting the oxygen dissociation curve to the left; acidosis also decreases cerebrospinal pH and could be responsible for the confusional state. Altered pH suppresses lymphocyte function; the chemotactic and phagocytic capacity of leukocytes is reduced, and the proinflammatory response of macrophages is increased, all of which sets the stage for the development of infections. The impact is also expressed in energy and enzymatic exhaustion, stimulating apoptosis and cell death. These mentioned alterations are of multifactorial origin in the context of sepsis, ischemia reperfusion, and AKI [61].

Not all acidosis is the same and it also depends on the disease that causes the acidosis, since the type of acid determines the risk of mortality. In an observational cohort study of 851 critically ill patients, it was identified that 64% developed acidosis and mortality was 45%. When the subgroup analysis was performed, mortality was higher in the lactic acidosis subgroup (56%) when compared to strong ion gap (SIG) acidosis (39%) and hyperchloremic acidosis (29%) [62].

The treatment of acidosis should be aimed at treating the cause that generates it. The administration of bicarbonate has the objective of reversing the deleterious effects of severe acidosis, and the complications related to its use must be weighed. Sodium bicarbonate is reported to cause a transient decrease in blood pressure and cardiac output and hypocalcemia, sensitizing the heart to abnormal electrical activity [63].

The use of sodium bicarbonate is a common medical practice in critically ill patients and has not demonstrated a clear benefit. Next, we will review the evidence that limits the general use of bicarbonate and is limited to particular cases (**Table 4**).

In a prospective, observational, multicenter study, 155 critically ill patients with severe acidemia (single metabolic acidemia or mixed respiratory and metabolic

Bicarbonate is indicated in patients with hyperlactatemia with circulatory shock with pH < 7.2 and AKI in the initial phase of resuscitation **(Level of evidence: B)**
In severe non-anion gap metabolic acidosis (NAGMA) **(Level of evidence: B).**
There is no evidence to recommend its use in a general way in cardiac arrest unless caused by hyperkalemia; there is no clear evidence for its use in diabetic ketoacidosis and rhabdomyolysis [64].

Table 4.
Recommendations for the use of bicarbonate IN different clinical scenarios.

acidemia) with pH values <7.2 within the first 24 hours of ICU admission were analyzed. It showed that the incidence of acidosis in the ICU was 6%; 90% of the patients studied required mechanical ventilation and vasopressors; 20% required KRT within the first 24 hours, and the mortality rate was 57%. In non-survivors, SOFA, SAPSII, anion gap, base excess, lactatemia scores and length of ICU stay were higher and associated with higher mortality ($p = <0.01$). Regarding the development of AKI or the need for KRT, there was no difference between survivors and non-survivors. Administration of bicarbonate at different concentrations in the first 24 hours did not improve prognosis [65]. Regarding the development of AKI or the need for KRT, there were no differences between the survivors and not survivors. The administration of bicarbonate in different concentrations in the first 24 hours did not improve the prognosis [65].

In the BICAR-ICU a multicenter, open-label, randomized controlled, phase 3 trial, a study of 389 patients, of whom 61% had sepsis (195 in the bicarbonate group and 194 in the control group), included patients within 48 hours of ICU admission presenting with severe acidemia (pH <7.2, PaCO2 ≤ 45 mm Hg, and sodium bicarbonate concentration ≤ 20 mmol/L) and an arterial lactate concentration of 2 mmol/L or more total Sequential Organ Failure Assessment (SOFA) score of 4 or more. The bicarbonate group received 125–250 ml in 30 min, with a maximum of 1000 ml within 24 h of inclusion. When assessing mortality on day 28 and failure of ≥1 organ on day 7 (primary composite outcome), there were no significant differences ($p = 0.24$) and in those who developed AKI on the AKIN 2 and 3 scale, the use of bicarbonate improved survival at 28 days ($p = 0.017$) and failure of ≥1 organ on day 7 ($p = 0.014$) and decreased the need for KRT ($p = 0.0283$). This study shows several weaknesses and requires a trial with a larger number of patients to obtain more conclusive results [49].

In another RCT of 1718 patients diagnosed with sepsis and metabolic acidosis (pH < 7.3 and bicarbonate <20 mmol/L) randomized into two groups, 500 patients in the bicarbonate group and 1218 patients in the control group, bicarbonate infusion had no effect in reducing mortality ($p = 0.67$), but it is beneficial in reducing mortality risk in patients with KIDGO AKI stage 2 or 3 and pH < 7.2 by 22% ($p = 0.032$) [66].

In two meta-analyses of five randomized controlled trials (RCTs) of AKI secondary to cardiac surgery (CSA-AKI) as a preventive measure, bicarbonate was administered at a bolus dose of 0.5 mmol/kg of body weight, diluted in 250 ml of dextrose to 5% for 1 hour immediately after induction of anesthesia and then continuous infusion of 0.15 mmol/kg/h diluted in 1000 ml of 5% dextrose for 23 hours. There were no differences in the development of CSA-AKI between the patients in the sodium bicarbonate group and the control group; there was no difference in mortality at 30 and 90 days, no differences in the need for KRT, nor in the days of stay in ICU between both groups. It should not be recommended for the prevention of CSA-AKI, and the perioperative infusion should be administered with caution due to the risk of fluid overload [67, 68].

It should be considered that the injury mechanisms in CSA-AKI and in sepsis are different and it is possible that the response and benefits of the use of bicarbonate are also different. We hope that future studies will make it possible to individualize the therapy in each group.

KRT is indicated for severe metabolic acidosis refractory to medical treatment in the setting of AKI. In a retrospective study of 1815 AKI patients undergoing CKRT who were assessed for pH trajectory in five groups during CKRT: 1st group normal pH; 2nd group, suboptimal pH trajectory of 7.3 initially and approached pH 7.4; the 3rd group, recovering from acidosis with pH 7.2 to 7.3; 4th group, tendency to worsen acidosis with pH 7.3 to 7.2; and 5th group, uncorrected pH trajectory and less than 7.2 despite CKRT. AKI due to sepsis was more common in the 3rd group; the SOFA and APACHE II scores, and the requirement for mechanical ventilation were higher in groups 4 and 5. In the multivariate analysis, mortality increased from the first to the fifth group, showing higher mortality from the 3rd to the 5th group (3rd group 74.2%, 4th group 78.2%, and 5th group 82.2%) despite the start of CKRT. The measurement of CRP values >30 mg/dl occurred in a greater proportion in the patients of groups 4 and 5 of metabolic acidosis. It is important to consider that the inflammatory response triggered by different pathways conditions the origin of oxidative stress, and mitochondrial and endothelial damage that can be a point of no return in patients with sepsis, septic shock, and AKI. We see that with the support of CKRT, mortality did not decrease. This work has several limitations, and randomized clinical trials are required to ascertain whether pH correction during CKRT improves the survival rate of patients with metabolic acidosis [69].

There is no consensus with which pH or bicarbonate value hemodialysis should be started. In the RCTs in recent years, they use different values. In the ELAIN and AKIKI study, they use a pH value <7.15 in the context of pure metabolic acidosis or mixed acidosis, and it represented 21% of the CKRT indications in the second study. In the IDEAL-ICU study, the cut-off value was pH < 7.15 and base deficit >5 mEq/l or $HCO3-$ < 18 mEq/l, and acidosis represented 13.4% of CKRT indications. In the STARRT-AKI study, the absolute criterion for CKRT was considered in the presence of severe acidemia and metabolic acidosis, with a pH ≤ 7.2 or $HCO3-$ < 12 mmol/l, and this criterion was present in 16.6% of those who required CKRT. Patients with severe metabolic acidosis and stage 2 or 3 AKI should be managed with bicarbonate with the based of delayed dialysis therapy that avoids complications associated with early dialysis therapy and which does not confer a survival benefit [55–58].

4.3 Fluid overload

The administration of intravenous fluids is one of the cornerstones of the resuscitation of critically ill patients, with the aim of optimizing hemodynamics, increasing stroke volume, improving organ perfusion, and supplying the O_2 supply. Fluid resuscitation has been empirical; there is no ideal administration strategy free of complications. The Surviving Sepsis Campaign recommends the use of a minimum of 30 mL/kg (ideal body weight) of intravenous crystalloids and was based on observational studies [70].

Fluid resuscitation carries a narrow line between insufficient resuscitation and fluid overload. In the past, hydration was based on clinical parameters and basic measurements ("blood pressure, edema, arterial blood gases, chest Rx, central venous pressure (CVP) and pulmonary capillary wedge pressure (PCWP)" which have low sensitivity, specificity and are late [71]. Currently, for a better assessment, dynamic tests are used to assess the change in stroke volume after a maneuver that increases or decreases venous return (preload) through echocardiography at the patient's bedside, pulse contour analysis (PCA), and trans-pulmonary thermodilution (TPTD). It is mentioned that only 50% [72] of hemodynamically unstable patients respond to volume; according to the Frank-Starling curve, increasing the preload allows the left ventricular (LV) stroke volume to be increased until the optimal preload is reached, achieving a stroke volume at a constant plateau. Resuscitation must be individualized and guided in order to improve preload and increase stroke volume with fluid challenge and avoid excessive use of fluids in nonresponders [73, 74].

% Fluid overload = (total fluid in − total fluid out) /admission body weight × 100)

Table 5.
% Fluid overload.

Fluid overload is the consequence of excess fluids in resuscitation, maintenance solutions, drug dilutions, nutrition, and use of blood products. Fluid overload (FO) was defined as the ratio between cumulative fluid balance (L) and initial body weight (kg) at admission and expressed as a percentage. It is considered that an FO > 10% at the time of AKI development has an adjusted odds ratio (OR) for associated death of 3.14 (95% CI, 1.18 to 8.33); for this reason, its importance in the assessment lies in the critical patients (**Table 5**) [75].

It is important to differentiate that the positive cumulative balance that reflects higher admissions than discharges without necessarily generating fluid overload; the fluid overload itself reflects the degree of fluid accumulation in tissues (pulmonary congestion and/or edema) and is expressed as a percentage [76].

The clinical condition with a positive cumulative fluid balance will have an impact with multiple adverse effects such as the development and progression of AKI, need for KRT, mechanical ventilation, intra-abdominal hypertension, and capillary leak syndrome and with a higher probability of overload-associated mortality (OR 2.07) [77].

How is fluid overload generated?

The development of FO is due to the close balance between a deterioration in cardiac function, the vasoplegic state that does not improve fluid supply, the AKI in a state of oliguria/anuria, the inflammatory response in sepsis or other proinflammatory clinical condition, and endothelial and glycocalyx damage, which are relevant factors in the development of FO.

A key component is the endothelium of all blood vessels; it is covered by glycocalyx or Endothelial Surface Layer (ESL), which is made up of a layer of polysaccharides that forms a network of molecules that generate a state of equilibrium between the vascular wall and the plasma [78].

The glycocalyx is made up of: (**Figure 3**)

1. **Proteoglycans:** These are centrally arranged proteins with a domain attached to the basement membrane through glypicans, syndecans, and other proteoglycans.

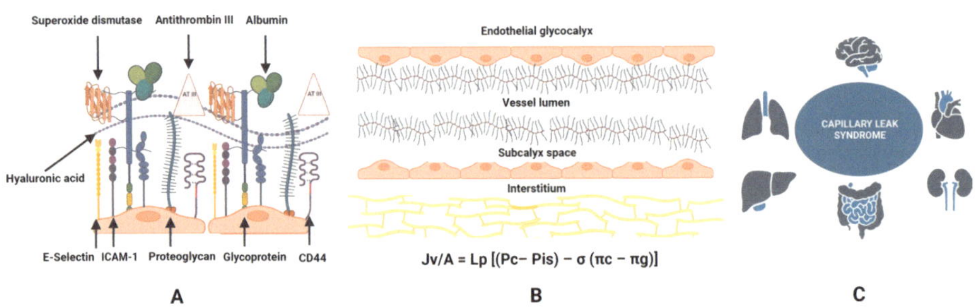

Figure 3.
Structure of the glycocalix—capillary leak syndrome. (A) Structure of the glycocalyx. (B) Modified Starling's law. (C) Capillary leak syndrome [78–80].

They are usually soluble and released into the bloodstream with mimecans, perlecan, and biglycan.

2. **Glycosaminoglycans:** It is a grid made up of multiple members such as: chondroitin sulfate heparan sulfate, dermatan sulfate, keratan sulfate, and hyaluronic acid; these are attached to the proteoglycans in the form of side chains and serve as binding sites for other proteins such as albumin, anticoagulant factors (antithrombin III, Heparin cofactor II, Thrombomodulin, and tissue factor pathway inhibitor), and antioxidants (superoxide dismutase).

   There are patterns of sulfation, deacetylation, and epimerization in the disaccharides that bind glycosaminoglycans, the structural variation of glycosaminoglycans, and their effect on binding to specific proteins generates a modification in glycocalyx function, thickness, charge modification, transcellular permeability, and paracellular.

3. **Glycoproteins:** They are of three types:

   - L and P type selectins that bind to leukocytes activated by cytokines (IL-1, TNF alpha, lipopolysaccharides).

   - Integrins that interact with laminin and fibronectin and subcellular matrix.

   - Immunogglogulins: I-CAM 1-2, V-CAM-1, PE-CAM-1 that increase the adhesion of leukocytes and platelets and allow diapedesis, respectively.

     Von Willebrand Factor platelet receptor: Allows the Ib-IX-V, VWF, and platelet complex union.

The glycocalyx plays an important role in homeostasis between the vascular wall and the blood, dampens shear forces, prevents albumin loss, prevents leukocyte and platelet adhesion, locally regulates coagulation, and has antioxidant properties (superoxide dismutase) and vasodilator (release of nitric oxide) [78].

The difference of the pressures of the hydraulic conductivity and the reflection coefficient of the proteins: $Jv/A = Lp[(Pc - Pi) - \sigma(\pi C - \pi i)]$, which, according to Starling's studies, shows that the hydrostatic pressure capillary (Pc) is 40 mm Hg and the capillary oncotic pressure (πc) is 25 mm Hg) at the arterial end of the capillaries, allowing fluid to leak from the endothelium into the interstitium; when the Pc (15 mm Hg) at the venous end will be less than πc, it will allow the reabsorption of liquid from the interstitium into the blood vessel. This theory has been modified, and the participation of the glycocalyx is incorporated through the subglycocalyx space located above a tight junction in the intercellular space, which has subglycocalyx hydrostatic pressure (Pg) and subglycocalyx oncotic pressure (πg) typical of the subglycocalyx space; the pressures that oppose liquid filtration toward the interstitium are $\pi C - \pi g$, which must be greater than πi, which equalizes the rate of lymphatic drainage and thus prevents interstitial edema (**Figure 3**). Alteration of the endothelial barrier allows albumin to move into the interstitium, increasing πi, and fluid moves into the interstitium of different organs. Crystalloids increase Pc and reduce πc, which translates into increased transcapillary filtration forces, while colloids also increase Pc but do not decrease πc. In inflammatory states, albumin allows better intravascular volume expansion, but it is not retained intravascularly and loses its oncotic effect, and its administration did not improve oxygenation in ARDS in a sustained manner, nor mortality (**Figure 3**) [79, 81].

In patients, sepsis, COVID-19, acute pancreatitis, and burned within the multiple etiologies, have a common denominator that is the inflammatory response, where TNF alpha, heparinase, hyaluronidase, thrombin, reactive oxygen species (ROS), metalloproteinase 15, and the Atrial Natriuretic Peptide (ANP) are described as molecules that damage the integrity of the glycocalyx, expose the selectins and integrins of the endothelium, allow the adhesion of leukocytes and platelets, and increase hypercoagulability and loss of endothelial integrity with capillary leakage, altering blood flow and altering the transport of oxygen to tissues and organs. In experimental studies syndecane-1, heparan sulfate are used as a biomarker of endothelial damage and disease severity [82].

Fluid overload has a negative impact on lung function due to the presence of extravascular water that alters gas exchange, increases the work of breathing, reduces compliance, decreases $PaO2/FiO2$, and decreases blood oxygen content. In a randomized study of 1000 patients, liberal vs. conservative hydration was compared in patients with acute respiratory distress syndrome (ARDS), where the cumulative balance was positive (6992 ± 502 ml) in the liberal strategy group and the conservative strategy (-136 ± 491) ($P < 0.001$). The restrictive strategy had more free days without mechanical ventilation (14.6 ± 0.5 vs. 12.1 ± 0.5) and shorter ICU stay, but no statistical differences were found in mortality [83].

Considering the deleterious effects of FO in a multisystemic way, in medical management, with the current evidence, the use of restrictive measures in fluid resuscitation is fundamental, and a strategy that should be used is the ROSE protocol and deresuscitation [77].

Similar results are found in a systematic review and a meta-analysis evaluating the efficacy of conservative fluid strategies in adults and children with ARDS, sepsis, or systemic inflammatory response syndrome (SIRS); there were no differences in mortality with the conservative strategy vs. liberal ($p = 0.83$); duration in days of ventilation was shorter in the conservative group (10.13 vs. 12.6 days, $p = < 0.05$). In the FACCT study, a multicenter, randomized, and controlled trial of 1000 ARDS patients who are intubated and receiving positive pressure ventilation, two hydration strategies are compared in two groups, the conservative group ($n = 503$) and the liberal group ($n = 497$); there were no differences in 60-day mortality ($P = 0.30$), the duration of mechanical ventilation was shorter (10.37 vs. 13.59 days ($P < 0.001$)), shorter ICU stay within the first month (1.4% vs. 11.2% ($P < 0.001$)), CV failure-free days within first week 3.9% vs. 4.2% ($P = 0.04$), and furosemide daily dose on day 7 is higher in the conservative group (137 mg vs. 87 mg) ($P < 0.001$). In a post hoc analysis of the FACTT study, Liu et al. show that the incidence of AKI is lower in the conservative strategy group and in only one study of this meta-analysis, it shows that the conservative strategy decreased the days of KRT dependence ($P < 0.05$) [83, 84].

In the REVERSE-AKI trial, a multinational, randomized, and controlled study of 100 critically ill patients with AKI according to KDIGO criteria who received fluid resuscitation was randomized into two groups, the restrictive fluid management group ($n = 49$) and the usual care group ($n = 51$). The primary outcome as cumulative fluid balance at 24 (-416 ml)($p = 0.004$) and 72 h was lower in the restrictive group (-1080 ml) ($p = 0.033$); cumulative fluid balance at ICU discharge /day 7 was less in the restrictive group (-2166 ml) ($p = 0–043$); fewer patients in the restrictive group required KRT (13% vs. 30%) ($p = 0.043$); there were no differences in the duration of AKI [85].

In a retrospective cohort of 172 patients of whom 21.8% had FO, the median fluid accumulation in the FO group was 8.6% (12,644 mL) versus 0–4% (5976 mL) in the non-FO group. In the multivariate analysis, the predictor variables for the development of FO were surgery prior to ICU admission (OR 2.35), septic shock (OR 2.05), need for mechanical ventilation on ICU admission (OR 1.56) and planned ICU admission (OR 1.70), baseline lactate (OR 1.28) on day 3 of admission to the ICU. The Random Forest and Boruta, Classification Decision Tree, and Fast and Frugal Tree models show that the highest risk of FO is found in patients with lactate ≥2.6 mmol/L, bicarbonate <19.0 mmol/L, surgery prior to admission, baseline creatinine >156 μmol/L (> 1.7 mg/dl), and APACHE IV of ≥36. This proposal of FO phenotypes based on the variables described is interesting, but it has limitations as it is a retrospective, single-center study with possible bias [76].

In recent years, pulmonary ultrasound has gained a lot of ground in the assessment at the patient's bedside and has been very useful in the diagnosis of pulmonary congestion. In a prospective cohort of 50 critically ill patients with different pathologies, 4 parasternal territories were evaluated with ultrasound (US) with a score of 0 to 32 according to the degree of pulmonary congestion, and extravascular lung water index (ELWI) measurements were also performed; a close correlation was observed between the ultrasound score and the EVLWI (Spearman's r = 0.91, P < 0.0001). A US score > 18.5 correlates with a severely increased EVLWI >15, with a sensitivity of 92.3% and a specificity of 94.6% (AUC ROC = 0.9636). The correlation of chest radiographs with the EVLWI was weak; therefore, US is an excellent alternative to evaluate FO in the ICU [86].

The harmful effect of FO on the kidneys begins with the use of unbalanced solutions rich in chlorine that generate the release of adenosine that causes vasoconstriction of the afferent arteriole; a decrease in renal perfusion is described, seen in magnetic resonance with the use of 0.9% saline [87]. FO causes interstitial edema in the kidneys when the lymphatic drainage capacity is exceeded, and the kidney, being an encapsulated organ, does not have space to expand, and an increase in intracapsular pressure is generated "renal tamponade," this alters tissue oxygenation, worsening of venous congestion which reduces the transrenal pressure gradient for renal blood flow (RBF) and reduces arterial blood flow affecting glomerular filtration rate and also impacts renal recovery [88]. Rapid infusion of solutions increases atrial pressure, allowing the release of ANP, which is described as one of many determinants in the degradation of endothelial glycocalyx-syndecan-1 [89].

Liberal resuscitation with crystalloids in terms of total volume as well as volume administration rate are risk factors in patients with sepsis, pancreatitis, burns, and polytraumatized patients for increased intra-abdominal pressure (IAP). When PIA values are ≥12 mmHg in a sustained manner, it is defined as intra-abdominal hypertension (IAH), and when sustained PIA values are >20 mmHg, it may or may not compromise the Abdominal Perfusion Pressure (APP = TAM-PIA); if the values of APP are <60 mmHg, it is associated with new organ dysfunction or failure, and this clinical situation is called abdominal compartment syndrome (ACS) [80].

The increase in intra-abdominal pressure elevates the diaphragm, which causes an increase in intrathoracic pressure, central venous pressure, and pulmonary capillary pressure, and reduces cardiac output (CO). The increase in CVP allows the increase in intracranial pressure, generating a decrease in cerebral blood flow. The IAH produces compression of the inferior vena cava; it also reduces renal blood flow and, together with the decrease in cardiac output, is factor for the development of AKI. The impact of AHI extends to the intestinal level with decreased intestinal capillary perfusion, causing ischemia, bacterial translocation, and increased release of cytokines [90].

The management of AHI/ACS has three pillars: measuring the magnitude of intra-abdominal pressure, identifying the development of organic dysfunction, and identifying the etiology. Management is focused on resolving the medical or surgical cause; the use of diuretics is a treatment option, but the decrease in cardiac output and resistance to diuretics are factors that limit their usefulness. KRT is an alternative and has an effect on the decrease in intra-abdominal pressure, described in a retrospective cohort study of nine critically ill patients where changes in IAP, global end-diastolic index (GEDVI), and EVLWI were evaluated through the PiCCO monitor in those receiving dialysis, Sustained low-efficiency daily diafiltration (SLEDD), or continuous veno-venous hemofiltration (CVVH) with the objective of achieving a negative cumulative balance. It was observed that Δ IAP decreased per dialysis session in a range of −1.4 mmHg ($p < 0.0001$); decrease in GEDVI after dialysis was 830 ml/m^2 (range 628 to 1199 ml/m^2) ($p = 0.008$). The reduction in EVLWI was very modest at 1 mL/kg or 65 mL for a mean fluid loss of 1.9 L. This slight reduction in EVLW is said to be due to greater extravascular water mobilization from other regions than from the lungs, and the presence of capillary leak syndrome perpetuates the movement of fluid into the pulmonary interstitium. There are many limitations to this work, ours being a small, heterogeneous group with cardiogenic and noncardiogenic pulmonary edema [88, 91].

The use of diuretics is an important alternative in the management of FO. In a multicenter, randomized, controlled trial of 59 fluid-overloaded adult patients admitted to the ICU (radiographic evidence of pulmonary edema, clinical signs of volume overload in association with elevated central venous pressure > 16 mm Hg or pulmonary wedge pressure capillary >16 mm Hg). They were randomized into two arms of furosemide administration, bolus group ($n = 27$) vs. continuous infusion group ($n = 32$); diuresis in 24 hours was similar 5.3 L vs. 5.4 L ($p = 0.64$); in the bolus group a higher dose of furosemide (24.1 mg/h) was required versus 9.2 mg/h in the infusion group ($p = 0.0002$) in the first 24 hours; and after 24 hours, there were no differences. Mean urine output per furosemide dose was higher in the continuous infusion group (31.6 ml/mg versus the 18 ml/mg bolus group) ($p = 0.014$) in the first 24 hours, and after 24 hours, there were no differences; the values in serum creatinine between the beginning and at the end of the therapy with furosemide did not have differences [92].

Extrapolating from the results of the DOSE study in patients with acute decompensated heart failure, we compare the administration of loop diuretics in continuous infusion versus intermittent bolus and low versus high doses in terms of achieving symptom improvement and deterioration of renal function at 72 hours. There were no statistically significant differences in the global assessment of symptoms in the intermittent bolus or continuous infusion groups, or between the low and high dose groups, and the high dose tended to be better than the low dose ($P = 0.06$). High-dose use resulted in an increase in creatinine >0.3 mg/dl at 72 hours as a positive effect of decongestion compared with the low-dose group, but there was no difference in kidney injury rates at 60 days (4 vs. 9%) [93].

In critical patients with resistance to loop diuretics, the dose can be increased exponentially or sequential blockade of the tubules with acetazolamine, thiazda, and/or spironolactone with the aim of improving the diuretic response, another option widely used empirically is the use of furosemide and human albumin [94, 95].

In a meta-analysis of 13 studies of heterogeneous quality, where they recruited 422 patients and the administration of furosemide with albumin increased the mean diuresis rate to 31.45 ml/hour (p = <0.01), and increased natriuresis by 1.76 mEq/hour (p = <0.01). In the subgroup analysis, it was observed that those with albumin values <2.5 gr/dl; the use of higher doses of albumin (>30gr) had a better effect in terms of diuresis and natriuresis. A trend of better diuresis is observed in eGFR lower than 60 ml/min/1.73 m2 without statistical relevance (p = 0.1) [96].

In cases of significant FO, acute pulmonary edema refractory to diuretics with PaO2/FiO2 < 300 mmHg, a resource in this clinical scenario, is Slow Continuous Ultrafiltration (SCUF) and/or CKRT depending on the clinical requirement, and these are alternatives that have been extensively studied with conflicting results. In a retrospective cohort study of 98 critically ill patients who required ECMO, 85% of them developed AKI, and of these, 49% required CKRT; in those who had FO > 10% 72 hours after connection to ECMO and developed severe AKI, 90-day mortality was higher when compared to those who did not develop AKI (HR 2.2; 95% CI, 1.3 to 3.8; P = 0.004) and those in the subgroup requiring CKRT had higher mortality (P = 0.029), and it is observed that CKRT does not ensure a negative fluid balance, but helps to achieve a less positive balance [97].

In the ELAIN study, fluid overload was defined as worsening pulmonary edema, PaO2/FiO2 < 300 mgHg or fluid balance >10% of body weight. In this study, the positive cumulative balance on the 3rd day after randomization was 2773 ml for the early group versus 2207 ml for the late group; these positive cumulative balances are similar to the restrictive hydration groups of other works, and these volumes could have little impact on mortality. The parameters used in the AKIKI study for fluid overload correspond to the presence of acute pulmonary edema due to fluid overload causing severe hypoxemia defined by the need for >5 L/min of oxygen to achieve SpO2 > 95%, or FiO2 requirement >50% in mechanically ventilated patients; these parameters can be subjective to define them at the bedside of the patient [55, 56].

In the IDEAL-ICU study, the definition of fluid overload corresponds, pulmonary edema due to fluid overload refractory to the use of diuretics; the accumulated positive balance on day 7 of hospitalization in the ICU in the early strategy group was 5570 $\pm$ 8761 (1%) and in the late strategy group 5878 $\pm$ 7472 (4%), and there were no differences in terms of 90-day mortality between both strategies [57].

In the STARRT-AKI in the accelerated group, the cumulative fluid balance was positive (2.7 L) at the start of dialysis, and 97% of the patients in this group received KRT. In the standard group, the balance was more positive (5.9 L), and only 62% received KRT. The most common reason for starting dialysis in the standard group was volume overload with a PaO2 /FiO2 < 200, and KRT did not impact on improved survival [58].

It is possible that in the AKIKI, IDEAL-ICU, and STARRT-AKI studies, FO is less than 10%, so that KRT has little impact on better survival regardless of the timing of the start of KRT. The use of an agreed definition of FO and the use of ultrasonographic evaluation methods or EVLWI measurement techniques will allow a better interpretation of this variable and a better evaluation of its impact on mortality.

4.4 Uremia

For many years, it has been defined as a "toxic syndrome due to kidney damage associated with changes in the tubular and endocrine function of the kidney, characterized by the retention of toxic metabolites and accompanied by changes in the volume and composition of body fluids and excess or deficiency of various hormones" [98].

Water-soluble compounds without protein binding (< 500 Da)	Protein-bound compounds (< 500 Da)	Intermediate molecules (>500 Da)
• ADMA1 • Guanidine • Uric acid • Guanidinosuccinate • Creatinine and urea • Dimethylglycine • N-Methyl-pyridone-carboxamide • Uric acid • Dimethylguanosine • Nitrosodimethylamine • Uridine • Erythritol	• Homocysteine • Indoxyl sulfate • p-Cresyl • Homocysteine • p-OH-hippurate • 2-Methoxyresorcinol • Indole-3-acetate • Pentosidine • 3-Deoxyglucosone • Phenol	• β2-Microglobulin • Atrial natriuretic peptide • Endothelin • Hepcidin • Interleukin-1β • Interleukin-6 • Tumor necrosis factor α • Interleukin-18 • Complement factor D

Table 6.
Classification of uremic toxins [101].

Urea measurement is not an ideal biomarker to assess uremia; it is a metric that is used as a proxy for authentic uremic toxins. The presence of uremic toxin has been extensively studied in CKD, but in AKI the evidence is scant.

Uremic toxins are metabolite products generated by the diet and are excreted by the kidneys under conditions of preserved renal function. AKI generates uremic toxins that rapidly affect nonrenal organs such as the brain, lungs, heart, liver, and intestines. Only 30% of CKD uremic toxins have been studied in AKI; these toxins have a biological effect with an impact on non-renal organs, renal recovery, and mortality [99]. AKI is characterized by reduced excretory capacity and leads to the accumulation of metabolic products that interact with the blood-brain barrier, intestinal microbiota, lung epithelium, and the cardiovascular system [100].

Uremic toxins are classified into three groups according to the European Working Group on Uremic Toxins (EuTox) (**Table 6**) [100].

5. Water-soluble compounds without protein binding

In AKI, dimethylarginine dimethylaminohydrolase (DDAH) activity decreases, which is an enzyme produced in renal tissue that degrades asymmetric dimethylarginine (ADMA), the latter is a competitive inhibitor of NO synthase (NOS), thus reducing the formation of nitric oxide (NO), which is expressed by a decrease in urinary sodium and nitrite/nitrate excretion [101]. The kidneys under normal conditions metabolize ≈260 μmol (≈50 mg) of ADMA and excrete ≈60 μmol, during AKI the increase between 1 and 3 μmol/L [100]. The increase in ADMA is associated with endothelial damage through the p38 MAPK/caspase-3 pathway that regulates the organization of the actin cytoskeleton and intercellular junctions by interrupting VE-cadherin [102] of the systemic vascular endothelium and at the in the lung there is severe epithelial hyperpermeability and pulmonary edema [103]; contractility and heart rate also decrease, and pulmonary artery pressure increases due to loss of NO vasodilator capacity [99]. In AKI, proximal tubule injury, heat shock protein 27 (MAPK/HSP 27) is released, which activates p38 protein kinase, which is involved in increased vascular permeability, epithelial edema, and pulmonary capillary congestion [104]. It also decreases contractility and heart rate and increases pulmonary artery pressure due to loss of NO vasodilator capacity [101].

The increase in uric acid is related to the reduced excretion due to decreased eGFR; it is described that uric acid has a vasoconstrictor effect on afferent arterioles and inhibits the release of NO in endothelial cells and proinflammatory activity because it induces the release of MCP-1, ROS and activation of NF-KB and p38-MAPK [100, 104].

6. Protein-bound compounds

In models of acute tubular necrosis, proximal tubular cell injury results in loss of expression of OAT1/3, which are transcellular transporters, and loss of protein-bound uremic toxin secretion and reabsorption function. Accumulation of protein-bound uremic toxins may continue despite renal recovery [105].

In recent years, the concept of the kidney-intestine axis has gained much importance, due to the fact that dysbiosis is generated in AKI with a decrease in Lactobacilli *Ruminococaceae* and an increase in *Enterobacteriaceae* and *Escherichia coli*, the latter being responsible for the generation of p-precursors cresol and indole sulfate, and intestinal permeability is altered, and the inflammatory response is amplified [105].

6.1 Indoxyl Sulfate (IS)

It is a product of tryptophan metabolism that is eliminated by secretion from the proximal tubule and accumulates in AKI. At the pulmonary level, it decreases the expression of Aquaporin-5 and Na/K+ ATPase, altering alveolar clearance mechanisms and causing thickening of interstitial lung tissue. IS blocks a K+ channel, delays cardiac repolarization, and prolongs the QT interval with an arrhythmogenic effect, and also causes endothelial progenitor cell dysfunction [100]. At the renal level, it increases the formation of ROS, stops the tubular cell cycle in the G2M phase, damages the DNA of tubular cells, and activates fibroblasts that induce progression to CKD, and there is a correlation with the severity of renal injury [105, 106].

6.2 P-cresol sulfate

It originates from the p-cresol precursor, which is formed by bacterial fermentation of proteins in the large intestine and which increases the adhesion of leukocytes to the vascular wall, increases vascular permeability, and is associated with decreased cardiac contractility [105].

Hyperhomocysteinemia has been described in AKI, which aggravates mitochondrial damage and may be a factor in increasing apoptosis of renal tubular epithelial cells and perpetuating the damage [100, 107].

7. Average molecular weight molecules

AKI during tubular injury, regardless of the etiology, cytokines are released by the tubules and this conditions the migration to renal tissue of immune cells such as neutrophils, monocytes, and lymphocytes; the increased immune response causes damage to renal tissue. The released cytokines weigh in a range of 5 and 20 kDa, and

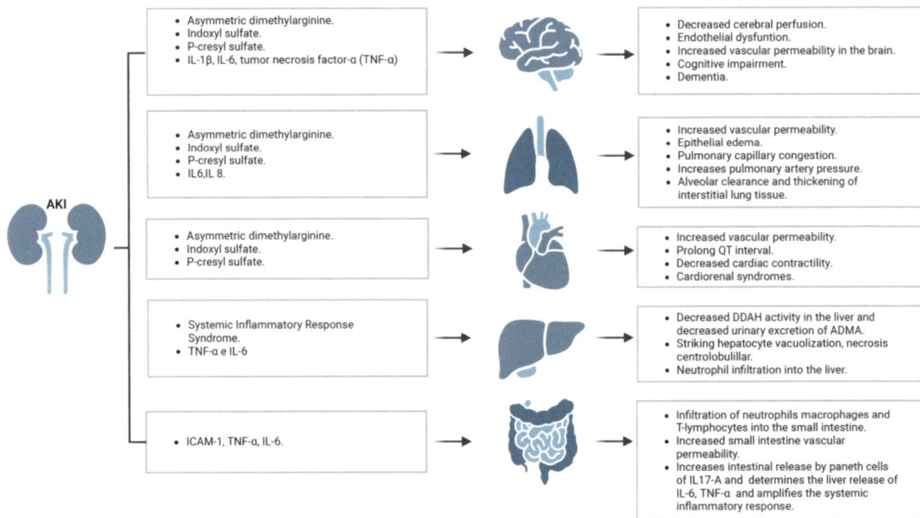

Figure 4.
Systemic effects of uremic toxins. AKI conditions retention of uremic toxins and has a deleterious effect at the multisystemic level [100, 101, 104–106].

there is controversy as to whether the proinflammatory state that impacts multiorgan damage should be considered as uremic toxins (**Figure 4**) [100].

8. Role of the gut microbiota in acute kidney injury and inflammation

In AKI, the inflammatory response of the parenchyma determines a remote signal that is expressed in the activation of neutrophils in the lamina propria of the intestine; this leads to the dedifferentiation of circulating monocytes and generates a proinflammatory macrophage phenotype at the intestinal level; this is accompanied by of inflammation, increased permeability of the intestinal wall, and bacterial or endotoxin translocation; a dysbiosis is generated with a decrease in Lactobacillus and an increase in Escherichia and Enterobacter, and this imbalance leads to the loss of short-chain fatty acids (SCFAs).) that under normal conditions fulfills pleiotropic functions in the integrity of the intestinal barrier, T-reg activation mediating immunomodulation and under dysbiosis conditions; it facilitates the activation of the innate immune response [108].

Through the increase of TGF-β and IL-6 and *E. coli*, Th17 lymphocytes are activated in the small and large intestine; it is also mentioned that the intestinal inflammatory response is expressed with increases in the mRNA of renal tumor necrosis factor (TNFα) and interferon (IFN-γ) and IL17, which is related to inflammatory amplification and greater severity of AKI [109]. TNFα, IFN, and IL-6 are elevated after ischemic and non-ischemic AKI these cytokines generate liver damage, which in turn amplifies the inflammatory response that impacts intestinal damage and induces IL-17A release [110].

The marker used to assess uremia for many years has been urea/BUN; the cut-off value of blood urea nitrogen (BUN) for CKRT onset originates from retrospective cohort studies of several studies in which high values or values considered as "late" onset for CKRT as values >94.5 mg/dl were related to higher mortality ($p < 0.0001$)

[110]. In another retrospective cohort study of patients with sepsis and AKI, those requiring KRT were defined as "early" onset with BUN <100 mg/dl and "late" onset with BUN values ≥100 mg/dl. In logistic regression analysis, those in the "late" group mortality at 14 days (OR 3.6, P = 0.001), 28 days (OR 2.6, P = 0.01), and 365 days (OR 3.5, P = 0.02) was higher [111]. Vin-Cent Wu et al. in another retrospective cohort study of critically ill patients with acute liver injury and AKI who required CKRT after major surgery, it was observed that those in the "late" dialysis group with BUN >80 mg/dl had higher mortality rate (P = 0.02) and lower rate of recovery of renal function (P = 0.02) compared to the "early" dialysis group [112].

In the PICARD study, a multicenter observational study of 243 patients, it was observed that in the group with high azotemia (BUN >76 mg/dl) adjusted by variables, the relative risk (RR) of death associated with the start of dialysis at a high BUN was of 1.85 (95% confidence interval: 1.16 to 2.96) [113].

In the RCTs, the urea values for the start of CKRT were taken from the reference values of retrospective cohort studies; in the ELAIN study, in the "late" start group, BUN >46.67 mg/dl had an outcome of higher mortality at 90 days, when compared to the "early" start (P = 0.03.). In the AKIKI study, the development of uremia was defined as a BUN >112 mg/dl, criteria for starting KRT in the late group; 60-day mortality did not have significant differences with the early start group (AKI KDIGO3). The AKIKI 2 study defines a limit of very late when BUN >112 mg/dl or oliguria is >72 hours. In the multivariable analysis, the risk of mortality is 65%. If we wait a long time for the decision to start KRT, this study gives us the waiting limit [48, 49, 114].

Future studies on risk assessment of AKI development, prevention measures, use of biomarkers or modulation of the inflammatory response, management of dysbiosis, and timely initiation of KRT will be important to make better decisions on AKI management in critically ill patients.

9. Evidence at the START of kidney replacement therapy

9.1 Randomized controlled trials (RCTs)

Controversy has been generated for many years at the start of KRT in AKI, with the desire to answer this question; from 2016, several RCTs were carried out in order to make better decisions and with better outcomes, then will describe the most relevant studies.

The ELAIN is a French study, with a single-center RCTs design, which included patients aged 18–90 years, with severe Sepsis with catecholamines (noradrenaline/adrenaline) at a dose >0.1 mcg/kg/min, with refractory fluid overload data (PaO2/FiO2 < 300 mgHg, FO >10% of body weight), with SOFA ≥2 and with Acute Kidney Injury - KDIGO stage 2 and NGAL >150 ng/dl. Two groups were randomized, when the "early" KRT onset (n = 112) was within 8 hours of AKI - KDIGO2 diagnosis and the "late" onset group (n = 119) within 12 hours of AKI-KDIGO3 diagnosis or when they met any of the absolute indications (Urea >100 mg/dl, oliguria <200 ml/12 hours or anuria, K > 6 and/or ECG abnormalities, magnesium >4 mmol, pH <7. 15, organ edema in the presence of AKI, resistance to diuretics). The primary outcome was mortality at 90 days showing lower mortality in the "early" group (39.3) vs. "late" (54.7%) with HR 0.66, and p = 0.03, in relation to secondary outcomes median duration of KRT, was lower in the "early" group (9 days) vs. "late" (25 days) (p = 0. 04); improved recovery of renal function at day 90 in the "early" group was 53.6% (p = 0.02) vs. 38.7% in the "late" group; median duration of mechanical ventilation was shorter in the early group (p = 0.02); the same group had shorter hospital stay (p = <0.001); in the rest of outcomes, there were no significant statistical differences. This is a single-center study with our patients mostly surgical; not all treatments were standardized, and it generates bias in internal validity. On a positive note, it is worth noting that CKRT was performed and then transitioned to SLED and intermittent haemodialysis. These results of the benefit in the "early" start are related to other similar results in patients operated on cardiac surgery, where the temporality is different with respect to other etiologies of AKI [55].

The AKIKI Trail, a French study, is a multicenter, unblinded, RCTs design, which included critically ill patients >18 years with invasive ventilation and/or catecholamine infusion, with AKI within 6 hours after validation of KDIGO stage 3 renal injury (defined by creatinine >354 μmol/liter or 3 times baseline, Anuria (<100 ml/day for >12 hours) and Oliguria (diuresis <0.3 ml/kg/h or < 500 ml/day for >24 hours) compatible with tubular necrosis. Two groups were randomized; the "early" KRT initiation group (n = 312) was within 6 hours after AKI-KDIGO3 diagnosis and the "late" KRT initiation group (n = 308) when they developed absolute indications (urea >40 mmol/L, K > 6 mmol/L, pH < 7.15; acute pulmonary edema with severe hypoxemia and oliguria/anuria >72 hours). The primary outcome was mortality at 60 days and there was no statistical difference between groups (p = 49); in the secondary outcome, the "early" group received KRT in 98% of patients unlike the other group (51%); there were more catheter-associated infections in the "early" group (10%) vs. 5% in the late group; in other outcomes analyzed, there were no significant statistical differences. A strength is that 49% of patients in the "late" group did not require KRT and recovered renal function (50). This work was not blinded, and this generates bias. It is noteworthy that 50% of the critical patients performed KRT in intermittent modality, and this is not a common practice in the clinical condition where 80% of the patients required vasoactive agents, and it is not a common practice in the country where the study was carried out. This study is not comparable to ELAIN, because a greater number of patients who were included in the AKIKI were medical causes of hospital admission and the most frequent cause of AKI was sepsis, which has a different pathophysiological context than the cardiac surgery patients in the ELAIN Trail [56].

In the IDEAL-ICU is another French study with a multicenter, unblinded RCTs design, which included adult patients with septic shock within 48 hours of vasopressor initiation and AKI defined and classified according to RIFLE criteria in grade F; randomization was performed in two branches: those who initiated KRT "early" (n = 239) within 12 hours of AKI-RIFLE(F) diagnosis and those who initiated KRT "late" (n = 238) was within 48 hours of AKI-RIFLE(F) diagnosis or in the presence of absolute indications (K > 6. 5 mmol/L, pH < 7.15, fluid overload refractory to diuretics). In mortality outcomes at 28 and 90 days, there were no significant statistical differences (p = 048 and p = 38, respectively), median days free of KRT, mechanical ventilation, vasopressors, and positive cumulative balance at 7th day; there were no differences between groups, but a higher incidence of hyperkalemia was identified in 4% (p = 0.03) in the "late" start group. Delayed onset allowed time for spontaneous recovery, and only 29% of this group did not require KRT [57].

STARRT-AKI Trail is a multinational RCTs with larger number of patients enrolled (n = 2927); participants were randomized 1:1 for accelerated versus standard KRT initiation. >18 years of age, admitted to an ICU with AKI defined as Cr > 100 umol/l in women and Cr > 130 umol/l in men and who have not decreased Cr by >27 umol/l in 48 hours and with evidence of severe AKI with at least 1 of the following 3 cases: >2-fold increase in creatinine from baseline, Cr > 354 umol/l and >27 umol/l above baseline creatinine and with urine output < 6 ml/kg in 12 hours. Two groups were randomized: "accelerated" (n = 1462) was termed when starting KRT within 12 hours after AKI-KDIGO3 diagnosis and the standard group(n = 1465), when AKI persists >72 hours from randomization and one or more of the classic indications: K > 6 mmol/L, pH < 7.2 or HCO3 < 12 mmol/L, acute pulmonary edema (P/F < 200). In the analysis of the outcomes, it is evident that in mortality at 90 days, there were no differences between both groups (p = 0.92); KRT dependence at 90 days was higher in the accelerated group (10.4%) vs. 6% (RR1.74), and adverse events such as hypotension and hypophosphatemia were higher in the accelerated group, all-cause mortality, KRT dependence at 90 days, MAKE, glomerular filtration, albuminuria, mechanical ventilation, and vasoactive-free days, no significant differences were found between the two groups. This study recruited the largest number of patients of all the RCTs and has internal and external validity, which is applicable to real-world life and has significant results at the time of decision making [58].

The AKIKI2 study is from the group of S. Gaudry et al. and is an unblinded, multicenter, prospective, randomized, and controlled trial. It included patients hospitalized in ICU who received mechanical ventilation and/or catecholamine infusion with AKI according to KDIGO definition. Randomization was performed in two groups, "delayed" group (n = 137) when KRT onset occurs with AKI-KDIGO3 with KDIGO with oliguria: diuresis <0.3 ml/kg/h or < 500 ml/d) or anuria (diuresis <100 ml/d) for >72 hours or azotemia: BUN >112 mg/dl (40 mmol/l) and 140 mg/dl (50 mmol/l) and the "more delayed" group (n = 141), those with absolute indications mentioned in the AKIKI or urea >140 mg/dl (50 mmol/l). In the primary outcome was number of days without KRT from randomization to day 28; there were no differences between groups (p = 0.93); in terms of ICU, in hospital mortality at 28 and 60 days, there were no statistical differences (p = 0.26, p = 0.71, respectively), the number of patients with renal recovery, days free mechanical ventilation, vasoactive agents, ICU-hospital stay time, dialysis dependency time, infection rates, and positive cumulative balance was similar in the two groups. In the multivariate analysis, the risk factors associated with 60-day mortality were more delayed initiation of KRT (HR 1.65), mechanical ventilation (HR 3.44), and SAPS III (HR 1.03). The strength of this study is that it places an "upper limit" for dialysis initiation as a mortality risk point [114].

9.2 Meta-analysis

In a systematic review and meta-analysis, they included 56 studies, and of these, 10 were RCTs; 4753 critically ill patients with severe AKI were included, where all-cause mortality was 45.5% in the accelerated group vs. 46.6% in the standard group (p = 0.46), without differences in mortality at 28 and 90 days; there were no differences in dependence between both groups (p = 0.08). In the analysis by subgroups, there was a greater dependence on KRT in early-onset patients with SOFA >11 and in mixed dialysis modality (CKRT and intermittent hemodialysis). The subgroup of surgical patients had lower mortality when receiving CKRT and less dialysis dependence than the subgroup of nonsurgical patients; the risk of dialysis dependence was increased in the accelerated KRT group when those patients used non-CKRT modality or had high SOFA scores. This meta-analysis was methodologically flawless and low in publication bias [115].

Another meta-analysis includes 18 RCTs with 2856 patients and focused on the timing of KRT initiation (accelerated vs. standard), and there were no differences in mortality (p = 0.9). In the subgroup of high-quality RCTs, there were no statistical differences (p = 0.7) and there were no differences in mortality at 28 and 90 days, mortality was similar in the CKRT and intermittent hemodialysis modalities, and mortality was similar in the AKI groups. In the community and in the ICU, it is reported that there was greater dependence on KRT in the accelerated start group and in four studies catheter-associated complications and infections were observed [116].

Wei-Ting Lin et al. report a meta-analysis of 11 RCTs assigned to early (n = 1131) and late (1111) groups; mortality at 28, 60, and 90 days was similar in both groups; in ICU and hospital mortality, there were no statistical differences. In four studies of surgical patients, mortality was lower in the early-onset group and is supported by other studies with similar results in the same population, but the dependence of KRT at 28 and 90 days was similar between groups and did not improve renal recovery either. Regarding adverse events, infections and hypophosphatemia were more frequent in the early-onset group. In this study, the heterogeneity of the studies was high [117]. In another meta-analysis of 15 RCTs, they included 5395 patients who showed similar results in that there were no significant differences in mortality at 28, 60, and 90 days, without differences in terms of ICU and hospital stay, with more episodes of hypotension and infections in the early-onset group [118].

Another meta-analysis of 14 RCTs where 5234 patients were recruited and compared early vs. late initiation of KRT, no differences were found in mortality at 30 (RR 1.0) and 90 days (RR 1.0); there was greater dependence on KRT; hypotension and hypophosphatemia in the early-onset group [119].

The current evidence supports the conservative approach of waiting for classic indications, considering a time limit of more than 3 days of anuria/oliguria or urea >240 mg/dl for the start of KRT, given that a longer delay increases the risk of mortality [114, 119].

10. Other non-classic indicators that should be considered when decisión making at the START of KRT

10.1 Patient severity

Patient severity influences the risk of developing AKI, as evidenced in a prospective cohort study of 33 surgical patients admitted to the ICU, 22 of whom had sepsis and AKI at different stages. The biomarkers SOFA, APACHE III and serum and urinary NGAL these last two biomarkers had an area under the curve (AUROC) of 0.98, AUROC of 0.885 respectively, the SOFA score together with serum and urinary NGAL reach an AUROC 0.963 to predict AKI and mortality [120].

It is a retrospective cohort of 90 patients who are divided into two groups: the survivors and the non-survivor group. In the non-survivor group at the start of KRT, the APACHE III value, vasoactive-inotropic score (VIS), and lactate were higher than in the survivor group; the APACHE III scores had an AUROC of 0.866 and the VIS AUROC of 0.796; the SOFA had an AUROC of 0.732, as predictors of mortality. In the multivariate analysis at the beginning of KRT, APACHE III had an OR 1.22, VIS an OR1.147, low MAP before KRT had OR 1.17, lactate before KRT had OR 1.55; time from diagnosis to "late" start of KRT reached OR 1.014; all were independent risk factors for mortality in AKI with KRT. Variables other than the classical ones are

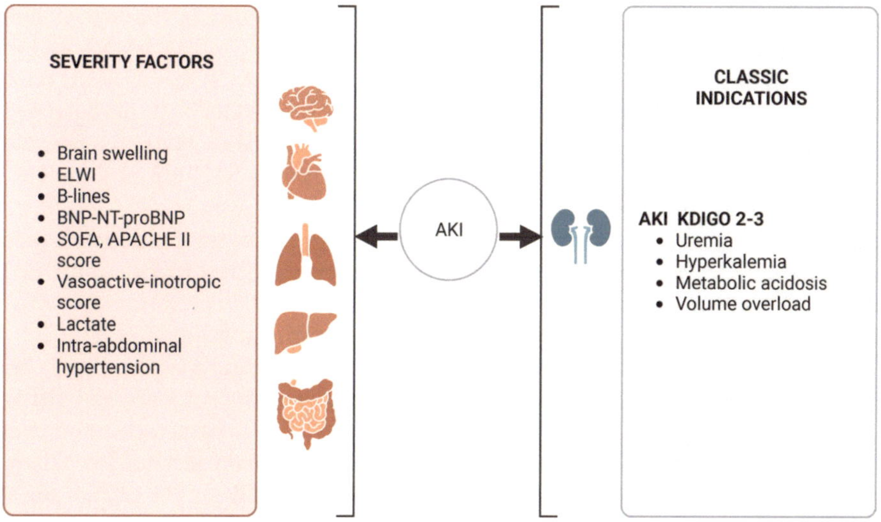

Figure 5.
Classic and severity criteria in the critically ill patient for initiation of KRT. Classically known indications for KRT are when complications are generated in severe AKI. We mention that AKI is a pathology with systemic impact and it is important to observe other severity factors in the critically ill patient that allow us to make the best decision on when to initiate KRT [120–122, 124–127].

possible (uremia, pH, bicarbonate and K) and should be considered and help to choose the moment to start KRT in critically ill patients [121]. Regarding VIS, a retrospective cohort showed in the multivariable logistic regression analysis that VIS was associated with postoperative AKI (OR 1.19) ($P < 0.001$) and with the need for KRT (OR: 1.29, $P = 0.007$). The VIS AUROC is a good predictor of postoperative AKI (AUROC: 0.84, $P < 0.001$) and predictor of the need for KRT (AUROC: 0.91, $P < 0.001$) [122]. Further studies are required to validate these data.

Lactate is a good biomarker to assess tissue perfusion and energetic-metabolic status; in different clinical circumstances, production may be normal or increased with defective or close to normal clearance. The increase in lactate has been widely studied as a predictor of mortality in sepsis and septic patients receiving KRT [123].

It is important to mention that lactate clearance is 1379 ml/min under normal conditions and the clearance capacity for a hemofilter is on average 24.2 ml/min, and the hemofilter represents <3% of lactate clearance, which is not sufficient in patients critical and should focus on treating the primary cause of decompensation (**Figure 5**) [128].

In a prospective cohort of 186 patients with sepsis and septic AKI (S-AKI) who received CKRT-CVVHDF, serum lactate value was assessed before initiation, 24 hours after CKRT, and percentage lactate clearance. They were divided into a group of survivors and non-survivors; in this last group lactate at the beginning, at 24 hours, it was significantly higher ($p = <0–001$), and lactate clearance was <10% ($p = 0.004$). The lactate value 24 hours after starting the CKRT is associated with early mortality (48 hours) with OR 1.72 and late mortality (28 days) with OR 2.35; in those in which clearance is >10%, it is associated with lower early mortality (OR 0.114) and late (OR 0.235); the AUROC values for lactate at 24 hours predict early mortality 0.87 and late mortality 0.82; the AUROC for lactate clearance as a predictor of early mortality was 0.72 and late mortality 0.70, respectively [124].

In a retrospective cohort of 342 patients divided into three groups: early recovery, early death group, and control group, the multivariate logistic regression analysis identified factors that can predict the recovery of renal function in the first 48 hours, such as the presence of diuresis. (AUROC 0.64), SOFA <10 (AUROC 0.67), and short duration (0.3 days) between ICU admission and initiation of CKRT (AUROC 0.68); all three factors predict recovery of renal function with AUROC 0.78. In the group with early mortality, they presented SOFA values >13, SAPSIII>74 points, neurological disease (OR 9.64), use of vasopressors (OR 3.68), lactate >3.6 mmol/L with a sensitivity of 88%, and a specificity of 67% (OR 1.19).), albumin <2.2 g/dl (OR 0.52) as predictors of mortality and capable of predicting a group of very seriously ill people who do not benefit from KRT [129]. In the post hoc study of the AKIKI and IDEAL-ICU clinical trials in the stratified analysis of thirds of the SOFA score, those with SOFA >10, the CKRT did not show a decrease in mortality at 60 days [125].

In a prospective cohort of 999 patients with S-AKI requiring dialysis, three patient phenotypes were identified through the Manhattan plot of the standardized differences of the clinical characteristics evaluated. Phenotype 1 is characterized by young patients, low Charlson comorbidity index (CCI), normal renal function, low Glasgow, low Po2, low PaO2/FiO2, high lactate and SOFA, APACHE III, unlike phenotype 2 with intermediate characteristics and phenotype 3 with older patients, altered renal function, and less severe acute disease with low lactate and SOFA. Phenotype 1 presented a higher risk of mortality 73.86% and when compared with group 2 (56.57%) and group 3 (46.22%) ($p < 0.001$); also, a lactate >3.3 mmol/L at the start of KRT is associated with mortality (HR 1. 34), and KRT-dependent (HR 0.69) could be a predictive biomarker for dialysis initiation or SA-AKI severity, and further research is required to confirm this hypothesis [126].

In a prospective cohort of 500 patients with type 1 cardiorenal syndrome (type 1 CRS) who required KRT, serum lactate measurement may be a marker of hemodialysis withdrawal and 90-day mortality. qSOFA values were higher (>1) in the mortality group and hemodialysis dependence group; lactate values >4.2 mmol/L were associated with higher 90-day mortality (p = <0.001) and lower probability of withdrawal of dialysis (p = <0.001) in the presence or absence of sepsis [127].

In relation to what has been reviewed, it should be considered that patients with diuresis, SOFA <10, and lactate <4.2 mmol/L, are likely to have early renal recovery and do not require KRT.

10.2 Furosemide stress test (FST)

Diuretic use has been controversial in AKI; Chawa et al. show in a retrospective, prospective cohort that administering a furosemide bolus of 1 mg/kg or 1.5 mg/kg in those receiving diuretics is one way to assess functional reserve.. In the presence of AKI, the use of FST with a value of <200 ml of diuresis in 2 hours is a predictive marker of AKI-AKIN III progression with AUC 0.87 ($p = 0.001$) with a sensitivity of 87.1% and a specificity of 84. 1% and as a predictor of the need for KRT with AUROC 0.86 and mortality with AUROC 0.70. Koyner et al. compare the use of FST and biomarkers or biomarkers alone to assess AKI progression; the combination of FST and biomarkers predicts progression to AKI-AKIN III with AUROC 0.90 and predicts the need for KRT with AUROC 0.91. This furosemide challenge is useful to differentiate those without functional reserve and consider initiation of KRT [52, 130].

In a randomized, multicenter, and controlled trial of 162 patients with ARF at any KDIGO stage without emergency indications and without contraindications, the use of FST allowed the evaluation of two groups, responders and nonresponders; the latter group was divided according to the time of KRT initiation into two groups: the early-onset group within 6 hours of ARF-KDIGO diagnosis 1,2,3 and the late-onset group when initiation is due to absolute indications. FST discriminates patients with AKI who may potentially require KRT; in nonresponders, early or late onset of KRT did not affect mortality [131].

The diagnostic accuracy of FST for AKI progression had an AUROC of 0.88 (sensitivity 0.81 and specificity 0.88); as a predictor for KRT initiation, it has an AUROC of 0.86 (sensitivity 0.84 and specificity 0.77); FST performs better as a predictor of need for KRT in AKI-KDIGO 1–2 compared to AKI-KDIGO 3 with a pooled diagnostic accuracy of 0.86 [132].

In a prospective, double-blind, and interventional cohort study of 187 patients admitted to the ICU with AKI undergoing FST, 37.5% of patients who responded to FST received CKRT, while 89.2% of patients who did not respond to FST received CKRT. On univariate analysis, platelet count was lower in the CKRT group ($p = 0.04$); more patients with acidosis were identified in the CKRT group ($p = < 0.05$); there were more patients with AKI-KDIGO 2 and 3 in the CKRT group and a higher number of stage 1 patients in the non-KRT group; urinary volume was lower in the CKRT group (35 ml, IQR 5–143. 75 vs. 400 ml, IQR 210–890; $P = 0.000$), SOFA and APACHE II were lower in the non-KRT group ($p = 0.000$); SOFA and APACHE II scores were higher in the CKRT group ($P < 0.05$); in multivariate analysis, negative FST (diuresis <200 ml in 2 hours) was a predictor of CKRT initiation ($P = 0.032$). Patients who did not respond to FST were 2.379 times more likely to initiate CKRT ($P = 0.000$). Post-STF urine volume of 156 ml had an AUROC of 0.966 (sensitivity 94.85%, specificity 98.04%, $p < 0.001$), and SOFA (>8) had an AUROC of 0.846 predictors of CKRT initiation [133].

In a prospective, observational study of 312 patients in a medical ICU, those who developed AKI according to KDIGO diuresis criteria were subjected to receive Sequential Nephron Blockade (SBN) with initial use of Furosemide at 1 mg/kg (maximum 60 mg), followed by a maintenance dose of 10 to 20 mg/hour; adequate diuretic response was termed >0.5 ml/kg/h or > 300 ml in 6 hours and 5 ml/kg/h or > 300 ml in 6 hours, if adequate diuretic response was not achieved (<0.5 ml/kg/h or < 300 ml in 6 hours). Metolazone 10 mg was administered; those nonresponders to SBN started KRT [134]. In multivariate logistic regression analysis, those with SOFA >9 (OR 4.5), those who achieved a positive cumulative balance of 4.2 L (OR 2.82), those who required KRT (OR 1.78), and those with negative diuresis (OR 0.45) had higher mortality [134].

It is important to mention that the SOFA score is a good predictor of AKI severity, poor diuretic response, and the need for KRT. More prospective studies with larger numbers of patients are required to confirm these data.

The combination of FST and elevated urine levels of the chemokine biomarker (C-C motif) ligand 14 (CCL14) had a high predictive value (AUC ROC 0.87) as a predictor of the need for CKRT, compared to FST alone (AUC ROC 0.79) or CCL14 (AUC 0.83), $P = <0.001$ [135].

I believe that negative FST and the use of biomarkers along with factors determining increased demands for critical illness may be useful at the time of decision making.

10.3 Kinetic eFG

It is known that creatinine is a late marker in AKI, and its value is influenced by various variables that underestimate (fluid overload, hyperbilirubinemia, malnutrition) or overestimate the value (cimetidine, fibrates, and sulfamethoxazole and trimethoprim). Determination of eGFR in the patient with AKI with the classic eGFR formulas in CKD requires a steady state of creatinine values, a condition that is not met in AKI.

The eFG kinetic (KeFG) is a formula proposed by Chen [136] incorporates the mass equilibrium principles (generation, distribution, excretion) together with an "elapsed time" factor to assign an eGFR to each value of Cr as long as the time elapsed since the last value is known. The KeFG evaluates sudden and rapid changes in eGFR, unlike the eGFR measured by Clearance calculated, where the decrease in GFR is gradual by the Crocoft, MDRD, and CKD-EPI formulas (**Figure 6**).

In a retrospective cohort of 2492 patients, the KeGFR was incorporated with or without UO criteria (diuresis) and added to the KDIGO classification with three modified stages:

Stage 1: KeGFR 45 to 60 mL/min/1.73 m^2 or urine output <0.5 mL/kg/h for 6 h.

$$KeGFR = \frac{baseline\,SCr\,X\,eGFR}{Mean\,SCr} \quad x\left[1-\frac{24x\Delta SCr}{\Delta Time(h)xMax\Delta SCr/day}\right]$$

Figure 6.
Modified see end of document. KeGFR. SSPCR is steady-state plasma creatinine; crcl is MDRD creatinine clearance. Mean PCR refers to the difference in plasma creatinine concentration. Δ time(h) is the interval in hours between two consecutive creatinine measurements and max delta pcr/day is the theoretical maximum change in plasma creatinine that can occur per day if renal function ceases completely. ΔPCr is defined as the initial creatinine subtracted from the final creatinine. MaxΔPCr/day, addresses the principle of creatinine mass balance by incorporating the volume of distribution factor (V d) [136].

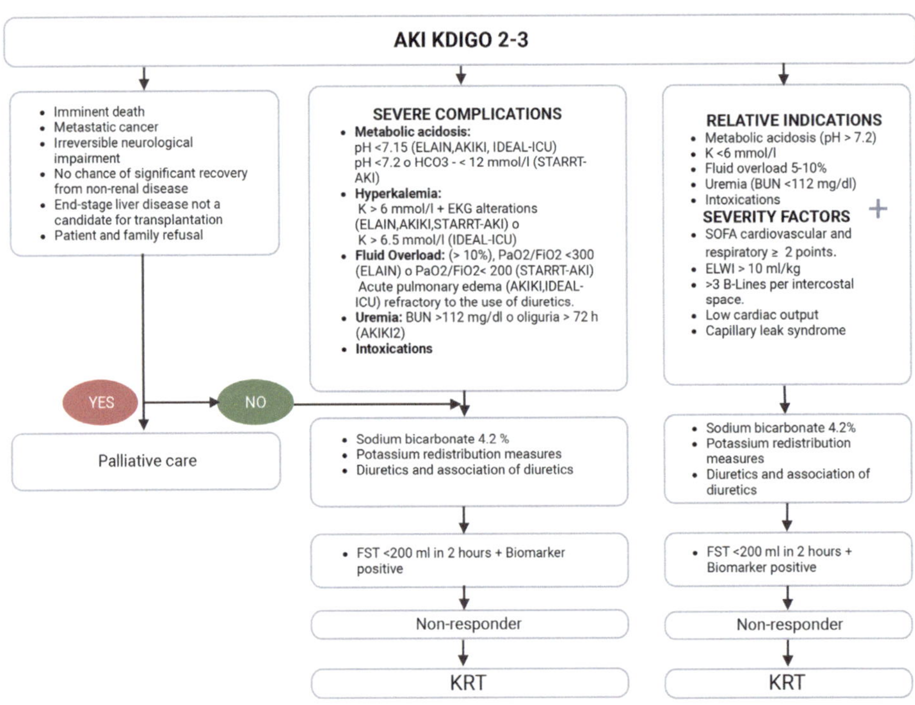

Figure 7.
Kidney replacement therapy initiation algorithm [137].

Stage 2: KeGFR 30 to 45 mL/min/1.73 m^2 or urine output <0.5 mL/kg/h for 12 hours.

Stage 3: KeGFR <30 ml/min/1.73 m^2 or diuresis <0.3 ml/kg/h for 12 h or anuria for 12 h.

In this study, the degree of agreement between KDIGO and KeGFR was very good (Cohen's kappa with square weights = 0.77). The sensitivity of the combined KeGFR and urine criteria compared to the KDIGO criteria was 93.2%, specificity 73.0%, and accuracy 85.7%, also allowing faster AKI recognition, where a time difference in recognition between KDIGO and KeGFR at stage 1 is 5.9 hours, stage 2 is 7.2 hours, and stage 3 is 4 hours. In the logistic regression model, the prediction of mortality at 28 days by KDIGO was AUROC 0.57 and for KeGFR, an AUROC 0.60; as a predictor of the need for KRT, the KDIGO had an AUROC 0.81 and for KeGFR, an AUROC 0.80. We see that the KeGFR allows a faster diagnosis of AKI using serial creatinine determinations at time intervals and with good ability to predict the severity of AKI, with the ability to predict the need for KRT and mortality. It is possible that the use of KeGFR, FST, and biomarkers provides complementary tools for the early diagnosis of AKI and allows better decisions to be made in choosing the right moment to start KRT (**Figure** 7) [138].

11. Conclusions

AKI leads to increased health care costs in each country, with higher morbidity and mortality. Detection of risk factors, early diagnosis, and use of severity classification systems and biomarkers are necessary for a timely preventive and therapeutic approach.

It is important to assess trends in creatinine elevation and consider the use of KeGFR along with KDIGO, the use of biomarkers, and FST as tools that give a clear scenario of renal capacity that may not be able to support the magnitude of severity of a critically ill patient.

The controversy generated about the ideal time to initiate KRT in critically ill patients is currently supported by evidence from RCTs and meta-analyses that support waiting in the classic "late" indications, taking into account the waiting limits suggested by the AKIKI trial 2.

Author details

Maiko Alejandro Tavera Diaz
Department of Nephrology, Univalle Hospital, Bolivia

*Address all correspondence to: taveradiaz@gmail.com

References

[1] Uchino S, Bellomo R, Goldsmith D, Bates S, Ronco C. An assessment of the RIFLE criteria for acute renal failure in hospitalized patients. Critical Care Medicine. 2006;**34**:1913-1917

[2] Bellomo R, Ronco C, Kellum JA, Mehta RL, Palevsky P, Acute Dialysis Quality Initiative workgroup. Acute renal failure-definition, outcome measures, animal models, fluid therapy and information technology needs: The second international consensus conference of the acute dialysis quality initiative (ADQI) group. Critical Care. 2004;**8**(4):R204-R212. DOI: 10.1186/cc2872 Epub 2004 May 24

[3] Mehta RL, Kellum JA, Shah SV, Molitoris BA, Ronco C, Warnock DG, et al. Acute kidney injury Network: Report of an initiative to improve outcomes in acute kidney injury. Critical Care. 2007;**11**(2):1-8. DOI: 10.1186/cc5713. PMID: 17331245; PMCID: PMC2206446

[4] Clinical Practice Guidelines for Acute Kidney Injury. 2012. Available from: http://www.kdigo.org/clinical_practice_guidelines/AKI.php

[5] Nash K, Hafeez A, Hou S. Hospital-acquired renal failure. American Journal of Kidney Diseases. 2002;**39**(5):930-936. DOI: 10.1053/ajkd.2002.32766

[6] Hsu RK, McCulloch CE, Dudley RA, Lo LJ, Hsu CY. Temporal changes in incidence of dialysis-requiring AKI. Journal of the American Society of Nephrology (JASN). 2013;**24**(1):37-42. DOI: 10.1681/ASN.2012080800 Epub 2012 Dec 6

[7] Uchino S, Kellum JA, Bellomo R, Doig GS, Morimatsu H, Morgera S, et al. Beginning and ending supportive therapy for the kidney (BEST kidney) investigators. Acute renal failure in critically ill patients: A multinational, multicenter study. NEVER. 2005; **294**(7):813-818. DOI: 10.1001/jama.294.7.813

[8] VA/NIH Acute Renal Failure Trial Network, Palevsky PM, Zhang JH, O'Connor TZ, Chertow GM, Crowley ST, et al. Intensity of renal support in critically ill patients with acute kidney injury. The New England Journal of Medicine. 2008;**359**(1):7-20. DOI: 10.1056/NEJMoa0802639 Epub 2008 May 20. Erratum in: N Engl J Med. 2009 Dec 10;361(24):2391

[9] Xue JL, Daniels F, Star RA, Kimmel PL, Eggers PW, Molitoris BA, et al. Incidence and mortality of acute renal failure in Medicare beneficiaries, 1992 to 2001. Journal of the American Society of Nephrology (JASN). 2006; **17**(4):1135-1142. DOI: 10.1681/ASN.2005060668 Epub 2006 Feb 22

[10] Hashemian SM, Jamaati H, Farzanegan Bidgoli B, Farrokhi FR, Malekmohammad M, Roozdar S, et al. Outcome of acute kidney injury in critical care unit, based on AKI network. Tanaffos. 2016;**15**(2):89-95

[11] Rizo-Topete LM, Rosner MH, Ronco C. Acute kidney injury risk assessment and the nephrology rapid response team. Blood Purification. 2017; **43**(1–3):82-88. DOI: 10.1159/000452402 Epub 2016 Dec 3

[12] Ostermann M, Zarbock A, Goldstein S, Kashani K, Macedo E, Murugan R, et al. Recommendations on acute kidney injury biomarkers from the acute disease quality initiative consensus conference: A consensus statement. JAMA Network Open. 2020;**3**(10):

e2019209. DOI: 10.1001/jamanetwork open.2020.19209 Erratum in: JAMA Netw Open. 2020;3(11):e2029182

[13] Roy JP, Forster CS. Clinical Progress note: Pediatric acute kidney injury. Journal of Hospital Medicine. 2019;**14**(9):552-554. DOI: 10.12788/jhm.3280

[14] Parsons FM, Hobson S, Blagg CR, Mcracken BH. Optimum time for dialysis IN acute reversible renal failure. The Lancet. 1961;**277**(7169): 129-134. DOI: 10.1016/s0140-6736(61) 91309-5

[15] KDIGO Clinical Practice Guideline for Acute Kidney Injury. Kidney International Supplements. 2012;**2**:1. DOI: 10.1038/kisup.2012.1

[16] Ostermann M, Joannidis M, Pani A, Floris M, De Rosa S, Kellum JA, et al. 17th acute disease quality initiative (ADQI) consensus group. Patient selection and timing of continuous renal replacement therapy. Blood Purification. 2016;**42**(3):224-237. DOI: 10.1159/000448506 Epub 2016Aug26

[17] Peng Q, Zhang L, Ai Y, Zhang L. Epidemiology of acute kidney injury in intensive care septic patients based on the KDIGO guidelines. Chinese Medical Journal (Eng). 2014;**127**(10): 1820-1826

[18] Dépret F, Peacock WF, Liu KD, Rafique Z, Rossignol P, Legrand M. Management of hyperkalemia in the acutely ill patient. Annals of Intensive Care. 2019;**9**(1):32. DOI: 10.1186/s13613-019-0509-8

[19] Libório AB, Leite TT, Neves FM, Teles F, Bezerra CT. AKI complications in critically ill patients: Association with mortality rates and RRT. Clinical Journal of the American Society of Nephrology. 2015;**10**(1):21-28. DOI: 10.2215/CJN.04750514 Epub 2014 Nov 5

[20] Kovesdy CP, Appel LJ, Grams ME, Gutekunst L, McCullough PA, Palmer BF, et al. Potassium homeostasis in health and disease: A scientific workshop sponsored by the National Kidney Foundation and the American Society of Hypertension. Journal of the American Society of Hypertension. 2017; **11**(12):783-800. DOI: 10.1016/j.jash.2017.09.011 Epub 2017 Oct 10

[21] Class CM, Carrero JJ, Ellison DH, Grams ME, Hemmelgarn BR, Jardine MJ, et al. Potassium homeostasis and management of dyskalemia in kidney diseases: Conclusions from a kidney disease: Improving global outcomes (KDIGO) controversies conference. Kidney International. 2020;**97**(1):42-61. DOI: 10.1016/j.kint.2019.09.018 Epub 2019 Oct 10

[22] McMahon GM, Mendu ML, Gibbons FK, Christopher KB. Association between hyperkalemia at critical care initiation and mortality. Intensive Care Medicine. 2012;**38**(11): 1834-1842. DOI: 10.1007/s00134-012-2636-7 Epub 2012 Jul 18

[23] Kovesdy CP, Matsushita K, Sang Y, Brunskill NJ, Carrero JJ, Chodick G. Serum potassium and adverse outcomes across the range of kidney function: A CKD prognosis consortium meta-analysis. European Heart Journal. 2018; **39**(17):1535-1542. DOI: 10.1093/eurheartj/ehy100

[24] Gao XP, Zheng CF, Liao MQ, He H, Liu YH, Jing CX, et al. Admission serum sodium and potassium levels predict survival among critically ill patients with acute kidney injury: A cohort study. BMC Nephrology. 2019; **20**(1):311. DOI: 10.1186/s12882-019-1505-9

[25] Li Q, Li Y, Zhou F. Association of serum potassium level with early and late mortality in very elderly patients with acute kidney injury. Journal of Intensive Medicine. 2022;**2**(1):50-55. DOI: 10.1016/j.jointm.2021.11.005

[26] Khanagavi J, Gupta T, Aronow WS, Shah T, Garg J, Ahn C, et al. Hyperkalemia among hospitalized patients and association between duration of hyperkalemia and outcomes. Archives of Medical Science. 2014;**10**(2): 251-257. DOI: 10.5114/aoms.2014.42577 Epub 2014 May 13

[27] Priori SG, Blomström-Lundqvist C, Mazzanti A, Blom N, Borggrefe M, Camm J, et al. ESC guidelines for the management of patients with ventricular arrhythmias and the prevention of sudden cardiac death: The task force for the Management of Patients with ventricular arrhythmias and the prevention of sudden cardiac death of the European Society of Cardiology (ESC). Endorsed by: Association for European Pediatric and Congenital Cardiology (AEPC). European Heart Journal. 2015;**36**(41):2793-2867. DOI: 10.1093/eurheartj/ehv316 Epub 2015 Aug 29

[28] Weiss JN, Qu Z, Shivkumar K. Electrophysiology of Hypokalemia and Hyperkalemia. Circulation. Arrhythmia and Electrophysiology. 2017;**10**(3): e004667. DOI: 10.1161/CIRCEP.116.004667

[29] Hunter RW, Bailey MA. Hyperkalemia: Pathophysiology, risk factors and consequences. Nephrology, Dialysis, Transplantation. 2019;**34**(Suppl. 3):iii2-iii11. DOI: 10.1093/ndt/gfz206

[30] Montague BT, Ouellette JR, Buller GK. Retrospective review of the frequency of ECG changes in hyperkalemia. Clinical Journal of the American Society of Nephrology. 2008; **3**(2):324-330. DOI: 10.2215/CJN.04611007 Epub 2008 Jan 30

[31] Montford JR, Linas S. How dangerous is Hyperkalemia? Journal of the American Society of Nephrology (JASN). 2017;**28**(11):3155-3165. DOI: 10.1681/ASN.2016121344 Epub 2017 Aug 4

[32] Raffee LA, Alawneh KZ, Ababneh MJ, Hijazi HH, Al Abdi RM, Aboozour MM, et al. Clinical and electrocardiogram presentations of patients with high serum potassium concentrations within emergency settings: A prospective study. International Journal of Emergency Medicine. 2022;**15**(1):23. DOI: 10.1186/s12245-022-00422-8

[33] Bianchi S, Rossi GM. Predicting hyperkalemia in patients with acute kidney injury: Time for a change of weaponry. Internal and Emergency Medicine. 2020;**15**(3):371-372. DOI: 10.1007/s11739-019-02245-7 Epub 2019 Dec 3

[34] Rossi E, Perazzoli F, Negro A, Sani C, Davoli S, Dotti C, et al. Acute effects of intravenous sodium chloride load on calcium metabolism and on parathyroid function in patients with primary aldosteronism compared with subjects with essential hypertension. American Journal of Hypertension. 1998; **11**(1 Pt 1):8-13. DOI: 10.1016/s0895-7061(97)00366-x

[35] Chávez-Íñiguez JS, Maggiani-Aguilera P, Aranda-García de Quevedo A, Claure-Del Granado R, Vega-Vega O, Lopez-Giacoman SR, et al. Serum potassium trajectory during AKI and mortality risk. Nephron. 17 Feb, 2023. DOI: 10.1159/000529588. Epub ahead of print. PMID: 36808092

[36] Yessayan L, Yee J, Frinak S, Szamosfalvi B. Continuous renal replacement therapy for the Management of Acid-Base and Electrolyte Imbalances in acute kidney injury. Advances in Chronic Kidney Disease. 2016;**23**(3):203-210. DOI: 10.1053/j.ackd.2016.02.005

[37] Moussavi K, Garcia J, Tellez-Corrales E, Fitter S. Reduced alternative insulin dosing in hyperkalemia: A meta-analysis of effects on hypoglycemia and potassium reduction. Pharmacotherapy. 2021;**41**(7):598-607. DOI: 10.1002/phar.2596 Epub 2021 Jun 1

[38] Bushinsky DA, Williams GH, Pitt B, Weir MR, Freeman MW, Garza D, et al. Patiromer induces rapid and sustained potassium lowering in patients with chronic kidney disease and hyperkalemia. Kidney International. 2015;**88**(6):1427-1433. DOI: 10.1038/ki.2015.270 Epub 2015 Sep 16

[39] Ballantyne F III, Davis LD, Reynolds EW Jr, et al. Cellular basis for reversal of hyperkalemic electrocardiographic changes by sodium. The American Journal of Physiology. 1975;**229**: 935-940

[40] Lindner G, Burdmann EA, Class CM, Hemmelgarn BR, Herzog CA, Małyszko J, et al. Acute hyperkalemia in the emergency department: A summary from a kidney disease: Improving global outcomes conference. European Journal of Emergency Medicine. 2020;**27**(5): 329-337. DOI: 10.1097/MEJ.0000000000000691

[41] Celebi Yamanoglu NG, Yamanoglu A. The effect of calcium gluconate in the treatment of hyperkalemia. Turkish Journal of Emergency Medicine. 2022;**22**(2):75-82. DOI: 10.4103/2452-2473.342812

[42] Liu M, Rafique Z. Acute Management of Hyperkalemia. Current Heart Failure Reports. 2019;**16**(3):67-74. DOI: 10.1007/s11897-019-00425-2

[43] Chothia MY, Halperin ML, Rensburg MA, Hassan MS, Davids MR. Bolus administration of intravenous glucose in the treatment of hyperkalemia: A randomized controlled trial. Nephron Physiology. 2014;**126**(1): 1-8. DOI: 10.1159/000358836 Epub 2014 Feb 22

[44] Harel Z, Kamel KS. Optimal dose and method of Administration of Intravenous Insulin in the Management of Emergency Hyperkalemia: A systematic review. PLoS One. 2016; **11**(5):e0154963. DOI: 10.1371/journal.pone.0154963

[45] Grandpa JG. Treatment of severe Hyperkalemia: Confronting 4 fallacies. Kidney International Reports. 2017;**3**(1): 47-55. DOI: 10.1016/j.ekir.2017.10.001

[46] Geng S, Green EF, Kurz MC, Rivera JV. Sodium bicarbonate administration and subsequent potassium concentration in hyperkalemia treatment. The American Journal of Emergency Medicine. Dec 2021;**50**:132-135. DOI: 10.1016/j.ajem.2021.07.032 Epub 2021 Jul 21

[47] Gutierrez R, Schlessinger F, Oster JR, Rietberg B, Perez GO. Effect of hypertonic versus isotonic sodium bicarbonate on plasma potassium concentration in patients with end-stage renal disease. Mineral and Electrolyte Metabolism. 1991;**17**(5):297-302

[48] Perkins GD, Graesner JT, Semeraro F, Olasveengen T, Soar J, Lott C, et al. European resuscitation council guidelines 2021: Executive summary. Resuscitation. 2021;**161**:1-60. DOI: 10.1016/j.resuscitation.2021.02.003

Epub 2021 Mar 24. Erratum in: Resuscitation. 2021 May 4; 163:97-98

[49] Jaber S, Paugam C, Futier E, Lefrant JY, Lasocki S, Lescot T, et al. Sodium bicarbonate therapy for patients with severe metabolic acidaemia in the intensive care unit (BICAR-ICU): A multicentre, open-label, randomized controlled, phase 3 trial. Lancet. 2018; **392**(10141):31-40. DOI: 10.1016/S0140-6736(18)31080-8 Epub 2018 Jun 14. Erratum in: Lancet. 2018 Dec 8; 392(10163):2440

[50] Mandelberg A, Krupnik Z, Houri S, Smetana S, Gilad E, Matas Z, et al. Salbutamol metered-dose inhaler with spacer for hyperkalemia: How fast? How safe? Chest. 1999;**115**(3):617-622. DOI: 10.1378/chest.115.3.617

[51] Elliott MJ, Ronksley PE, Class CM, Ahmed SB, Hemmelgarn BR. Management of patients with acute hyperkalemia. CMAJ. 2010;**182**(15): 1631-1635. DOI: 10.1503/cmaj.100461 Epub 2010 Sep 20

[52] Chawla LS, Davison DL, Brasha-Mitchell E, Koyner JL, Arthur JM, Shaw AD, et al. Development and standardization of a furosemide stress test to predict the severity of acute kidney injury. Critical Care. 2013;**17**: R207

[53] Meaney CJ, Beccari MV, Yang Y, Zhao J. Systematic review and meta-analysis of Patiromer and sodium zirconium Cyclosilicate: A new armamentarium for the treatment of Hyperkalemia. Pharmacotherapy. 2017; **37**(4):401-411. DOI: 10.1002/phar.1906 Epub 2017 Mar 10

[54] Batterink J, Cessford TA, Taylor RA. Pharmacological interventions for the acute management of hyperkalaemia in adults. Cochrane Database of Systematic Reviews. 2015;**10**(10):CD010344. DOI: 10.1002/14651858.CD010344.pub2

[55] Zarbock A, Kellum JA, Schmidt C, Van Aken H, Wempe C, Pavenstädt H, et al. Effect of early vs delayed initiation of renal replacement therapy on mortality in critically ill patients with acute kidney injury: The ELAIN randomized clinical trial. JAMA. 2016; **315**(20):2190-2199. DOI: 10.1001/jama.2016.5828

[56] Gaudry S, Hajage D, Schortgen F, Martin-Lefevre L, Pons B, Boulet E, et al. Initiation strategies for renal-replacement therapy in the intensive care unit. The New England Journal of Medicine. 2016; **375**(2):122-133. DOI: 10.1056/NEJMoa1603017 Epub 2016 May 15

[57] Barbar SD, Clere-Jehl R, Bourredjem A, Hernu R, Montini F, Bruyère R, et al. IDEAL-ICU trial investigators and the CRICS TRIGGERSEP Network. Timing of renal-replacement therapy in patients with acute kidney injury and sepsis. The New England Journal of Medicine. 2018; **379**(15):1431-1442. DOI: 10.1056/NEJMoa1803213

[58] STARRT-AKI Investigators, Canadian Critical Care Trials Group, Australian and New Zealand Intensive Care Society Clinical Trials Group, United Kingdom Critical Care Research Group, Canadian Nephrology Trials Network, Irish Critical Care Trials Group. Timing of initiation of renal-replacement therapy in acute kidney injury. The New England Journal of Medicine. 2020;**383**(3):240-251. DOI: 10.1056/NEJMoa2000741 Erratum in: N Engl J Med. 2020 Jul 15

[59] Coppola S, Caccioppola A, Froio S, Chiumello D. Sodium bicarbonate in different critically ill conditions: From physiology to clinical practice.

Anesthesiology. 2021;**134**(5):774-783. DOI: 10.1097/ALN.0000000000003733

[60] Schotola H, Toischer K, Popov AF, Renner A, Schmitto JD, Gummert J, et al. Mild metabolic acidosis impairs the β-adrenergic response in isolated human failing myocardium. Critical Care. 2012; **16**(4):R153. DOI: 10.1186/cc11468

[61] Kraut JA, Madias NE. Metabolic acidosis: Pathophysiology, diagnosis and management. Nature Reviews. Nephrology. 2010;**6**(5):274-285. DOI: 10.1038/nrneph.2010.33 Epub 2010 Mar 23

[62] Gunnerson KJ, Saul M, He S, Kellum JA. Lactate versus non-lactate metabolic acidosis: A retrospective outcome evaluation of critically ill patients. Critical Care. 2006;**10**(1):R22. DOI: 10.1186/cc3987

[63] Yagi K, Fujii T. Management of acute metabolic acidosis in the ICU: Sodium bicarbonate and renal replacement therapy. Critical Care. 2021;**25**(1):314. DOI: 10.1186/s13054-021-03677-4

[64] Wardi G, Holgren S, Gupta A, Sobel J, Birch A, Pearce A, et al. A review of bicarbonate use in common clinical scenarios. The Journal of Emergency Medicine. 2023. DOI: 10.1016/j.jemermed.2023.04.012

[65] Jung B, Rimmele T, Le Goff C, Chanques G, Corne P, Jonquet O, et al. Severe metabolic or mixed acidemia on intensive care unit admission: Incidence, prognosis and administration of buffer therapy. A prospective, multiple-center study. Critical Care. 2011;**15**(5):R238. DOI: 10.1186/cc10487 Epub 2011 Oct 13

[66] Zhang Z, Zhu C, Mo L, Hong Y. Effectiveness of sodium bicarbonate infusion on mortality in septic patients with metabolic acidosis. Intensive Care Medicine. 2018;**44**(11):1888-1895. DOI: 10.1007/s00134-018-5379-2 Epub 2018 Sep 25

[67] Kim JH, Kim HJ, Kim JY, Hs A, Ahn IM, Choe WJ, et al. Meta-analysis of sodium bicarbonate therapy for prevention of cardiac surgery-associated acute kidney injury. Journal of Cardiothoracic and Vascular Anesthesia. 2015;**29**(5):1248-1256. DOI: 10.1053/j.jvca.2015.03.007 Epub 2015 Mar 5

[68] Tie HT, Luo MZ, Luo MJ, Zhang M, Wu QC, Wan JY. Sodium bicarbonate in the prevention of cardiac surgery-associated acute kidney injury: A systematic review and meta-analysis. Critical Care. 2014;**18**(5):517. DOI: 10.1186/s13054-014-0517-x

[69] Lee J, Kim SG, Yun D, Kang MW, Kim YC, Kim DK, et al. Longitudinal trajectory of acidosis and mortality in acute kidney injury requiring continuous renal replacement therapy. BMC Nephrology. 2022;**23**(1):411. DOI: 10.1186/s12882-022-03047-4

[70] Oczkowski S, Alshamsi F, Belley-Cote E, Centofanti JE, Hylander Møller M, Nunnaly ME, et al. Surviving sepsis campaign guidelines 2021: Highlights for the practicing clinician. Polish Archives of Internal Medicine. 2022;**132**(7-8):16290. DOI: 10.20452/pamw.16290 Epub 2022 Jul 6

[71] Frank Peacock W, Soto KM. Current technique of fluid status assessment. Congestive Heart Failure. 2010;**16** (Suppl. 1):S45-S51. DOI: 10.1111/j.1751-7133.2010.00166.x

[72] Legrand M, Le Cam B, Perbet S, et al. Urine sodium concentration to predict fluid responsiveness in oliguric ICU patients: A prospective multicenter observational study. CritCare.

2016;**20**:165. DOI: 10.1186/s13054-016-1343-0

[73] Marik PE, Monnet X, Teboul JL. Hemodynamic parameters to guide fluid therapy. Annals of Intensive Care. 2011; **1**(1):1. DOI: 10.1186/2110-5820-1-1

[74] Koratala A, Ronco C, Kazory A. Diagnosis of fluid overload: From conventional to contemporary concepts. Cardiorenal Medicine. 2022;**12**(4): 141-154. DOI: 10.1159/000526902 Epub 2022 Sep 12

[75] Bouchard J, Soroko SB, Chertow GM, Himmelfarb J, Ikizler TA, Paganini EP, et al. Program to improve Care in Acute Renal Disease (PICARD) study group. Fluid accumulation, survival and recovery of kidney function in critically ill patients with acute kidney injury. Kidney International. 2009;**76**(4): 422-427. DOI: 10.1038/ki.2009.159 [Epub 2009 May 13]. PMID: 19436332

[76] Messmer AS, Moser M, Zuercher P, Schefold JC, Müller M, Pfortmueller CA. Fluid overload phenotypes in critical illness-A machine learning approach. Journal of Clinical Medicine. 2022;**11**(2):336. DOI: 10.3390/jcm11020336

[77] Malbrain MLNG, Van Regenmortel N, Saugel B, De Tavernier B, Van Gaal PJ, Joannes-Boyau O, et al. Principles of fluid management and stewardship in septic shock: It is time to consider the four D's and the four phases of fluid therapy. Annals of Intensive Care. 2018;**8**(1):66. DOI: 10.1186/s13613-018-0402-x

[78] Reitsma S, Slaaf DW, Vink H, van Zandvoort MA. Oude Egbrink MG. The endothelial glycocalyx: Composition, functions, and visualization. Pflügers Archiv. 2007; **454**(3):345-359. DOI: 10.1007/s00424-007-0212-8 Epub 2007 Jan 26

[79] Thin GS, Zanders S, Baker JK. Recent advances in the understanding of endothelial barrier function and fluid therapy. Postgraduate Medical Journal. 2018;**94**(1111):289-295. DOI: 10.1136/postgradmedj-2017-135125 Epub 2018 Jan 26

[80] De Laet IE, Malbrain MLNG, De Waele JJ. A Clinician's Guide to Management of Intra-abdominal Hypertension and Abdominal Compartment Syndrome in critically ill patients. Critical Care. 2020; **24**(1):97. DOI: 10.1186/s13054-020-2782-1

[81] Kuper M, Gunning MP, Halder S, Soni N. The short-term effect of hyperoncotic albumin, given alone or with furosemide, on oxygenation in sepsis-induced acute respiratory distress syndrome. Anesthesia. 2007;**62**(3): 259-263. DOI: 10.1111/j.1365-2044.2007.04941.x

[82] Iba T, Levy JH. Derangement of the endothelial glycocalyx in sepsis. Journal of Thrombosis and Haemostasis. 2019; **17**(2):283-294. DOI: 10.1111/jth.14371 Epub 2019 Feb 3

[83] National Heart, Lung, and Blood Institute Acute Respiratory Distress Syndrome (ARDS) Clinical Trials Network, Wiedemann HP, Wheeler AP, Bernard GR, Thompson BT, Hayden D, et al. Comparison of two fluid-management strategies in acute lung injury. The New England Journal of Medicine. 2006;**354**(24):2564-2575. DOI: 10.1056/NEJMoa062200 Epub 2006 May 21

[84] Silversides JA, Major E, Ferguson AJ, Mann EE, McAuley DF, Marshall JC, et al. Conservative fluid management or deresuscitation for patients with sepsis or acute respiratory distress syndrome following the resuscitation phase of

critical illness: A systematic review and meta-analysis. Intensive Care Medicine. 2017;**43**(2):155-170. DOI: 10.1007/s00134-016-4573-3

[85] Vaara ST, Ostermann M, Bitker L, Schneider A, Poli E, Hoste E, et al. Restrictive fluid management versus usual care in acute kidney injury (REVERSE-AKI): A pilot randomized controlled feasibility trial. Intensive Care Medicine. 2021;**47**(6):665-673. DOI: 10.1007/s00134-021-06401-6 Epub 2021 May 7

[86] Enghard P, Rademacher S, Nee J, Hasper D, Engert U, Jörres A, et al. Simplified lung ultrasound protocol shows excellent prediction of extravascular lung water in ventilated intensive care patients. Critical Care. 2015;**19**(1):36. DOI: 10.1186/s13054-015-0756-5

[87] Chowdhury AH, Cox EF, Francis ST, Lobo DN. A randomized, controlled, double-blind crossover study on the effects of 2-L infusions of 0.9% saline and plasma-lyte® 148 on renal blood flow velocity and renal cortical tissue perfusion in healthy volunteers. Annals of Surgery. 2012;**256**(1):18-24. DOI: 10.1097/SLA.0b013e318256be72 Erratum in: Ann Surg. 2013 Dec;258(6):1118

[88] Ding X, Cheng Z, Qian Q. Intravenous fluids and acute kidney injury. Blood Purification 2017;43(1-3):163-172. DOI: 10.1159/000452702. Epub 2017 Jan 24

[89] Chappell D, Bruegger D, Potzel J, Jacob M, Brettner F, Vogeser M, et al. Hypervolemia increases release of atrial natriuretic peptide and shedding of the endothelial glycocalyx. Critical Care. 2014;**18**(5):538. DOI: 10.1186/s13054-014-0538-5

[90] Molitoris BA. Low-flow acute kidney injury: The pathophysiology of prerenal Azotemia, abdominal compartment syndrome, and obstructive Uropathy. Clinical Journal of the American Society of Nephrology. 2022;**17**(7):1039-1049. DOI: 10.2215/CJN.15341121 Epub 2022 May 18

[91] De Laet I, Deeren D, Schoonheydt K, Van Regenmortel N, Dits H, Malbrain ML. Renal replacement therapy with net fluid removal lowers intra-abdominal pressure and volumetric indices in critically ill patients. Annals of Intensive Care. 2012;**2**(Suppl 1):S20. DOI: 10.1186/2110-5820-2-S1-S20 Epub 2012 Dec 20

[92] Ostermann M, Alvarez G, Sharpe MD, Martin CM. Frusemide administration in critically ill patients by continuous compared to bolus therapy. Nephron. Clinical Practice. 2007;**107**(2):c70-c76. DOI: 10.1159/000108641 Epub 2007 Sep 20

[93] Felker GM, Lee KL, Bull DA, Redfield MM, Stevenson LW, Goldsmith SR, et al. NHLBI Heart failure clinical research Network. Diuretic strategies in patients with acute decompensated heart failure. The New England Journal of Medicine. 2011;**364**(9):797-805. DOI: 10.1056/NEJMoa1005419

[94] Novak JE, Ellison DH. Diuretics in states of volume overload: Core curriculum 2022. American Journal of Kidney Diseases. 2022;**80**(2):264-276. DOI: 10.1053/j.ajkd.2021.09.029 Epub 2022 Feb 19

[95] Cox ZL, Sarrell BA, Cella MK, Tucker B, Arroyo JP, Umanath K, et al. Multinephron segment diuretic therapy to overcome diuretic resistance in acute Heart failure: A single-Center experience. Journal of Cardiac Failure.

2022;**28**(1):21-31. DOI: 10.1016/j.cardfail.2021.07.016 Epub 2021 Aug 14

[96] Lee TH, Kuo G, Chang CH, Huang YT, Yen CL, Lee CC, et al. Diuretic effect of co-administration of furosemide and albumin in comparison to furosemide therapy alone: An updated systematic review and meta-analysis. PLoS One. 2021;**16**(12):e0260312. DOI: 10.1371/journal.pone.0260312

[97] Gunning S, Kutuby F, Rose R, Trevino S, Song T, Koyner JL. Fluid overload and mortality in patients with severe acute kidney injury and extracorporeal membrane oxygenation. Kidney360. 2020;**1**(4):232-240. DOI: 10.34067/KID.0000402019

[98] Niwa T. Uremic Toxins. 1st ed. Japan: Wiley; 2012

[99] Herget-Rosenthal S, Glorieux G, Jankowski J, Jankowski V. Uremic toxins in acute kidney injury. Seminars in Dialysis. 2009;**22**(4):445-448. DOI: 10.1111/j.1525-139X.2009.00598.x

[100] Lara-Prado JI, Pazos-Pérez F, Méndez-Landa CE, Grajales-García DP, Feria-Ramírez JA, Salazar-González JJ, et al. Acute kidney injury and organ dysfunction: What is the role of uremic toxins? Toxins (Basel). 2021;**13**(8):551. DOI: 10.3390/toxins13080551

[101] Chebotareva N, Bobkova I, Shilov E. Heat shock proteins and kidney disease: Perspectives of HSP therapy. Cell Stress & Chaperones. 2017;**22**(3): 319-343. DOI: 10.1007/s12192-017-0790-0 Epub 2017 Apr 13

[102] Sukhovershin RA, Gilinskiĭ MA. The role of asymmetric dimethylarginine in the regulation of nitric oxide level in rats with acute renal injury. Ross Fiziol Zh Im IM Sechenova. Apr 2012;**98**(4): 497-505. Russian. PMID: 22834339

[103] Vallance P, Leiper J. Cardiovascular biology of the asymmetric dimethylarginine:Dimethylarginine dimethylaminohydrolase pathway. Arteriosclerosis, Thrombosis, and Vascular Biology. 2004;**24**(6): 1023-1030. DOI: 10.1161/01.ATV.0000128897.54893.26 Epub 2004 Apr 22

[104] Wang LY, Zhang DL, Zheng JF, Zhang Y, Zhang QD, Liu WH. Apelin-13 passes through the ADMA-damaged endothelial barrier and acts on vascular smooth muscle cells. Peptides. 2011;**32** (12):2436-2443. DOI: 10.1016/j.peptides.2011.10.001 Epub 2011 Oct 6

[105] Chen JH, Chiang CK. Uremic toxins and protein-bound therapeutics in AKI and CKD: Up-to-date evidence. Toxins (Basel). 2021;**14**(1):8. DOI: 10.3390/toxins14010008

[106] Caillard P, Bennis Y, Six I, Bodeau S, Kamel S, Choukroun G, et al. The role of gut-derived, protein-bound uremic toxins in the cardiovascular complications of acute kidney injury. Toxins (Basel). 2022;**14**(5):336. DOI: 10.3390/toxins14050336

[107] Zhang M, Dong R, Da J, Yuan J, Zha Y, Long Y. Hyperhomocysteinemia exacerbates acute kidney injury via increased mitochondrial damage. Frontiers in Physiology. 2022;**13**:967104. DOI: 10.3389/fphys.2022.967104

[108] Jo SK. Kidney-gut crosstalk in AKI. Kidney360. 2021;**2**(5):886-889. DOI: 10.34067/KID.0007722020

[109] Yang J, Kim CJ, Go YS, Lee HY, Kim MG, Oh SW, et al. Intestinal microbiota control acute kidney injury severity by immune modulation. Kidney

International. 2020;**98**(4):932-946. DOI: 10.1016/j.kint.2020.04.048 Epub 2020 May 26

[110] Gettings LG, Reynolds HN, Scalea T. Outcome in post-traumatic acute renal failure when continuous renal replacement therapy is applied early vs. beats. Intensive Care Medicine. 1999;**25**(8):805-813. DOI: 10.1007/s001340050956

[111] Carl DE, Grossman C, Behnke M, Sessler CN, Gehr TW. Effect of timing of dialysis on mortality in critically ill, septic patients with acute renal failure. Hemodialysis International. 2010;**14**(1): 11-17. DOI: 10.1111/j.1542-4758.2009.00407.x

[112] Wu VC, Ko WJ, Chang HW, Chen YS, Chen YW, Chen YM, et al. Early renal replacement therapy in patients with postoperative acute liver failure associated with acute renal failure: Effect on postoperative outcomes. Journal of the American College of Surgeons. 2007;**205**(2): 266-276. DOI: 10.1016/j.jamcollsurg.2007.04.006 Epub 2007 Jun 21

[113] Liu KD, Himmelfarb J, Paganini E, Ikizler TA, Soroko SH, Mehta RL, et al. Timing of initiation of dialysis in critically ill patients with acute kidney injury. Clinical Journal of the American Society of Nephrology. 2006;**1**(5): 915-919. DOI: 10.2215/CJN.01430406 Epub 2006 Jul 6

[114] Gaudry S, Hajage D, Martin-Lefevre L, Lebbah S, Louis G, Moschietto S, et al. Comparison of two delayed strategies for renal replacement therapy initiation for severe acute kidney injury (AKIKI 2): A multicentre, open-label, randomized, controlled trial. Lancet. 2021;**397**(10281): 1293-1300. DOI: 10.1016/S0140-6736(21)00350-0

[115] Pan HC, Chen YY, Tsai IJ, Shiao CC, Huang TM, Chan CK, et al. Accelerated versus standard initiation of renal replacement therapy for critically ill patients with acute kidney injury: A systematic review and meta-analysis of RCT studies. Critical Care. 5 Jan, 2021; **25**(1):5. DOI: 10.1186/s13054-020-03434-z. PMID: 33402204; PMCID: PMC7784335

[116] Zhang L, Chen D, Tang X, Li P, Zhang Y, Tao Y. Timing of initiation of renal replacement therapy in acute kidney injury: An updated meta-analysis of randomized controlled trials. Renal Failure. 2020;**42**(1):77-88. DOI: 10.1080/0886022X.2019.1705337

[117] Lin WT, Lai CC, Chang SP, Wang JJ. Effects of early dialysis on the outcomes of critically ill patients with acute kidney injury: A systematic review and meta-analysis of randomized controlled trials. Scientific Reports. 2019; **9**(1):18283. DOI: 10.1038/s41598-019-54777-9

[118] Li Y, Zhang Y, Li R, Zhang M, Gao X. Timing of initiation of renal replacement therapy for patients with acute kidney injury: A meta-analysis of RCTs. Therapeutic Apheresis and Dialysis. 2023;**27**(2):207-221. DOI: 10.1111/1744-9987.13914 Epub 2022 Aug 30

[119] Bhatt GC, Das RR, Satapathy A. Early versus late initiation of renal replacement therapy: Have we reached the consensus? An Updated Meta-Analysis. Nephron. 2021;**145**(4):371-385. DOI: 10.1159/000515129 Epub 2021 Apr 29

[120] Lee CW, Kou HW, Chou HS, Chou HH, Huang SF, Chang CH, et al. A combination of SOFA score and biomarkers gives a better prediction of

septic AKI and in-hospital mortality in critically ill surgical patients: A pilot study. World Journal of Emergency Surgery (WJES). 2018;**13**:41. DOI: 10.1186/s13017-018-0202-5

[121] Han H, Wen Z, Wang J, Zhang P, Gong Q, Ge S, et al. Prediction of short-term mortality with renal replacement therapy in patients with cardiac surgery-associated acute kidney injury. Frontiers in Cardiovascular Medicine. 2021;**8**: 738947. DOI: 10.3389/fcvm.2021.738947

[122] Hou K, Chen Q, Zhu X, Shen X, Zou L, Mu X, et al. Correlation between vasoactive-inotropic score and postoperative acute kidney injury after cardiovascular surgery. The Heart Surgery Forum. 2021;**24**(2):E282-E292. DOI: 10.1532/hsf.3537

[123] Nguyen HB, Rivers EP, Knoblich BP, Jacobsen G, Muzzin A, Ressler JA, et al. Early lactate clearance is associated with improved outcome in severe sepsis and septic shock. Critical Care Medicine. 2004;**32**(8):1637-1642. DOI: 10.1097/01.ccm.0000132904.35713.a7

[124] Passos RDH, Ramos JGR, Gobatto A, Mendonça EJB, Miranda EA, Dutra FRD, et al. Lactate clearance is associated with mortality in septic patients with acute kidney injury requiring continuous renal replacement therapy: A cohort study. Medicine (Baltimore). 2016;**95**(40):e5112. DOI: 10.1097/MD.0000000000005112

[125] Gaudry S, Grolleau F, Barbar S, Martin-Lefevre L, Pons B, Boulet É, et al. Continuous renal replacement therapy versus intermittent hemodialysis as first modality for renal replacement therapy in severe acute kidney injury: A secondary analysis of AKIKI and IDEAL-ICU studies. Critical Care. 2022;**26**(1):93. DOI: 10.1186/s13054-022-03955-9

[126] Lai CF, Liu JH, Tseng LJ, Tsao CH, Chou NK, Lin SL, et al. Unsupervised clustering identifies sub-phenotypes and reveals novel outcome predictors in patients with dialysis-requiring sepsis-associated acute kidney injury. Annals of Medicine. 2023;**55**(1):2197290. DOI: 10.1080/07853890.2023.2197290

[127] Pan HC, Huang TM, Sun CY, Chou NK, Tsao CH, Yeh FY, et al. Predialysis serum lactate levels could predict dialysis withdrawal in type 1 cardiorenal syndrome patients. EClinicalMedicine. 2022;**44**:101232. DOI: 10.1016/j.eclinm.2021.101232

[128] Levraut J, Ciebiera JP, Jambou P, Ichai C, Labib Y, Grimaud D. Effect of continuous venovenous hemofiltration with dialysis on lactate clearance in critically ill patients. Critical Care Medicine. 1997;**25**(1):58-62. DOI: 10.1097/00003246-199701000-00013

[129] Kawarazaki H, Uchino S, Tokuhira N, Ohnuma T, Namba Y, Katayama S, et al. JSEPTIC (Japanese Society for Physicians Trainees in intensive care) clinical trial group. Who may not benefit from continuous renal replacement therapy in acute kidney injury? Hemodialysis International. 2013;**17**(4):624-632. DOI: 10.1111/hdi.12053 Epub 2013 May 7

[130] Koyner JL, Davison DL, Brasha-Mitchell E, Chalikonda DM, Arthur JM, Shaw AD, et al. Furosemide stress test and biomarkers for the prediction of AKI severity. Journal of the American Society of Nephrology (JASN). 2015;**26**(8): 2023-2031. DOI: 10.1681/ASN.2014060535 Epub 2015 Feb 5

[131] Lumlertgul N, Peerapornratana S, Trakarnvanich T, Pongsittisak W, Surasit K, Chuasuwan A, et al. Early versus standard initiation of renal replacement therapy in furosemide

stress test non-responsive acute kidney injury patients (the FST trial). Critical Care. 2018;**22**(1):101. DOI: 10.1186/s13054-018-2021-1

[132] Chen JJ, Chang CH, Huang YT, Kuo G. Furosemide stress test as a predictive marker of acute kidney injury progression or renal replacement therapy: A systemic review and meta-analysis. Critical Care. 2020;**24**(1):202. DOI: 10.1186/s13054-020-02912-8

[133] Zhang K, Zhang H, Zhao C, Hu Z, Shang J, Chen Y, et al. Hebei key Laboratory of Critical Disease Mechanism and Intervention. The furosemide stress test predicts the timing of continuous renal replacement therapy initiation in critically ill patients with acute kidney injury: A double-blind prospective intervention cohort study. European Journal of Medical Research. 2023;**28**(1):149. DOI: 10.1186/s40001-023-01092-9

[134] Samprathi A, Padmakumar AV, Parekh A. Sequential nephron blockade in acute kidney injury in critically ill patients. Research Square. 2022. DOI: 10.21203/rs.3.rs-1366526/v2

[135] Meersch M, Weiss R, Gerss J, Albert F, Gruber J, Kellum JA, et al. Predicting the development of renal replacement therapy indications by combining the furosemide stress test and chemokine (C-C motif) ligand 14 in a cohort of postsurgical patients. Critical Care Medicine. 29 Mar 2023. DOI: 10.1097/CCM.0000000000005849. Epub ahead of print. PMID: 36988335

[136] Chen S. Retooling the creatinine clearance equation to estimate kinetic GFR when the plasma creatinine is changing acutely. Journal of the American Society of Nephrology (JASN). 2013;**24**(6):877-888. DOI: 10.1681/ASN.2012070653 Epub 2013 May 23

[137] Bagshaw SM, Wald R. Strategies for the optimal timing to start renal replacement therapy in critically ill patients with acute kidney injury. Kidney International. May 2017;**91**(5): 1022-1032. DOI: 10.1016/j.kint.2016.09.053. Epub 2017 Feb 17. PMID: 28222898

[138] Lijović L, Pelajić S, Hawchar F, Minev I, da Silva BHCS, Angelucci A, et al. Diagnosing acute kidney injury ahead of time in critically ill septic patients using kinetic estimated glomerular filtration rate. Journal of Critical Care. 2023;**75**:154276. DOI: 10.1016/j.jcrc.2023.154276 Epub 2023 Feb 10

Chapter 5

Role of RRT in Adult Patients with Hyperammonemia

Randah Dahlan and Ali Alkatheeri

Abstract

Hyperammonemia is not uncommonly encountered in adult critically ill patients in the intensive care unit (ICU). Although it often occurs in patients with underlying liver disease, it may also occur in patients with no evidence of acute or chronic liver disease. Hyperammonemia can cause serious complications, including acute brain injury (sometimes called hyperammonemia-induced encephalopathy). Hyperammonemia-induced encephalopathy often carries a poor prognosis and may even lead to death. Nephrologists may get involved in the management of hyperammonemic patients (with or without acute kidney injury) for consideration of renal replacement therapy (RRT) as an intervention to lower the ammonia level. This chapter will discuss the role of RRT in adult patients with hyperammonemia.

Keywords: ammonia, hyperammonemia, hemodialysis, renal replacement therapy, hyperammonemic encephalopathy

1. Introduction

The term hyperammonemia denotes an elevated ammonia level in the blood, however, it is often used in clinical practice to refer to a toxic accumulation of ammonia in the blood with its associated serious complications. The normal reference range of ammonia level in adults is 10 to 80 mcg/dL or 6 to 47 μmol/L (SI units) [1], but this range may vary slightly among different laboratories. Ammonia is most damaging to the brain, and this applies to both acute and chronic hyperammonemia [2, 3]. Cerebral edema and brain herniation are more common in patients with acute hyperammonemia, but patients with chronic hypernatremia (e.g., chronic liver disease patients) may develop encephalopathy and have a different mechanism of neurotoxicity caused by hyperammonemia [2, 3]. This serious and potentially fatal condition must be promptly recognized, evaluated, and treated. Although the role of RRT in the management of patients with hyperammonemia is more evident in the pediatric population [4], it is less clear in the adult population. This chapter will give a brief overview of hyperammonemia pathophysiology, causes, manifestations, and general management, but will discuss in detail the available data about the role of RRT in adult patients with hyperammonemia.

2. Pathophysiology of hyperammonemia

Ammonia is normally produced *via* the metabolism of nitrogen-containing compounds [2]. The main sites of ammonia production in the body are the intestine, and to a lesser extent, the kidneys and the muscles [2]. In the intestine, the ammonia is produced *via* the digestion and metabolism of dietary proteins by the mucosal bacteria, *via* urease-producing bacteria and microbial proteolysis, as well as *via* the uptake of glutamine from the systemic circulation with subsequent deamination to glutamate and ammonia [2]. In the kidneys, ammonia is produced by the catabolism of glutamine in the proximal convoluted tubules (ammoniagenesis) [2]. In the muscles, ammonia is the product of muscle metabolism, and this production is increased in certain situations such as seizures, intense exercise, or in catabolic states [2].

The liver is responsible for clearing 90% of the ammonia in the body, and it converts ammonia to urea *via* the urea cycle [2]. If the liver fails or becomes overwhelmed by the excess production of ammonia, the kidneys will decrease the ammonia production in the proximal tubules, and will also increase the urinary excretion of ammonia. Additionally, the brain and the muscles will try to help by metabolizing ammonia to glutamine [2].

Ammonia metabolism is regulated by the extracellular pH, potassium level, and mineralocorticoids and glucocorticoid secretion in the body [2].

With severe hyperammonemia, the osmotic stress is increased in the astrocytes of the brain, which may lead to astrocyte swelling with subsequent cerebral edema and brain herniation. Additionally, the accumulation of glutamine in the astrocytes will affect the energy delivery to neurons, increase oxidative stress, and increase the production of inflammatory cytokines. Together will lead to cellular apoptosis, dysfunction of neurotransmitters, mitochondrial dysfunction, neuronal irritability, and alteration of blood-brain barrier [2]. All cell types of the brain are affected by these changes [2].

3. Causes of hyperammonemia in adults

Hyperammonemia occurs when there is increased production or decreased clearance of ammonia. In the adult population, liver failure is responsible for the majority of cases of hyperammonemia, while non-hepatic causes are rare and account for the minority of cases [2, 5–8]. With non-hepatic causes of hyperammonemia, there is excessive production of ammonia which may exceed the handling capacity of the liver or may bypass the liver to enter directly into the systemic circulation [5–8].

The causes of hyperammonemia in adults are summarized in **Table 1**.

4. Clinical manifestations

In mild cases, symptoms may include headache, vomiting, irritability, behavioral changes, ataxia, and gait abnormalities [2, 7, 8]. Severe hyperammonemia may present with seizures, encephalopathy, coma, and even death [2, 7, 8].

In addition to the severity of hyperammonemia, the clinical manifestations depend on the onset (acute versus chronic). Patients with chronic hyperammonemia (e.g., chronic liver disease patients) have a gradual accumulation of ammonia, allowing for compensatory mechanisms to decrease osmolarity. Additionally, patients with chronic hyperammonemia may have compensatory increase in the ammonia metabolism by other organs (e.g., muscles), which may blunt some of the symptoms.

Hepatic:	
• Most common cause in adults.	
• In chronic liver disease; it is precipitated by gastrointestinal bleeding, infection, electrolytes disturbance, or/and constipation.	
• Also, in patients with acute hepatic failure.	
Non-Hepatic:	
Increased production	**Decreased clearance**
Catabolic states: e.g., burn, trauma, starvation	**Late-onset urea-cycle disorders:** precipitated by a stressful condition
Nutritional: e.g., total parenteral nutrition	**Bariatric surgery**: e.g., gastric bypass
Infection: e.g., by urease-producing organisms	**Anatomic:** e.g., porto-systemic shunts, urinary diversion
Muscular: e.g., seizure, intense exercise	**Anti-epileptics:** e.g., valproate, topiramate, carbamazepine
Malignancy: e.g., multiple myeloma	**Analgesics:** e.g., gabapentin, salicylates
Drugs: e.g., steroids, 5-Fluorouracil, Cytarabine	**Other drugs:** tacrolimus, cyclosporine, acetazolamide, haloperidol
Others: gastrointestinal bleeding, hemolysis, organ transplantation	**Others:** organ transplantation

Table 1.
Causes of hyperammonemia in adults.

Therefore, they are less like to present with cerebral edema and herniation than patients with acute conditions [5, 8].

5. General management

When managing a patient with hyperammonemia, several factors should be taken into consideration, including the onset (acute vs. chronic), presence or absence of symptoms, degree or severity of the hyperammonemia, and the underlying cause. Acute severe hyperammonemia carries the highest risk of adverse outcomes and is potentially fatal. Thus, all measures must be taken to lower the ammonia level rapidly [9]. The following are essential lines of general management [2, 8–10]:

- Ensure that the result is not falsely positive. If the blood sample was kept at room temperature for a long time, it will lead to *in vitro* deamination and falsely elevated ammonia levels. Therefore, in cases of hyperammonemia, the first step is to repeat the test with a sample taken without a tourniquet and placed on ice immediately at the bedside, and then processed within 30 to 60 minutes maximum [5, 9].

- In addition to monitoring ammonia levels, blood gases, and requesting appropriate neurological images, investigating for the underlying cause is important. For example, investigating for underlying liver disease by sending liver function tests, coagulation profile, alcohol and acetaminophen levels, viral serology, and liver ultrasound with the duplex study. Additionally, looking for a source of infection, especially infection with urease-producing organisms, is very crucial.

If hyperammonemia is still not explained, one needs to consider investigating for underlying urea cycle disorders as soon as possible. As mentioned above, some of the cases of non-hepatic hyperammonemia in adults could be related to undiagnosed urea cycle disorder, which becomes unmasked under stressful conditions. Therefore, it might be prudent to involve a biochemical geneticist (metabolic) physician early on to provide some guidance on further investigations and management.

Nutritional	Stop all sources of protein (enteral and parenteral) for 48 hours only.
	Start high-rate IVF as D10%, 0.45 NS. Do not stop for any reason.
	For hyperglycemia, start insulin infusion.
	Contact the pharmacy to prepare lipid emulsion IV 2–3 g/kg.
Antibiotics	To treat any underlying infection and prevent superinfection.
	It may also alter gut flora and reduce the metabolizing intestinal bacteria.
	It is particularly important for immunocompromised patients.
	Consider both parenteral and enteral antibiotics
Laxatives	Use lactulose and other laxatives to decontaminate the gut.
	They reduce the production of ammonia by intestinal bacteria.
	Also, they promote the growth of non-urease-producing lactobacilli.
	Particularly important for patients with liver diseases.
Zinc	Check zinc level and give daily zinc supplementation.
	Zinc deficiency is common in alcoholics, malabsorption, or urinary loss.
	Zinc is a cofactor for urea cycle enzymes.
	So, it speeds up the urea formation from amino acids and ammonia.
Avoid	Valproic acid as it decreases urea cycle function.
	Steroids as they increase the protein turnover.
	Mannitol (ineffective in managing cerebral edema caused by hyperammonemia).
Empirical treatment for undiagnosed cases (functional deficiency or late-onset urea cycle disorder)	
L-carnitine	It stimulates the synthesis of urea as it favors mitochondrial respiration.
	Start levocarnitine IV/PO 100 mg/kg/day divided q 6–8 h,
	Also give hydroxycobalamin 1 mg IM/IV/PO, and biotin 10 mg IV/PO
L-Arginine	It is a urea cycle enhancer and should be given in all cases of unknown etiology.
	Available as oral and intravenous.
Sodium phenylacetate + sodium benzoate	It promotes ammonia degradation through "alternate" metabolic pathways.
	Give IV KCL as it may cause hyperchloremic hypokalemic metabolic acidosis.
	To be considered when the ammonia level is >150 μmol/L
	Use with caution in hepatic and renal insufficiency, and watch for toxicity
N-carbamylglutamate	Give 100 mg/kg through NG once followed by 50 mg/kg q 6 h.
	Once appropriate enzymatic deficiency is excluded, it should be stopped.

Table 2.
General and initial lines of management for hyperammonemia.

- Treating the underlying cause of hyperammonemia is also the best strategy to prevent the recurrence. But other strategies to lower the ammonia level should not be delayed if immediate management of the underlying cause is not feasible.

- Aim for a physiological pH between 7.35 and 7.44 and avoid alkalemia. Alkalemia will further increase the ammonia level by converting ammonium ion to ammonia. Hypokalemia must also be corrected as it may increase renal ammonia production.

- Ammonia level varies based on the patient's age and there is no consensus about which level needs immediate action. However, a level above 100 μmol/L in adult patients is considered serious and requires immediate attention.

- **Table 2** summarizes the non-dialysis lines of management, which are used to lower the ammonia level.

6. Role of renal replacement therapy

6.1 Ammonia clearance by dialysis

In general, solute-related factors that may affect the extent of its removal by dialysis include its molecular size, its water solubility, its volume of distribution, and its protein binding. Ammonia is a small molecule with a molecular mass of 17 mg/mmol, it is water soluble, has a volume of distribution that is considered to be equal to the total body water, and is not significantly protein-bound [11]. Therefore, it is highly dialyzable.

Hemodialysis prescription-related factors affecting the clearance of ammonia include the blood flow rate (Qb), the dialysate flow rate (Qd), and the dialyzer surface area [12]. This is supported by an *in vitro* study of the clearance of ammonia with single-pass dialyzers, which showed that ammonia clearance by dialysis is between 62% and 99% and could approach that of the liver [12]. In this study, ammonia clearance was directly dependent on the blood flow rate, which was modulated by the dialysate flow rate. For example, when the dialysate flow rate is 300 ml/min, an increase in ammonia clearance was observed with an increase in blood flow until a plateau was reached at 200 ml/min. When the dialysate flow is 500 ml/min, the same was observed but it plateaued at a blood flow rate of 300 ml/min [12]. At a dialysate flow rate of 800 ml/min, a further degree of ammonia clearance was observed with increasing blood flow rate but no plateau was observed within the range of the blood flow rate used. In other words, with a blood flow rate of 200 to 300 ml/min and a dialysate flow rate of 800 ml/min, a rate of ammonia extraction of up to 99% can be seen if there is no ongoing generation of ammonia [12, 13]. The influence of the dialyzer surface area on ammonia clearance depends on the blood flow rate. With a blood flow rate of 500 ml/min and a large surface area dialyzer (2.1 m^2), ammonia clearance may approach 450 ml/min. However, the ammonia clearance was not affected when using large surface area dialyzers at a blood flow rate of 100–200 ml/min. Of note, hemodialysis removes urea and glutamine, which may magnify the ammonia-lowering effects and benefits of hemodialysis [12].

6.2 Is dialysis indicated?

When coming to the role of RRT in the management of adult patients with hyperammonemia, it is important to remember that data reporting the clinical outcomes of this intervention and supporting its usefulness are limited. One retrospective review of adult patients in the intensive care unit (ICU) with hyperammonemia not due to liver failure showed that the requirement of dialysis was not a predictor of mortality [5]. However, this retrospective study of a small sample size does not inform us when to start RRT for such patients. It is difficult to have well-established evidence-based guidelines for managing adult patients with this condition with the rarity and heterogeneous nature of available data. One guideline discussing the acute management of hyperammonemia patients suggested starting RRT for adult patients when the ammonia level exceeds 200 µmol/L [9]. Nevertheless, the level of evidence to support this recommendation was low, and most of the recommendations in this guideline were based on extrapolated data from pediatric patients [9]. However, this extrapolation is of limited value because of different patients' demographics, and different distribution of underlying causes of hyperammonemia. The following are the summaries of recommendations from different reports based on the authors' opinions:

- Long et al. supported a more conservative initiation of RRT for ammonia levels >150 µmol/L (or > 200–250 µmol/L for adult cases of urea cycle disorder), for hyperammonemic encephalopathy, coma, or seizures, or for rising ammonia in the face of other therapy. If early and rapid clearance is necessary (e.g., impending brain herniation), plasmapheresis could be considered followed by CRRT [2]. This opinion was based mainly on case reports of patients with late-onset urea cycle disorders.

- Boer et al. suggested that dialysis should be considered in all patients with acute kidney injury and severe hyperammonemia when other treatment modalities fail to lower ammonia levels within hours [14]. This was the author's opinion, and the definition of severe hyperammonemia was not clarified in his report.

- Alfadhel and Häberle J et al. published guidelines and suggested that RRT to be the first-line therapy in the case of adult patients with acute hyperammonemia when the ammonia level exceeds 200 µmol/L [9, 15]. However, this suggestion was based on the low level of evidence (case reports, case series, and expert opinion) from patients with urea cycle disorders.

- Stergachis et al. presented a retrospective study of adult patients with noncirrhotic hyperammonemia and reported that RRT was utilized with an ammonia level above 250 µmol/L (range 322 to 4530 µmol/L) [16]. No clear-cut recommendations or outcomes were reported.

- Gupta et al. reviewed the available literature on the role of RRT for patients with hyperammonemia, and the limited data in adult patients was acknowledged [10]. The conclusion was that the clinical judgment of the treating physician as to when to initiate RRT is important [10].

- Bélanger-Quintana et al. provided recommendations for the management of hyperammonemia in the adults and pediatric patients, and the initiation of RRT was recommended when the ammonia level is >150–200 µmol/L [17].

With the lack of strong evidence, and thus the lack of consensus recommendations, the decision about initiating RRT for adult patients with hyperammonemia needs to be individualized. This must take into consideration if other treatment modalities failed to lower ammonia levels or not, the presence of neurological consequences of hyperammonemia, and the ammonia level (more than 150 μmol/L). The role of RRT in some of the identifiable causes of hyperammonemia is discussed below.

6.3 Continuous renal replacement therapy (CRRT) vs. intermittent hemodialysis

If the decision was made to start renal replacement therapy for the management of hyperammonemia, the next decision to make is whether to start intermittent hemodialysis or CRRT. To decide about this, a few points must be remembered:

- At the beginning of dialysis, the production of ammonia is likely more than the elimination, until the levels reach a steady state [11].

- Intermittent hemodialysis can lower blood ammonia levels rapidly and efficiently [6, 11, 12]. In fact, *in vitro* data of a single-compartment dialysis model showed that ammonia was decreased by 80% during the first half an hour of hemodialysis [12]. This rapid onset of action is very important to prevent brain injury. However, ammonia has a high volume of distribution, and once conventional hemodialysis is stopped, it diffuses back from the extravascular space. This rebound effect is considered a major disadvantage of intermittent hemodialysis, especially if ammonia generation is continued [11].

- On the other hand, CRRT will provide a steady removal of ammonia, and its continuous nature will address the issue of rebound increase in ammonia level seen with intermittent HD. However, it provides a slow rate of ammonia clearance compared to intermittent hemodialysis., and it will take a longer time to reach a steady state [11].

A scoping review of 28 studies looking at ammonia clearance by RRT in adult and pediatric patients concluded that intermittent hemodialysis provides the highest ammonia clearance followed by CRRT and, at very low levels, peritoneal dialysis [6]. In this review, clearance correlated with Qb and Qd in the case of intermittent hemodialysis, and with the effluent flow rate in CRRT [6].

Therefore, it might be prudent to start with conventional hemodialysis to ensure rapid reduction in ammonia level, followed by CRRT to prevent the rebound increase in ammonia level. However, this decision needs to be individualized and must take into consideration the advantage and disadvantages of each modality of RRT, the available resources, patient's condition, ammonia generation and metabolism in each specific case, and various organ functions (e.g., kidneys, liver, muscles, intestine, and brain) [11].

Of note: ammonia is osmotically active, yet, its rapid removal by dialysis is not associated with dialysis disequilibrium syndrome [18]. This is because the contribution of ammonia (even in the case of severe hyperammonemia) to plasma osmolality is negligible [17]. Additionally, the rapid equilibration of ammonia across the cell membrane will minimize any risk of dialysis disequilibrium syndrome.

6.4 Dialysis prescription

Dialysis prescription need to be tailored according to the patient's condition and diagnosis. The main aim is to provide a rapid reduction of ammonia levels, and then attempt to prevent ammonia rebound to prevent irreversible neurological damage.

Considering all the above-discussed points, below is a suggested prescription of RRT for adult patients with acute hyperammonemia [11, 14].

Initially, consider starting with a session of intermittent hemodialysis with the following details:

- Blood flow (Qb) of 400 to 450 mL/min.
- Dialysate flow (Qd) of 800 mL/min.
- If the patient is hemodynamically unstable or then developed new onset symptoms suggestive of cerebral edema, Qb could be decreased to 250 mL/min and Qd to 500 or 600 mL/min.
- Session length of 4 to 6 hours.

After the completion of the first session of intermittent hemodialysis, CRRT should be immediately started:

- Mode: continuous venovenous hemofiltration (CVVH). It is acceptable to use continuous venovenous hemodialysis (CVVHD) instead and adjust the dialysate flow rate accordingly.
- Blood flow (Qb) of 250 mL/minute.
- Replacement: replacement fluid (RF) at a rate of 50 ml/kg/hour.
- If circuit anticoagulation is used, citrate should be avoided in patients with liver disease.
- Monitor ammonia level Q 12 to 24 hours.
- If the ammonia level continues to rise, increase the Qb to a maximum of 300 mL/min and the replacement fluid to a maximum of 80 mL/kg/hour. If the patient developed alkalemia, the rate of the replacement fluid could be lowered again.

Continue monitoring the patient's ammonia level and arterial blood gases, and perform frequent neurological assessments. If the ammonia level does not improve or it continues to rise, the following options could be considered:

- Repeat the cycle of intermittent hemodialysis followed by CRRT.
- Consider using an ultra-high dose of continuous venovenous hemodiafiltration (CVVHDF) after a session of intermittent hemodialysis. This method was successful in one case report of a woman with refractory hyperammonemia (caused by acute liver failure, AKI, pelvic hematoma, and uterine necrosis) and cerebral

edema complicating an emergency cesarean section [14]. In this case, they used intermittent hemodialysis with Qb of 400 ml/min, and Qd of 500 ml/min, for a duration of 4 hours, followed by immediate start of CVVHDF with 2 CRRT machines, resulting in an ultra-high effluent rate (100 mL/kg/hour). For each of the CRRT machines, the Qb was 160 mL/min; RF rate was 1400 mL/h; and Qd was 2800 mL/h. This strategy was successful to restore the patient's baseline neurological condition [14].

Dialysis could be discontinued if the patient is back to the baseline neurological status, the ammonia level has decreased or stabilized, and if no improvement in the neurological status despite 48 hours of maximum therapy and decreasing ammonia level. In the latter situation, a new CT or MRI of the brain should be considered.

6.5 Dialysis and cause-specific situations

6.5.1 Liver disease

In patients with chronic liver disease; the rise in serum ammonia is slow and gradual [19]. As mentioned before, this slow rise will allow for compensatory mechanisms to decrease the osmolarity, and also for compensatory increase in the ammonia metabolism by other organs [5, 8, 19]. Therefore, hemodialysis in chronic liver disease patients (who may already have chronic hyponatremia) may worsen cerebral edema due to the rapid reduction of osmolality, rapid change in the blood pH, and the effect of the bicarbonate-based solution on increasing CO_2 production and cerebral vasodilatation [19]. Therefore, RRT for the sole purpose of hyperammonemia in chronic liver disease patients is not indicated, and there is insufficient data to support its use in such a setting [19]. If RRT is used for the conventional indications in the setting of AKI, CRRT with its slow nature of clearance is less likely to worsen cerebral edema, especially with lower Qb rates [11, 19].

In adult patients with acute liver failure and hyperammonemia, CRRT provides significant ammonia clearance and this clearance was shown to be correlated with the ultrafiltration rate [20]. In one retrospective analysis of adult patients with hyperammonemia and acute liver failure, early start of CRRT (likely for hyperammonemia rather than for conventional indication of AKI) was associated with prevention of worsening hyperammonemia, which in turn, was associated with increased transplant-free survival [21]. However, ICU mortality was nearly four times higher in this group of patients [21]. Another retrospective review showed that the early start of CRRT in patients with acute liver failure and hyperammonemia resulted in reduced ammonia concentration, and this effect was related to the cumulative dose of dialysis [22]. However, most patients in this study did not demonstrate obvious neurologic recovery during the initial 5 days of ICU management despite the reduction in ammonia level [22]. There is also some evidence to support the use of high-volume plasma exchange in this group of patients [23, 24].

To summarize, the early start of RRT for hyperammonemia (level > 100 μmol/L) may have a beneficial role in patients with acute liver failure. CRRT is preferred over intermittent hemodialysis in patients with liver diseases.

6.5.2 Multiple myeloma

Patients with multiple myeloma may develop hyperammonemia, which may lead to encephalopathy or even death. The mechanism of hyperammonemia in multiple myeloma is unknown, but possible mechanisms are: the production of ammonia by myeloma cells as a result of amino acid metabolism, the Infiltration of the liver by plasma cells or amyloid leading to systemic-portal shunt, and the interference with urea metabolism, and some subtypes of multiple myeloma might undergo leukemic changes which would predispose these patients to hyperammonemia [25].

Treatment of hyperammonemia in such patients is by treating the underlying multiple myeloma, which will lead to a sustained and rapid reduction in the ammonia level as well as an improvement in the mental status [8, 13, 26]. Data about the role of RRT suggests that dialysis plays only a minor role in lowering ammonia in this patient population [26]. Some data showed that patients who received hemodialysis without concurrent therapy of the underlying myeloma had no response [25]. However, if definitive treatment cannot be immediately instituted for any reason, RRT could be considered depending on the severity and clinical status. In one report of severe cases of hyperammonemia in the setting of multiple myeloma, simultaneous hemodialysis and CVVHD were successfully used to augment ammonia clearance, allowing for definitive treatment to be administered [13].

6.5.3 Valproic acid-induced hyperammonemia

Therapeutic concentration of valproic acid is between 50 and 100 mg/L (350–700 μmol/L). Valproic acid-associated hyperammonemia may occur after acute overdose or chronic use and does not necessarily result in clinical encephalopathy [27]. Hyperammonemia in this setting is because valproic acid and its metabolites inhibit enzymes and cofactors necessary for normal functions of urea cycle. Valproic acid is primarily metabolized in the liver. In case of toxicity, management is usually supportive (e.g., protection of airway, cardiovascular stabilization, and supplementation with L- carnitine). Valproic acid has a small molecular mass of 144 Dalton, a small volume of distribution, and is highly protein bound [27]. At therapeutic levels, RRT has little impact on the elimination of valproic acid because of its high degree of protein binding, which limits the amount of free drug available for diffusion. In case of overdose, protein-binding sites become saturated and more free drug is available for elimination by RRT. Therefore, in the case of valproic acid intoxications associated with hyperammonemic encephalopathy, dialysis serves a definitive role in correcting hyperammonemia. This is regardless of the underlying renal function.

RRT is recommended in the following situations [27]:

- Serum valproic acid concentration is more than 1300 mg/L (9000 μmol/L),
- Cerebral edema, or
- Shock attributed to valproic acid toxicity.

RRT is suggested if any of the following is present [27]:

- Serum valproic acid concentration > 900 mg/L (6250 μ mol/L).
- Coma or respiratory depression requiring mechanical ventilation.
- Acute hyperammonemia.
- pH is less than 7.10.

Intermittent hemodialysis is the preferred method of RRT in such cases, followed by CRRT if intermittent hemodialysis is not feasible. RRT can be discontinued when [27]:

- The valproic acid is between 50 and 100 g/L (350 to 700 micromol/L).
- There is clinical improvement like improvement in hemodynamics, or improvement in mental status.
- Improvement in electrolytes and acid-base abnormalities.

6.5.4 Organ transplantation and hyperammonemia

Hyperammonemia is a rare but serious complication following solid-organ transplantation. The most common occurrence is after lung transplantation, and to a lesser extent after other solid-organ transplant transplantations [28]. The mechanisms of hyperammonemia in transplant recipients are not well understood. The mortality is usually high in such patients; therefore, prompt recognition and treatment are necessary [28]. Conservative therapy is usually ineffective, and RRT is often required in most patients [28]. The RRT modality depends on the patient's condition and hemodynamic status.

6.5.5 Seizure

It is difficult to differentiate if hyperammonemia is caused by seizure or *vice versa* [2]. If seizure is unlikely to be caused by hyperammonemia, then traditional investigations and management of seizure need to be instituted. Hyperammonemia caused by seizure is more common in patients with generalized tonic-clonic seizures [29]. It is usually self-limiting and rarely requires RRT. In such cases, ammonia clearance is usually rapid over 3–8 hours [29]. In all cases, it is important to closely monitor the ammonia level and decide accordingly.

6.5.6 Urea cycle disorders

Adult patients with urea cycle disorders may present as already-diagnosed cases, with hyperammonemia being part of the acute relapse presentation. Less commonly, they may manifest for the first time in adulthood when they are exposed to stressful conditions [2]. It is important in known cases, or in undiagnosed non-hepatic cases of hyperammonemia, to immediately start all previously mentioned lines of management (see **Table 2**). These are specifically important as empiric therapies when the ammonia is more than 100 μmol/L. Consultation with a genetic specialist is important to guide further investigation and therapies [2]. The level at which RRT is initiated varies between guidelines and recommendations [2, 17]. In adult patients, ammonia level > 150–200 μmol/L or > 200–250 μmol/L have been suggested [2, 17]. However, other previously mentioned indications (e.g., hyperammonemic encephalopathy, coma, seizures, or rising ammonia despite conservative therapy) should also be considered when deciding about RRT. Intermitted hemodialysis is the preferred modality in such cases, and sometimes can be followed by CRRT.

7. Peritoneal dialysis and hyperammonemia

Data suggest that peritoneal dialysis (PD) is insufficient to achieve adequate ammonia clearance compared to other modalities of RRT [6]. A scoping review of data addressing the ammonia clearance by PD indicated a low rate of clearance (less than 40 mL/min). Unfortunately, studies about the effectiveness of PD in the management of adult patients with hyperammonemia are limited. PD might be considered when other effective forms of RRT are not readily available.

8. Conclusions

Hyperammonemia is a serious condition and must be considered in all patients with unexplained alterations in neurological status. Hyperammonemia in adult patients is usually caused by liver diseases, and non-hepatic causes are uncommon. Treatment of non-hepatic causes of hyperammonemia includes general supportive measures, as well as investigating and treating the underlying cause. Data about the role of RRT in the management of adult patients with hyperammonemia are limited. In such cases, many factors must be taken into consideration, including the clinical condition of the patient, severity of hyperammonemia, underlying cause, and response to supportive therapy. If RRT is considered, the choice of modality and the dialysis prescription depend on the patient's condition and available resources. Intermittent hemodialysis provides the highest and the most rapid degree of ammonia clearance, followed by CRRT, then PD.

Conflict of interest

The authors declare no conflict of interest.

Author details

Randah Dahlan* and Ali Alkatheeri
King Abdullah Medical City, Makkah, Saudi Arabia

*Address all correspondence to: randahdahlan@gmail.com

References

[1] Pagana K, Pagana T, Pagana T. Ammonia Level. Mosby's Diagnostic and Laboratory Test Reference. 12th ed. Mosby Elsevier; 2014. p. 47. ISBN: 9780323225762

[2] Long MT, Coursin DB. Undifferentiated non-hepatic hyperammonemia in the ICU: Diagnosis and management. Journal of Critical Care. 2022;**70**:154042

[3] Ali R, Nagalli S. Hyperammonemia. 2022 Aug 8. In: StatPearls [Internet]. Treasure Island (FL): StatPearls Publishing; 2023

[4] Raina R, Bedoyan JK, Lichter-Konecki U, Jouvet P, Picca S, Mew NA, et al. Consensus guidelines for management of hyperammonaemia in paediatric patients receiving continuous kidney replacement therapy. Nature Reviews. Nephrology. 2020;**16**(8):471-482

[5] Sakusic A, Sabov M, McCambridge AJ, Rabinstein AA, Singh TD, Mukesh K, et al. Features of adult Hyperammonemia not due to liver failure in the ICU. Critical Care Medicine. 2018;**46**(9):e897-e903

[6] Naorungroj T, Yanase F, Eastwood GM, Baldwin I, Bellomo R. Extracorporeal ammonia clearance for Hyperammonemia in critically ill patients: A scoping review. Blood Purification. 2021;**50**(4-5):453-461

[7] Van Son J, Rietbroek RC, Vaz FM, Hollak CEM. Bizarre behavior and decreased level of consciousness in an adult patient. The Netherlands Journal of Medicine. 2019;**77**(1):25-28

[8] Laish I, Ben AZ. Noncirrhotic hyperammonaemic encephalopathy. Liver International. 2011;**31**(9):1259-1270

[9] Alfadhel M, Mutairi FA, Makhseed N, Jasmi FA, Al-Thihli K, Al-Jishi E, et al. Guidelines for acute management of hyperammonemia in the Middle East region. Therapeutics and Clinical Risk Management. 2016;**12**:479-487

[10] Gupta S, Fenves AZ, Hootkins R. The role of RRT in Hyperammonemic patients. Clinical Journal of the American Society of Nephrology. 2016;**11**(10):1872-1878

[11] Fenves A, Schwartz J. Intermittent dialysis and continuous modalities for patients with hyperammonemia. In: Berns J editor. UpToDate. Waltham, MA: UpToDate; 2023 [Accessed: 20 May 2023]

[12] Cordoba J, Blei AT, Mujais S. Determinants of ammonia clearance by hemodialysis. Artificial Organs. 1996;**20**(7):800-803

[13] Brucculeri M, Gabbard W, Masson J, Jooma N. Simultaneous double hemodialysis for the control of refractory hyperammonemia. The International Journal of Artificial Organs. 2013;**36**(2):135-138

[14] Boer DP, Mourik SL, van den Hoogen MWF, Langendonk JG, de Geus HRH. Successful treatment of severe Hyperammonaemia with ultra-high dose continuous Veno-venous Haemodiafiltration. Blood Purification. 2019;**48**(3):283-285

[15] Häberle J, Boddaert N, Burlina A, Chakrapani A, Dixon M, Huemer M, et al. Suggested guidelines for the diagnosis and management of urea cycle disorders. Orphanet Journal of Rare Diseases. 2012;**7**:32

[16] Stergachis AB, Mogensen KM, Khoury CC, Lin AP, Peake RW,

Baker JJ, et al. A retrospective study of adult patients with noncirrhotic hyperammonemia. Journal of Inherited Metabolic Disease. 2020;**43**(6):1165-1172

[17] Bélanger-Quintana A, Arrieta Blanco F, Barrio-Carreras D, Bergua Martínez A, Cañedo Villarroya E, García-Silva MT, et al. Recommendations for the diagnosis and therapeutic Management of Hyperammonaemia in paediatric and adult patients. Nutrients. 2022;**14**(13):2755

[18] Wiegand C, Thompson T, Bock GH, Mathis RK, Kjellstrand CM, Mauer SM. The management of life-threatening hyperammonemia: A comparison of several therapeutic modalities. The Journal of Pediatrics. 1980;**96**(1):142-144

[19] Kamboj M, Kazory A. Expanding the boundaries of combined renal replacement therapy for non-renal indications. Blood Purification. 2019;**47**(1-3):69-72

[20] Slack AJ, Auzinger G, Willars C, Dew T, Musto R, Corsilli D, et al. Ammonia clearance with haemofiltration in adults with liver disease. Liver International. 2014;**34**(1):42-48

[21] Warrillow S, Fisher C, Tibballs H, Bailey M, McArthur C, Lawson-Smith P, et al. Australasian Management of Acute Liver Failure Investigators (AMALFI). Continuous renal replacement therapy and its impact on hyperammonaemia in acute liver failure. Critical Care and Resuscitation. 2020;**22**(2):158-165

[22] Warrillow S, Fisher C, Bellomo R. Correction and control of Hyperammonemia in acute liver failure: The impact of continuous renal replacement timing, intensity, and duration. Critical Care Medicine. 2020;**48**(2):218-224

[23] Larsen FS, Schmidt LE, Bernsmeier C, Rasmussen A, Isoniemi H, Patel VC, et al. High-volume plasma exchange in patients with acute liver failure: An open randomized controlled trial. Journal of Hepatology. 2016;**64**(1):69-78

[24] Clemmesen JO, Kondrup J, Nielsen LB, Larsen FS, Ott P. Effects of high-volume plasmapheresis on ammonia, urea, and amino acids in patients with acute liver failure. The American Journal of Gastroenterology. 2001;**96**(4):1217-1223

[25] Pham A, Reagan JL, Castillo JJ. Multiple myeloma-induced hyperammonemic encephalopathy: An entity associated with high in-patient mortality. Leukemia Research. 2013;**37**(10):1229-1232

[26] Tamayo J, Palom X, Sarrá J, Gasch O, Isern V, Fernández de Sevilla A, et al. Multiple myeloma and hyperammonemic encephalopathy: Review of 27 cases. Clinical Lymphoma & Myeloma. 2008;**8**(6):363-369

[27] Ghannoum M, Laliberté M, Nolin TD, MacTier R, Lavergne V, Hoffman RS, et al. Extracorporeal treatment for valproic acid poisoning: Systematic review and recommendations from the EXTRIP workgroup. Clinical Toxicology (Philadelphia, Pa.). 2015;**53**(5):454-465

[28] Seethapathy H, Fenves AZ. Pathophysiology and Management of Hyperammonemia in organ transplant patients. American Journal of Kidney Diseases. 2019;**74**(3):390-398

[29] Hung TY, Chen CC, Wang TL, Su CF, Wang RF. Transient hyperammonemia in seizures: A prospective study. Epilepsia. 2011;**52**(11):2043-2049

Chapter 6

Advanced Treatment of Refractory Congestive Heart Failure by Peritoneal Ultrafiltration with Icodextrin in Patients without End-Stage Renal Disease

Božidar Vujičić, Koraljka Benko, Ana Petretić, Nenad Nemarnik, Matko Spicijarić, Dean Markić, Matej Bura, Fabio Kadum, Sanjin Rački and Alen Ružić

Abstract

In patients with Congestive Heart Failure (CHF), neurohormonal activation leads to fluid overload that can be treated with high doses of furosemide unless diuretic resistance and hyponatremia develop. End-stage CHF, including patients with normal or slightly deteriorated kidney function, can resist medical treatment. In some cases of refractory CHF, ultrafiltration (UF) is required. To manage a refractory CHF population, extracorporeal UF is commonly used as an emergency treatment, but peritoneal UF should be considered a follow-up therapy option. This method offers potential advantages over extracorporeal therapies, including better preservation of residual renal function, tighter control of sodium balance, less neurohumoral activation, and the possibility of daily treatment in the home environment. Using glucose as an osmotic agent leads to the deterioration of the peritoneal membrane. The UF properties of icodextrin depend on the dwell time, whereby the maximum effect of icodextrin concerning glucose is achieved at a prolonged dwell time. Icodextrin may offer improved peritoneal membrane biocompatibility compared with conventional glucose-based dialysates by decreasing glucose exposure, iso-osmolarity, and reduced carbonyl stress. The proper anesthesia technique and surgical approach for peritoneal dialysis (PD) catheter placement in CHF patients must be based on the patient's characteristics, available equipment, and surgeon's experience. An open procedure using a transversus abdominis plane block for PD catheter placement in patients with CHF is strongly recommended.

Keywords: chronic heart failure, heart failure treatment, peritoneal catheter placement, peritoneal ultrafiltration, refractory chronic heart failure

1. Introduction

Congestive Heart Failure (CHF) is a severe and common disease affecting up to 10% of adults. In patients with CHF, neurohormonal activation leads to fluid overload that can be treated with high doses of furosemide unless diuretic resistance and hyponatremia develop. End-stage CHF, including patients with normal or slightly deteriorated kidney function, can resist medical treatment. This patient group requires frequent hospitalizations for electrolyte imbalance dyspnea, orthopnea, and oliguria. In some cases of refractory CHF (RCHF), ultrafiltration (UF) is required. To manage an RCHF population, extracorporeal UF is commonly used as an emergency treatment, but peritoneal UF (PUF) should be considered a follow-up therapy option.

Schneierson first reported using PUF successfully in heart failure (HF) [1]. Mailloux et al. concluded that PUF may be helpful in cardiac patients with concomitant renal impairment, electrolyte imbalance, preparation for cardiac surgery, and rapid deterioration of a previously stable cardiac state [2]. It has been known that PUF does not alter the course of HF but improves the congestive condition by correcting electrolyte imbalance, re-responsiveness to diuretics, weight loss, and overall clinical improvement [2]. A prospective non-randomized study including 20 patients with New York Heart Association (NYHA) class IV showed regression to NYHA class I, left ventricular systolic function recovery, a significant reduction in hospitalization days, and first-year mortality lower than expected [3]. Another prospective non-randomized study from 2010 enrolled 17 patients with RCHF initially treated with extracorporeal UF and PUF. All patients improved their NYHA functional status within the first 3 months, and hospitalization days significantly decreased after 1 year [4]. Using an intraperitoneal solution such as icodextrin promotes a slow and efficient PUF that cardiac patients tolerate better, is less invasive, improves residual renal function, and improves quality of life and clinical symptoms.

Therefore, proposing PUF for long-term outpatient treatment of RCHF seems reasonable.

2. Congestive heart failure

HF or CHF is an inadequate ability of the heart to meet patients' metabolic demands. According to the current guidelines (European Society of Cardiology, 2021), it is defined as a complex clinical syndrome presenting with typical symptoms (fatigue, breathlessness, and ankle swelling) that can go together with signs (elevated venous pressure, pulmonary crackles, or peripheral edema). HF is caused by structural and/or functional heart abnormalities, which lead to high intracardiac pressures and/or reduced cardiac output [5].

The definition should involve elevated natriuretic peptide levels (brain natriuretic peptide—BNP, or N-terminal pro-brain natriuretic peptide—NTproBNP), which are a group of hormones produced by the myocardium cells and are released in the bloodstream in response to the wall stress [6].

The incidence of HF increases because of population aging and has become a leading cause of hospitalizations among patients over 65 [5].

Many conditions can cause HF. This includes high blood pressure, coronary artery disease (CAD), valvular heart disease (VHD), cardiomyopathies, arrhythmias, myocarditis, congenital heart disease, thyroid disease, chronic kidney disease (CKD), anemia, or toxic myocardium damage (alcohol, heavy metals, and chemotherapeutics).

2.1 Classification

The most used HF classification is based on left ventricular ejection fraction (EF). There are traditionally three phenotypes: HF with reduced ejection fraction (EF ≤ 40, heart failure with reduced ejection fraction (HFrEF)), HF with a mildly reduced ejection fraction (EF 41–49%, heart failure with mildly reduced and preserved ejection fraction (HFmrEF)), and HF with preserved EF (EF ≥ 50%, HFpEF) (**Figure 1**). EF is usually obtained by echocardiography. The explanation for this classification lies in many clinical treatment trials that showed different outcomes and heterogeneity between phenotypes.

Classification based on symptom severity and physical activity is the NYHA classification. NYHA has four functional classes (I–IV). Patients in class I have no limitation of physical activities, and there are no HF symptoms in ordinary physical activity. In contrast, patients in NYHA class IV have severe symptoms at rest and during minimal activity (**Figure 2**).

There are two main presentations of HF: acute and chronic. Acute heart failure (AHF) is a rapid or gradual onset of symptoms that require medical attention and/or hospitalization. AHF can be the new onset of HF (first manifestation, newly diagnosed) or, more often, decompensation of known chronic HF [5]. Besides left ventricular failure, there can be right ventricular failure (RVF). It is primarily due to left heart disease with secondary pulmonary hypertension, but there are some conditions in which RVF is isolated (arrhythmogenic right ventricular cardiomyopathy, RV myocardial infarction, etc.) [5].

Many HF patients worsen over time and progress into advanced HF. It is defined as persistent symptoms despite optimal therapy. Those patients often have systemic or peripheral congestion that requires high doses of diuretics or procedures like renal replacement therapy (RRT).

The incidence of advanced HF is increasing due to the aging of the population, a growing number, and better survival of HF patients. The criteria needed to define advanced HF include severe HF symptoms (NYHA III-IV) despite optimal medical therapy (OMT), severe cardiac dysfunction (defined by at least one of the following:

Type of HF	HFrEF	HFmrEF	HFpEF
	Symptoms with/without signs	Symptoms with/without signs	Symptoms with/without signs
	LVEF ≤ 40%	LVEF 41 – 49%	LVEF ≥ 50%
			Evidence of cardiac structural and/or functional abnormalities Raised natriuretic peptides

HF – heart failure, HFrEF – heart failure with reduced ejection fraction, HFmrEF – heart failure with mildly reduced ejction fraction, HFpEF – heart failure with preserved ejection fraction, LVEF – left ventricular ejection fraction

Figure 1.
Chronic heart failure definition and classification based on ejection fraction.

Heart failure classification based on symptoms severity and physical activity

NYHA class	
I	No limitation of physical activities and no heart failure symptoms in ordinary physical activity
II	Mild symptoms and slight limitation during ordinary activity
III	Marked limitation in activity due to symptoms, even during less-than-ordinary activity. Comfortable only at rest
IV	Severe limitations, symptoms even while at rest. Mostly bedbound patients

NYHA – New York Heart Classification

Figure 2.
Chronic heart failure classification based on symptoms severity and physical activity.

EF ≤ 30%, isolated RVF, severe and non-operable valve abnormalities, severe and non-operable congenital abnormalities, persistently high natriuretic peptides levels, and severe left ventricular diastolic dysfunction), episodes of congestion (systemic or pulmonary, requiring the use of high dose intravenous diuretics), attacks of low output states (requiring inotropes or vasoactive agents) or malignant arrhythmias causing more than one hospitalization in the last year, and severe impairment of exercise capacity (**Figure 3**). Further classification of advanced HF patients and assessment

All of the following despite optimal medical treatment
1. NYHA III or NYHA IV functional class
2. Severe cardiac disfunction; at least one of the following: - LVEF ≤ 30% - isolated RV failure (e.g., ARVC) - non-operable severe valve abnormalities or non-operable severe congenital abnormalities - high (or increasing) BNP or NT-proBNP values and severe LV diastolic dysfunction or structural abnormalities (according to the definitions of HFpEF)
3. Pulmonary or systemic congestion that requires high-dose i.v. diuretics (or diuretic combinations) or episodes of low output requiring inotropes/vasoactive drugs - malignant arrhythmias causing >1 unplanned visit or hospitalization in the last 12 months
4. Severe impairment of exercise capacity with inability to exercise

NYHA – New York Heart Association, LVEF – left ventricular ejection fraction, RV – right ventricular, ARVC-arrhythmogenic right ventricular cardiomyopathy, BNP = B-type natriuretic peptide, NT-proBNP = N-terminal pro-B-type natriuretic peptide, HFpEF – heart failure with preserved ejection fraction

Figure 3.
Advanced heart failure definition creteria (ESC2021).

of advanced therapy can be done using the Interagency Registry for Mechanically Assisted Circulatory Support (INTERMACS) profiles [5].

2.2 Pathophysiology

Pathophysiologically, HF is defined as the inability of the heart as a pump to maintain the metabolic needs of the human body (failure to maintain adequate cardiac output). In this context, HF can be divided into systolic and diastolic dysfunction and left-sided and right-sided HF.

The most common cause of systolic dysfunction is ischemic heart disease. Other causes include dilated cardiomyopathy, chronic volume and pressure overload, chronic pulmonary diseases, and heart rhythm disorders. Diastolic dysfunction is most commonly due to pressure overload conditions causing pathological hypertrophy, not allowing the ventricle to relax. Common causes include hypertension, aortic stenosis, hypertrophic, and restrictive cardiomyopathy [7]. Cardiac output results from stroke volume and heart rate. Stroke volume is dependent on cardiac contractility (the inotropic state of the heart), preload (stretching of the cardiac myocytes before contraction), and afterload (the pressure that the heart needs to overcome to eject blood) [8].

In systolic dysfunction, the cardiac contractility is impaired, causing a decrease in stroke volume and, subsequentially, a reduction in cardiac output, resulting in global hypoperfusion. At the same time, left ventricular end-diastolic pressure is elevated, resulting in increased left atrial pressure and causing a rise in pulmonary capillary pressure. These changes lead to pulmonary venous congestion.

Diastolic dysfunction is characterized by the inability of the left ventricle to adequately relax in diastole due to abnormal stiffness of the left ventricular wall. The result is an increased ventricular filling pressure with a subsequent increase in the pulmonary circulation pressure. Systolic function is usually maintained; however, in the setting of chronic pressure overload, it can also be impaired.

Right-sided HF is most commonly a result of left-sided HF; however, it can also develop as an isolated entity, secondary to pulmonary diseases ("cor pulmonale") and due to increased right ventricular afterload. The main clinical presentation, in this case, is systemic venous congestion with minimal to no pulmonary congestion [9].

2.3 Prognostic factors

Despite the new therapeutic options (mainly for HFrEF), HF remains a progressive disease with a poor prognosis and a five-year survival rate of nearly 50% [10].

Prognostic factors related to higher mortality rates are advanced age (especially >75 y/o), male sex, and comorbidities such as diabetes, CKD, peripheral artery disease, atrial fibrillation, higher body mass index (BMI), lower systolic blood pressure, and chronic obstructive pulmonary disease [11].

Studies have shown that the mortality rate also increases with the number and duration of hospitalizations for HF. Regarding EF, HFpEF patients generally have a better survival rate than HFrEF patients. Transition in EF can also occur, and patients who progress to a lower EF have worse outcomes than those who remain stable or progress to a higher EF [5].

Laboratory tests such as natriuretic peptides, C-reactive protein (CRP), and serum sodium levels are also helpful in assessing patient prognosis. Serial natriuretic peptide measurements are used not only as a diagnostic tool but also to determine the efficacy of HF treatment and to evaluate prognosis. Patients with elevated levels of NT-proBNP and CRP correlate with worse clinical outcomes than those without elevation of both markers. Hyponatremia (serum sodium level of less than 135 mmol/L) is linked with increased mortality rates in HF patients. Diabetes is associated with worse clinical outcomes and greater hospitalization rates [12].

3. Chronic kidney disease

CKD is classified into five stages according to the degree of kidney damage or glomerular filtration rate (GFR). Thus, patients with stage five CKD have a GFR of less than 15 ml/min/1.73 m^2 and are in the terminal stage of the disease: end-stage renal disease (ESRD). A better understanding of CKD, accompanied by the technological and scientific assumptions of dialysis techniques and kidney transplantation, has significantly improved the prognosis and survival of patients with ESRD. Despite the improvement of technology and clinical and scientific progress in treatment with RRT methods, the frequency of non-renal complications that significantly affect the morbidity and mortality of patients is increasing. The most important are cardiovascular complications, which impact treatment outcomes the most. Cardiovascular diseases are frequent in CKD, especially in ESRD, and are responsible for 40–60% of mortality in that population, according to data from national registries. The importance of cardiovascular diseases has been increasing in recent years with the appearance of an increasing number of elderly patients in whom diabetes and vascular diseases have led to CKD. In recent years, we have witnessed significant progress in understanding the causes and pathophysiology of cardiovascular diseases (CVD) and the possibilities of diagnosis, treatment, and prevention. Knowledge of the pathogenesis of cardiovascular complications, modern diagnostic options, methods of recognition, and treatment of these complications is of great importance to nephrologists and other doctors who care for ESRD patients.

Cardiovascular risk factors appear in the earlier stages of CKD and become more frequent in patients who begin treatment with renal replacement therapy. Risk factors for cardiovascular disease in patients with CKD include those that favor the development of ischemic heart disease, CHF, and left ventricular hypertrophy. Numerous risk factors, of which only general ones present in the general population, cannot explain the high incidence of cardiovascular diseases in patients with CKD. Timely diagnosis of CKD and effective treatment can delay the progression of CKD and the onset of ESRD. In the first and second stages of CKD, patients are usually checked by their family doctor. In the third stage of CKD, it is necessary to pay attention to the early metabolic complications of the disease. The fourth stage of CKD is the introduction to ESRD, and at that stage, the patient needs to be thoroughly familiarized with the RRT methods. Kidney and heart disease interaction manifests in the cardiorenal syndrome, which could significantly cause the worsening of both diseases. The clinical course of CKD is accompanied by numerous complications: renal anemia, mineral-bone disorders, progression of atherosclerosis, deterioration of CHF, development of protein-energy wasting, dyslipidemia, CVD, infections, diseases of the immune system, gastrointestinal disorders, neurological disorders, and others.

4. Cardiorenal syndrome and chronic heart failure treatment

4.1 Cardiorenal syndrome: classification and pathophysiology

Cardiorenal syndrome (CRS) results from inadequate heart and kidney function. It is caused by acute or chronic dysfunction of one of the mentioned organs, which then leads to acute or chronic dysfunction of another organ. The heart and kidneys jointly aim to regulate numerous processes in the human body, such as blood pressure, electrolyte and fluid homeostasis, and endocrine functions through natriuretic peptide, renin, erythropoietin, and vitamin D3. Because of the above, it is unsurprising that one organ's dysfunction leads to another's disorder. The term CRS itself was mentioned in 1951, and since then, numerous papers have been written to explain the pathophysiological mechanisms of the syndrome [13]. One of the most significant works on the mentioned topic was published in 2009. It resulted from the consensus conference of the Acute Dialysis Quality Initiative [14]. The paper above describes five subtypes of the syndrome, depending on whether it is caused by a primary disorder of the heart or the kidneys, and whether the onset is acute or chronic or is a result of a secondary process. Types 1 and 2 imply an acute or chronic heart disorder that leads to kidney dysfunction. Types 3 and 4 represent the opposite situation when acutely or chronically impaired kidney function leads to cardiac dysfunction. Type 5 represents a systemic process that leads to dysfunction of both organs.

Many authors have used observational and retrospective studies as precious sources to determine the epidemiological data of the syndrome. Uduman concluded that CRS type 1 is the most common. Given the lack of data sources, it is tough to distinguish the frequency of chronic types 2 and 4 [15]. A group of authors in India concluded with a cross-sectional study that around half of the observed patients with CRS had type 1, type 2, and type 4 prevalences of around 20% each. Representation of types 3 and 5 was only a few percent [16].

Recent papers by American scientists show how CKD affects 15–20% of adults globally. The leading cause of death in that population is CVD [17]. Also, a group of authors from Japan in the prospective cohort study called CKD-ROUTE have shown that the prevalence of CVD among CKD patients is around 26.8% [18]. The British authors did a similar study called CRISIS, presenting a slightly higher prevalence of 47.2% [19]. Vice versa, studies have shown that the prevalence rate of CKD in HF patients is 11 times higher than in the general population [20].

4.1.1 Type 1: acute CRS

CRS type 1 represents an acute worsening of heart function caused by AHF, acute coronary syndrome (ACS), or cardiogenic shock, leading to kidney injury and/or dysfunction [14]. All treatment strategies are explained in ESC guidelines, depending on the event's cause. Avoiding all potential nephrotoxins, such as contrast solution, and carefully monitoring cardiac and renal biomarkers is very important. The studies have shown that almost 30% of the patients hospitalized due to AHF had worsening renal function, which led to a higher number of deaths, complications, and longer length of stay [21]. One of the most important mechanisms leading to acute kidney injury (AKI) is lower kidney perfusion due to lower cardiac output and activation of the renin-angiotensin-aldosterone system (RAAS) [22]. Also, the critical mechanism is diuretic resistance of the kidneys, probably caused by sodium retention and the already-mentioned contrast-induced nephropathy.

4.1.2 Type 2: chronic CRS

Chronic CRS is caused by CHF, which leads to kidney injury or dysfunction. This mechanism has several causes, including chronic hypoperfusion of the kidneys, venous congestion, endothelial dysfunction, subclinical inflammation, and rapid atherosclerosis. Management strategy of this type is the same as the previous one: treat the primary cause of HF according to ESC guidelines and avoid nephrotoxins and prerenal factors that can lead to AKI. Due to CHF as a cause, kidney injury or dysfunction often progresses to CKD. As mentioned before, sometimes it is tough to distinguish the primary cause of CRS, whether CHF or CKD arose and caused CRS type 2 or 4. In some cases, cardiac re-synchronization or RRT can be used. A critical study was published in 2007 in the prestigious American Journal of Cardiology. In this clinical trial, almost 8000 patients with CKD were divided into two groups, depending on their EF. The patients were divided into systolic and diastolic HF subgroups; the cut-off value was EF 45%. The study has shown that CKD-associated mortality was higher in those with diastolic than systolic HF. Precisely, in the diastolic HF group, extra deaths per 10,000 person-years were 71% higher [23].

4.1.3 Type 3: acute renocardiac syndrome

In types 3 and 4 CRS, as the word order tells, the worsening of the kidney function leads to heart injury and/or dysfunction. Type 3 represents an acute worsening of kidney function or AKI. According to Kidney Disease: Improving Global Outcomes (KDIGO) foundation guidelines, the criteria for AKI are an absolute 0.3 mg/dL rise within 48 hours or a 50% relative rise in serum creatinine over 7 days. It is essential to mention that KDIGO was established by the National Kidney Foundation of the United States, and the mentioned guidelines are from 2012 [24]. The causes of AKI are numerous, and some of them are acute pyelonephritis, glomerular or tubular diseases, hypoperfusion of the kidneys, and obstruction of the urinary tract. Consequences of AKI can be fluid and sodium retention, a disorder of electrolytes or humoral mediators and toxemia. All mentioned could cause ACS, cardiac arrhythmias, or AHF. Sometimes, it is hard to determine whether the heart or kidney acute dysfunction appeared first. An excellent example of the connection between types 1 and 3 is called cardiac surgery-associated AKI. The probable etiology of AKI is renal hypoperfusion during the procedure, as well as hemodilution, hypothermia, and inflammatory responses, which cause constriction of afferent arterioles. After the procedure, a low cardiac output state with persistent hypotension worsens the patient's condition. It leads to CRS type 1 [25]. Consequently, AKI leads to fluid overload, which causes further deterioration of cardiac dysfunction or CRS type 3.

4.1.4 Type 4: chronic renocardiac syndrome

In some patients, CKD leads to heart disease, injury, and dysfunction. It is described as type 4 CRS. As mentioned before, the leading cause of death in patients with CKD is CVD, and the prevalence of CVD correlates with the stage of CKD. It is essential to define the criteria for CKD as abnormalities of kidney structure or function for more than 3 months. Cause, GFR, and albuminuria categories must be classified [26]. Very often, CKD has a place in cardiology guidelines together with arterial hypertension and diabetes. Those three chronic conditions coexist in most patients, leading to vascular stiffness, cardiac and renal fibrosis, left ventricular hypertrophy, sodium, and volume overload. Another important mechanism is anemia in CKD, which can cause peripheral ischemia and activation of RAAS and, consequently, sodium and volume retention. Vascular stiffness is one of the leading causes of CVD. It results from numerous events such as chronic inflammation and oxidative stress of the vessel, mineral and bone disorder, chronic uremia, and hyperphosphatemia, which causes soft tissue calcification.

4.1.5 Type 5: secondary CRS

The last type of CRS is caused by a systemic condition that leads to heart and kidney injury and/or dysfunction. That condition can be acute or chronic. Some causes are sepsis, amyloidosis, diabetes, and systemic lupus erythematosus. Recently, published papers have shown that sepsis-associated AKI (S-AKI) is a frequent complication with 12% up to 33% incidence [27, 28]. As expected, patients with S-AKI had much worse outcomes. A group of Chinese authors published a systematic review and meta-analysis, which included 47 observational studies and more than 55 thousand patients [29]. The study has shown that 20 factors were statistically significant as predisposing for S-AKI. Some are septic shock, hypertension, diabetes mellitus, abdominal infection, vasopressor administration, etc. Type 5 is probably the most complex type to determine because chronic conditions, such as hypertension, diabetes, or amyloidosis, can be a part of some other CRS subtype. Similar to previous types, to prevent *circulus vitiosus,* the aim is to cure the primary cause.

4.2 Treatment of heart failure with reduced ejection fraction (HFrEF)

The main goals of treatment of HFrEF (EF $\leq$ 40%) are reduction in overall mortality, prevention of recurrent hospitalizations, and improvement in quality of life. The cornerstone of treatment consists of pharmacological therapy that should be applied before other interventions, according to the 2021 European Society of Cardiology Guidelines for diagnosing and treating acute and chronic HF and the 2022 AHA/ACC/HFSA Guideline for the Management of Heart Failure.

Renin-angiotensin-aldosterone system (RAAS) blockers, beta-blockers (BB), and mineralocorticoid receptor antagonists (MRA) are recommended as the baseline treatment for these patients. In addition to this therapy, the sodium-glucose cotransporter two inhibitors (SGLT2I) are recommended to reduce cardiovascular and all-cause mortality due to worsening HF regardless of diabetes status. A general recommendation is to titrate all these drugs to maximally tolerated doses to improve outcomes (**Figure 4**). Loop diuretics are recommended for the reduction of symptoms and improvement in clinical status. Diuretics reduce the number of hospitalization days but do not decrease the risk of death in these patients. Angiotensin-converting enzyme (ACE) inhibitors are the first group of drugs that reduced mortality in clinical trials, including patients with HFrEF. The primary mechanism of action is a reduction in afterload, preload, and sheer stress on the myocardial wall, which results in increased cardiac output and renal blood flow and a reduction in myocardial remodeling. Angiotensin-receptor blockers (ARB) are recommended to reduce cardiovascular mortality and hospitalizations related to HF in patients intolerant to ACE inhibitors. However, according to clinical trials, ARBs did not show a decrease in all-cause mortality.

In addition to ACE inhibitors with diuretics, BB substantially decreases mortality and morbidity and improves quality of life. It should be initiated immediately in

BB	ACE – I/ARB/ARNI	MRA	SGLT2I

BB - beta-blocker, ACE – I - angiotensin-converting enzyme inhibitor, ARB - angiotensin receptor blocker, ARNI - angiotensin receptor-neprilysin inhibitor, MRA - mineralocorticoid receptor antagonist, SGLT2I - sodium- glucose co-transporter 2 inhibitor

Figure 4.
Treatment of HFrEF for all patients - to reduce mortality.

hemodynamically stable, euvolemic patients. Bisoprolol, carvedilol, and metoprolol succinate are three BBs that reduce mortality and the number of hospitalization days. MRA, alongside ACE inhibitors and BB, also reduce the mortality risk of hospitalization days and improves symptoms; therefore, they should also be initiated as the first-line treatment in patients with reduced EF, but with caution in patients with impaired renal function and elevated serum potassium. Eplerenone is preferred because of its fewer side effects.

Newer clinical studies with angiotensin-receptor-neprilysin inhibitors, in comparison with ACE inhibitors, showed high superiority in reduction of cardiovascular and all-cause mortality, the number of hospitalizations due to worsening of HF, as well as improvement in clinical status and possible diuretic reduction [30].

Another significant approach to managing HFrEF is cardiac device treatment and rhythm control (**Figures 5** and **6**). Some antiarrhythmic drugs reduce sudden death rates but do not reduce all-cause mortality. Some may even increase mortality in primary prevention of sudden cardiac death (SCD); implantable cardioverter defibrillators (ICD) are used instead to reduce all-cause mortality and prevent SCD in patients with reduced EF, which are expected to survive for more than 1 year with good functional status [31].

In primary prevention, ICD is indicated in patients with symptomatic HF of ischemic etiology and EF of 35% and lower despite OMT in 3 months or more to

Diuretics
ICD, CRT – P, CRT – D

ICD - implantable cardioverter-defibrillator; CRT – P - cardiac resynchronization therapy pacemaker, CRT – D - cardiac resynchronization therapy with defibrillator

Figure 5.
Treatment of HFrEF for selected patients -to reduce hospitilisation/mortality.

Atrial fibrillation	Anticoagulation, PVI, digoxin
Coronary artery disease	Revascularization – PCI, CABG
Valvular heart disease (AS, MR)	TAVI, MV repair

PVI – pulmonary vein isolation, PCI – percutaneous coronary intervention, coronary artery bypass graft, AS – aortic stenosis, MR – mitral regurgitation, TAVI – transcatheter aortic valve implantation

Figure 6.
Management of comorbidities.

reduce all-cause mortality. The same criteria should be considered in other etiologies of HF as clinical trials in those patients also showed a reduction of all-cause mortality with significant evidence but with lower absolute benefit because patients with non-ischemic cardiomyopathy have a lower risk of SCD.

In secondary prevention, it is recommended to use ICD in patients who suffer from a ventricular arrhythmia causing hemodynamic instability unless there is a reversible cause or a recent myocardial infarction occurred in the last 48 hours before arrhythmia. Cardiac resynchronization therapy (CRT) implies the implantation of a three-electrode pacemaker or implantable defibrillator (one electrode for the right atrium and two for each ventricle) that improves cardiac function and quality of life. This type of therapy showed a reduction of morbidity and mortality in selected patients with vast QRS complexes who are symptomatic and have low EF (<35%) despite optimal medical therapy. In case of high-degree atrioventricular (AV) block and indication for ventricular pacing, CRT is preferred rather than right ventricular pacing, and in patients with worsening HF with EF of 35% and lower who already have implanted pacemaker or ICD, an upgrade to CRT device should be considered [5].

4.3 Treatment of heart failure with mildly reduced and preserved ejection fraction (HFmrEF and HFpEF)

Although there are no specific clinical trials in patients with mildly reduced EF, considering that these patients have some similar clinical characteristics to patients with reduced EF, equal medical treatment can be deemed to act on further myocardial remodeling, prevent worsening HF, and reduce hospitalizations related to HF. There are some retrospective trials in which HFrEF treatment in these patients was potentially beneficial, but more tests are required to draw evidence-based conclusions.

In the DELIVER trial, dapagliflozin (SGLT2I) reduced the combined risk of worsening HF or cardiovascular death in patients with an EF of 40% and more [32].

In the case of HFpEF (EF $\geq$ 50%), no specific treatment showed a reduction in all-cause mortality. Besides dapagliflozin, empagliflozin reduced the combined risk of the primary outcome (first hospitalization and cardiovascular mortality) in HFpEF patients, mainly due to reduced risk of hospitalization related to HF despite diabetes status [33].

Loop diuretics are used to reduce symptoms of congestion and improve quality of life, but they do not reduce overall mortality. Moreover, in HFpEF patients, there is a general emphasis on screening for comorbidities and reducing and managing underlying risk factors.

4.4 Advanced heart failure management

Management of advanced HF includes pharmacological therapy, RRT, short- and long-term mechanical circulatory support (MSC), and heart transplantation (HTx) (**Figure 7**). Regarding pharmacological treatment, inotropes (milrinone, dobutamine) and inodilatators (like levosimendan) may improve symptoms, hemodynamics, and cardiac output. It can help improve heart, lung, and kidney perfusion [34]. They can also be used in chronic settings as palliative therapy in patients with no other therapeutic options.

Advanced HF is often characterized by worsening kidney function and diuretic resistance. Sometimes, high doses of intravenous potent diuretics (even in combination, like furosemide with acetazolamide, hydrochlorothiazide, indapamide,

Short-term MCS (BTR, BTD)
Long-term MCS as DT
HTx

MCS – mechanical circulatory support, BTR – bridge to recovery, BTD – bridge to destination, DT – destination therapy, HTx – heart transplantation

Figure 7.
Treatment for selected advanced heart failure patients.

or mineralocorticoid antagonists) are needed to commence diuresis with relief of symptoms and signs of congestion. When failure of pharmacological therapy occurs, RRT should be considered. It can be used in patients with or without kidney disease. The most used modality of RRT is UF, either by central venous catheter (extracorporeal therapy) or by peritoneal catheter. Extracorporeal treatment is used more in acute settings, and central venous catheters can be placed in the internal jugular, subclavian, or femoral, usually with ultrasound guidance using the Seldinger technique. PUF is a chronic treatment modality in selected patients with resistant congestion, either as destination therapy (in patients not candidates for MCS or HTx) or in patients waiting for MCS or HTx.

In terms of insertions, MCS can be percutaneous, intracorporeal, or extracorporeal, and considering the time of their use, they can be short- and long-term support. Percutaneous MCS are intra-aortic balloon pumps, the Impella family of devices, Tandemheart, and extracorporeal membrane oxygenation (ECMO). ECMO is also considered extracorporeal MCS and can be placed peripherally or centrally. Intracorporeal MCSs are left ventricular assist devices (LVAD), right ventricular assist devices (RVAD), or biventricular assist devices (BiVAD). They are surgically placed.

Short-term MCS is used in a few clinical scenarios in patients that require urgent circulatory support (cardiogenic shock, primarily refractory to medical therapy). It can be used as a bridge to recovery, bridge to bridge, or bridge to decision. Long-term MCS, such as LVAD, can be used as a bridge to HTx, a bridge to candidacy for HTx, or as destination therapy [5].

HTx is the gold standard for treating advanced HF [5]. There must be no contraindication for HTx. Post-transplantation survival is around 90%, with improved quality of life and physical status.

Management of advanced HF is complex, challenging, and expensive. It requires dedicated expertise in highly specialized centers. There must always be a plan for stopping procedures when they become futile due to disease trajectory and disease progression with conversion to symptom control in dignified end-of-life care (palliative care).

5. Extracorporeal ultrafiltration

Extracorporeal UF is a mechanical pump-driven therapy that emerged as an option to overcome diuretic resistance. With this procedure, the volume and fluid removal rate is customized by clinicians to the needs and clinical characteristics of the patients.

Asymptomatic CHF patients have reduced sodium excretion in response to volume expansion compared to normal subjects. This abnormal fluid state leads to physiological abnormalities in multiple organ systems. Increased water in the myocardium can lead to ischemia and reduced contractility [35]. Hypervolemia may be related to a reduced excretion capacity or increased salt and water retention in the presence of decreased adequate circulating blood volume. The most common causes are endothelial damage, protein retention capacity, loss of plasma oncotic pressure, and reduced renal perfusion due to impaired cardiac function. Disturbed neurohormonal activation, excessive tubular sodium reabsorption, change in hemodynamics, oxidative stress, inflammation, and use of nephrotoxic drugs are essential factors of adverse cardiorenal interactions in CHF patients [36]. Diuretic agents remain the primary treatment for fluid overload. Although effective early in HF, diuretics become ineffective in the progression of the disease due to the development of unresponsiveness [37].

UF could safely improve hemodynamics in HF patients as an alternative sodium and water removal method. Some isolated schedules of UF may be too aggressive and result in severe hemodynamic instability. That is why continuous extracorporeal techniques have been applied to patients with excellent clinical outcomes. A stable hemodynamic state, good cardiovascular response, and adequate diuresis are the most common effects of continuous extracorporeal fluid removal methods. Hemodynamic instability is the driving factor behind the physician's decision to initiate extracorporeal UF, and the treatment was postponed until it became indispensable. This has been overcome with the development and availability of better-tolerated treatment modalities such as continuous RRT. Earlier intervention should always be considered because it is not justified to wait until the appearance of severe symptoms [38].

The UF process produces water from plasma in response to a transmembrane pressure gradient across a semipermeable membrane. The sieving capacity of UF membranes is responsible for the UF of crystalloids but not of cells or colloids. When hydrostatic pressure exceeds oncotic pressure, iso-osmotic ultrafiltrate is generated.

UF is performed from the patient's blood and then returned to the patient through separate access to the venous circulation. Adequate UF rates are needed for extracellular fluid to refill the intravascular space and gradually maintain sufficient blood volume. If the UF rate is too high, there is a decrease in intravascular volume, reflecting the reduction in total blood volume. Maintaining circulating blood volume, accurately determining the amount of fluid to be removed, and optimizing the fluid removal speed are essential for the success of the therapy [39]. Different techniques can be used for the hypervolemic patient to achieve an adequate fluid balance: UF, hemofiltration, and dialysis together with UF. Pure UF is only a fluid removal technique; others can simultaneously purify the blood. According to their frequency and duration, the treatments are classified as acute (single session up to 4 h), intermittent (single sessions up to 4 h repeated daily or three times a week), or continuous (24 h/day or as required).

5.1 Isolated intermittent ultrafiltration

Intermittent isolated UF is carried out several hours daily to remove a desired amount of excess volume (1–2 L) [40]. The procedure can be repeated daily and uses standard hemodialysis (HD) equipment without dialysis fluid. Considering the short duration of the therapy, the effectiveness of this technique is in a higher UF rate. Sometimes, the UF rate may be too high, leading to significant hemodynamic instability. Many patients respond to diuretics again after one or more treatments with this method.

5.2 Slow continuous ultrafiltration

Its primary aim is to safely and effectively manage fluid overload in refractory edema without overt acute renal failure (ARF). This technique is mainly applied in patients with CHF NYHA IV. Slow continuous ultrafiltration (SCUF) can be performed with low blood flow rates (50–200 mL/min) in the veno-venous modality. The UF rate is usually 100–300 mL/h, according to fluid balance needs. The frequent complications from arterial cannulation are the primary reason the arterio-venous modality is rarely used. It is required to control the UF rate to maintain the desired volume status. Otherwise, higher UF rates would require fluid resuscitation. No fluids are administered as dialysate or replacement fluids, as the primary purpose of treatment is to achieve volume control. However, isolated UF is not a blood purification modality and solute clearance is irrelevant. UF in SCUF is iso-osmotic and isonatric, and water and sodium removal cannot be dissociated. That is possible because sodium elimination is linked to the sodium plasma water concentration. A small surface area filter can be used with reduced heparin doses to maintain the effectiveness of the therapy because low UF and blood flow rates are required. Removing myocardial depressant factors in the ultrafiltrate, reduction in preload, and modulation of the RAAS axis seem to be possible pathophysiological mechanisms underlying clinical improvement [41].

5.3 Continuous veno-venous hemofiltration

Continuous veno-venous hemofiltration (CVVH) produces a large ultrafiltrate volume across a high-permeability membrane. The advantages of CVVH include liberal fluid management, optimal clearance of uremic toxins, including middle molecules, and hemodynamic stability. The ultrafiltrate produced during CVVH is wholly or partly replaced with appropriate replacement solutions to achieve desired therapeutic goals. Replacement fluid can be infused before (predilution) and/or after (postdilution) the hemofilter. The decision on when to start CVVH should be based on the severity of organ failure and ARF. Early initiation should be considered at oliguric ARF and/or a steep rise in serum creatinine despite adequate fluid resuscitation. This method removes fluid with considerable solute clearance and blood purification [42]. The hemodynamic response is inimitable due to the possibility of dissociating water from sodium removal. In CVVH, the composition of ultrafiltrate is similar to plasma water, but sodium concentration in the replacement solution significantly affects the sodium balance.

5.4 Continuous hemodialysis/hemodiafiltration

The principal advantage of continuous hemodialysis/hemodiafiltration (CVVHD/HDF) is the ability to remove large volumes of fluid, avoiding the hypotensive episodes caused by intermittent HD. It is indicated for managing patients with ARF who are hemodynamically unstable and/or must receive large volumes of fluid or both. UF volumes are optimized to exceed the desired volume of excess water. Solute removal is both diffusive and convective. To perform a successful CVVHD/HDF, optimal clinical tolerance to fluid removal is critical. In a setting of too aggressive UF, blood volume may decrease due to a too-slow intravascular refilling, leading to severe hemodynamic instability [43].

6. The peritoneal dialysis catheter placement in patients with chronic heart failure: anesthesiology and surgical perspective

Adequately positioned peritoneal dialysis (PD) catheter is necessary for successful long-term PUF [44]. PD catheter insertion can be performed using different surgical methods, such as open approach, laparoscopy, and peritoneoscopy, or percutaneously [45, 46]. For all of these procedures, some anesthesia is required. The anesthesia techniques used for PD catheter placement are general (most utilized), spinal, regional, and local anesthesia [47].

6.1 Anesthetic considerations, including transversus abdominis plane block

PD catheter placement using an open approach usually requires general, neuraxial, and rarely local anesthesia. Local anesthesia is preferable for patients with significant comorbidities. However, the local infiltration of an anesthetic can produce edema and bleed at the incision site, which disturbs the surgical field. In most patients, especially obese ones, local anesthetic infiltration must be repeated, which can be connected with the patient's fear and anxiety. General anesthesia is usually required for laparoscopic PD catheter placement [46].

The CHF patients represent a group with an increased risk for anesthetic procedures, especially general anesthesia. For this reason, less invasive methods and

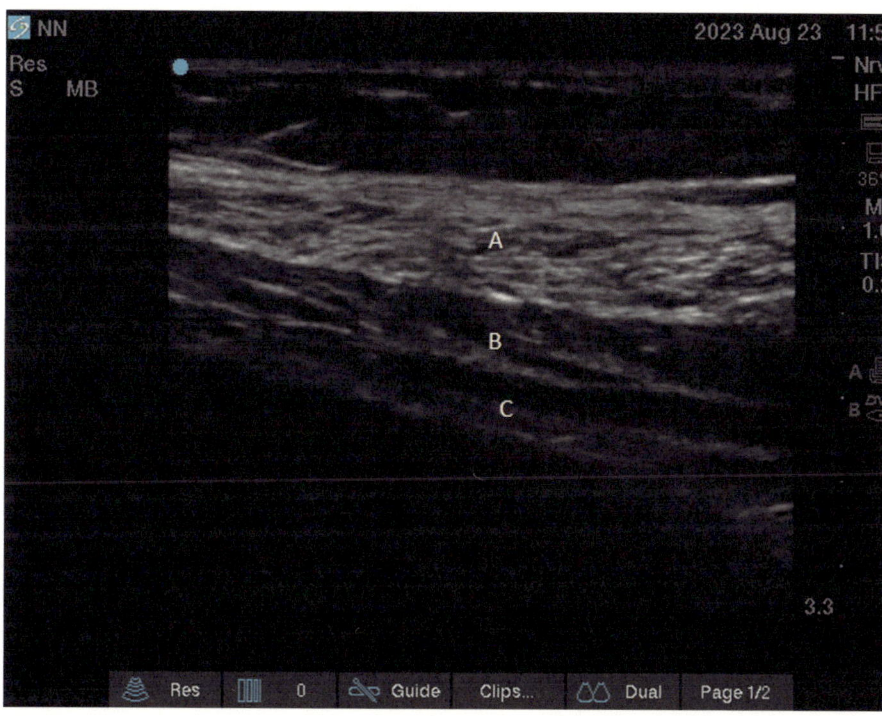

Figure 8.
Ultrasound image (linear ultrasound probe)visualised all three muscles of the abdominal wall:external oblique (A), Internal oblique (B). and trasversus abdonimis muscle(C). The space between the ineer oblique and transversus advominis muscles (transeversus abdominis plane) is a tareget area for applying a local anaesthetic. (Author's archive).

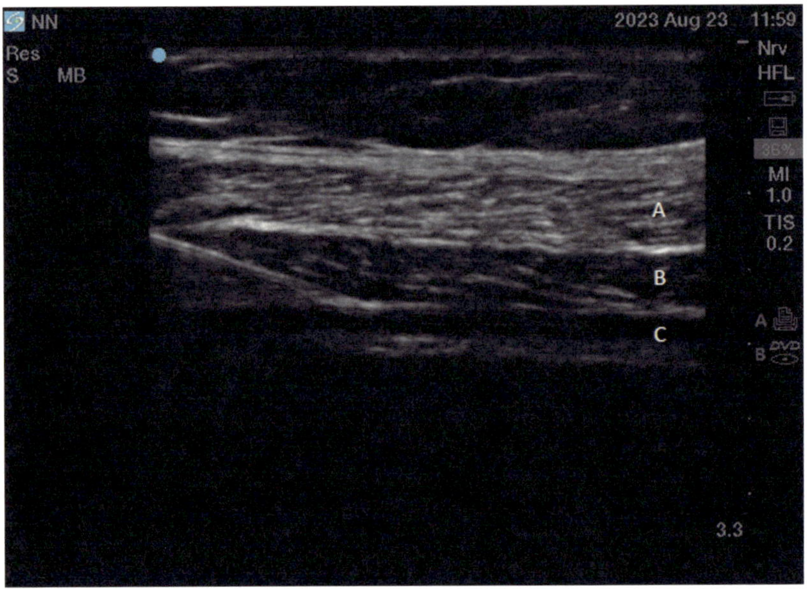

Figure 9.
Ultrasound image (linear ultrasound probe) showing a plane needle and needle tip positioned in the transversus abdominis plane just before injecting the loal anaesthetic. All three muscles of the abdominal wall are visualised: external oblique (A), interanl oblique (B) and transversus abdomimis muscle (C). (Author's archive).

techniques are being used. One of these is the transversus abdominis plane (TAP) block. It is a newer regional anesthesia technique, more precisely, a type of peripheral nerve block. The target area is a fascial layer between the transversus abdominis and internal oblique muscles. In this plane are situated thoracolumbar nerves (T7-L1), which supply the anterolateral abdominal wall (**Figures 8** and **9**). Using a TAP block, analgesia from the skin to the parietal peritoneum is achieved, and recently, a TAP block was used for PD catheter surgery [48, 49].

We recommended a combined ultrasound-guided subcostal and posterior approach using a linear, high-frequency probe (6–15 MHz) as we described previously [48, 49]. Briefly, when the TAP is identified, the needle is advanced in the targeted area, and local anesthetic is injected. In most patients, 30 mL of 0.25% levobupivacaine hydrochloride or 30 mL of 0.75% ropivacaine is used. Standard equipment used for patient monitoring includes an oxygen saturation probe, a non-invasive blood pressure monitor, and an electrocardiogram. Cold and pain sensation tests (pinprick) are used before the operation. About 30 minutes after the TAP block, a skin incision is possible. Just before the skin incision, all patients received additional drugs, such as sufentanil (10 mcg) and/or propofol (0.1–0.2 mg/kg), for a better analgesic/sedation effect [48, 49].

6.2 Preoperative management

As for any surgical procedure, patients must sign informed consent before the operation. Preoperatively, thromboprophylaxis (low molecular weight heparin) and antibiotics (cefazolin) were administered in all patients. The patient's position depends on the surgical approach, but a supine position is mainly used. The skin is disinfected with an antiseptic solution.

6.3 Open approach

The patient is in the supine position. In our institution, in concordance with the patient's will, we put the PD catheter on the side of the patient's dominant hand (most often the right side). We use a vertical paramedian, infraumbilical skin incision 3–4 cm long for all patients. The incision includes skin, subcutaneous tissue, anterior and posterior rectus sheath, preperitoneal tissue, and parietal peritoneum. The PD catheter (Tenckhoff type, two cuffs) is inserted in the peritoneal cavity. Both cuffs must be outside the peritoneum. The deep cuff is usually tied with the suture, which closes the peritoneum. After completing all the layers, the PD catheter is tunneled (inverse U shape), with an exit site different from the incision site. The proximal cuff is situated in the subcutaneous tissue, and the distal cuff is preperitoneally. The skin suture for the PD catheter's fixation is unnecessary because the catheter is fixed with sutures, including a deep cuff and peritoneum [48].

6.4 Laparoscopic approach

The patient is supine, with the surgeon on the right side (if the right-sided implantation is planned) and the assistant on the left side. The scrub nurse is on the side of the surgeon. The monitor is usually opposite the surgeon or near the legs. A periumbilical incision is used to create a pneumoperitoneum. In most cases, three trocars are used. One is in the camera's periumbilical position (10 mm), and two are in both lower abdominal quadrants. Through the left lower abdominal quadrant, a 5-mm trocar is placed usually for grasper, and on the right lower quadrant, the specially designed trocar (the so-called "Čala's trocar" according to his inventor). Čala's trocar is a metal trocar, with the possibility to be dismantled and through its internity, the PD catheter could be inserted (**Figure 10**) [45]. After trocar placement, the patient is placed in the Trendelenburg position, and the whole abdomen is explored. Via the Čala's trocar, a PD catheter is inserted in the peritoneal cavity using grasper for directed catheter deep in the pelvis. During catheter insertion, the deep cuff must be placed in a preperitoneal position, not in the peritoneal cavity. The Čala's trocar is dismantled and removed, and the catheter must be clamped to prevent exufflation of the peritoneal cavity. A subcutaneous tunnel is made with the finger, and a skin exit site is created. PD catheter is fixed to the skin in its exit site. After PD catheter fixation, the exufflation of CO_2 is performed, the trocars are removed, and their exit sites are closed.

Another trocar is placed when the deep cuff goes inside outside the peritoneal cavity. A suture is put laparoscopically to decrease the hole in the peritoneum and prevent migration of the deep cuff, which stays in an extraperitoneal position. If the patient has intrabdominal adhesions, adhesiolysis must first be performed using ultrasound or bipolar scissors.

6.5 Peritoneoscopic approach

This approach is partly similar to laparoscopic and is made under local anesthesia and in the supine position. First, the pneumoperitoneum is created. The guide is then inserted through the small skin incision through the abdominal wall in the peritoneal cavity with the optical control using a small diameter endoscope (peritoneoscope). After verification of proper position, the channel is dilated, and the catheter is inserted into the abdominal cavity.

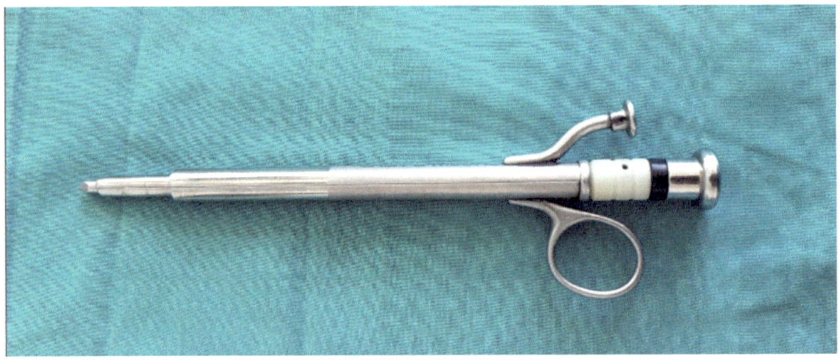

A

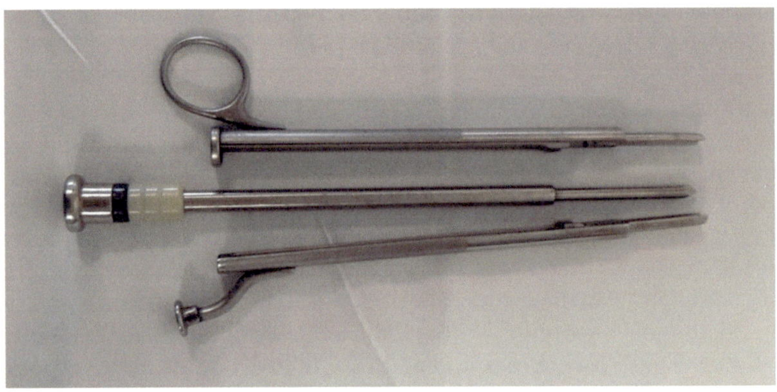

B

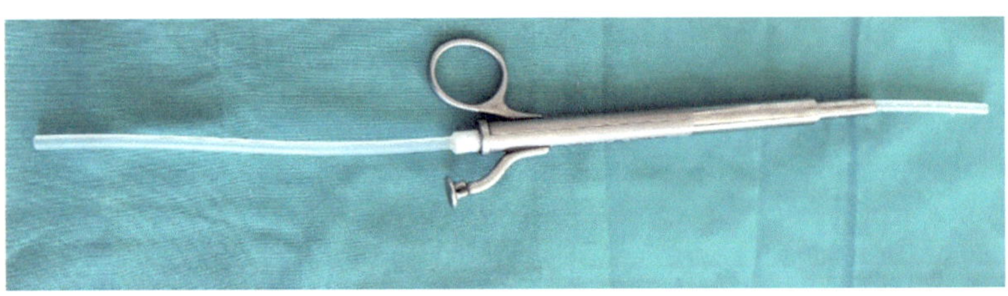

C

Figure 10.
Cala's trocar is a metal trocar (A), with the possibility to be dismanted (B) and through its internity, the PD catheter could be inserted (C). (Author's archive).

6.6 Selecting the best method for PD catheter insertion

CHF patients have substantially more comorbid conditions than the general population, leading to higher mortality in this group of patients. General anesthesia impacts the pulmonary and cardiovascular systems contrary to peripheral nerve block and local anesthesia, whose influence is negligible. For this reason, peripheral nerve block and local anesthesia can be recommended for placing PD catheters in patients with CHF, especially those with significant comorbidities. The guideline for choosing a PD catheter insertion approach is shown in **Table 1** [50].

Compared to general anesthesia, a TAP block has increased anesthetic induction time and requires additional equipment (ultrasound), performance time, and technical skill. A TAP block provides a longer duration and better quality of analgesia

Patient's characteristics	Previous major intraabdominal surgery and peritonitis	No last major intraabdominal surgery and peritonitis
Patient suitable for general anesthesia	1. Laparoscopic approach 2. Open approach	1. Laparoscopic approach 2. Percutaneous approach (x-ray) 3. Open approach or peritoneo-scopic approach 4. Percutaneous approach (with-out x-ray)
Patient non-suitable for general anesthesia (reconsider TAP block or local anesthesia)	1. Open approach	1. Percutaneous approach (x-ray) 2. Open approach or peritoneo-scopic approach 3. Percutaneous approach (without x-ray)

The table is modified according to the International Society of Peritoneal Dialysis (ISPD) guidelines [50].

Table 1.
Guideline for selecting a PD catheter insertion approach.

compared to local anesthesia [51]. In our institution, the TAP block is used as a primary anesthetic technique for PD catheter surgery for all patients, but especially for elderly patients and patients with significant comorbidities. Complications from a TAP block are rare and include nerve injury, injection site bruising, infection, allergic reaction, and liver laceration [52]. Contraindications for TAP block include infection at the injection site, patient refusal or inability to cooperate, allergy to local anesthetics, and coagulopathy [53]. An elevated BMI index was not a barrier to a successful TAP block [48, 49].

6.7 Outcomes of different PD catheter placement approaches

The two most common methods for PD catheter placement are open and laparoscopic approach [54]. Catheter malfunction is lower in the laparoscopic approach (13%) than in open surgery (35%). The one-year catheter survival rate was higher in the laparoscopic group compared to the open surgery group, but in the other study, this difference was not found [51, 55]. Dialysate leakage, exit-site infection, and peritonitis incidence between the laparoscopic and open surgery groups were similar [56].

The successful implantation of a PD catheter using a TAP block as a primary anesthetic method is from 82.2 to 94.2% in ESRD patients [48, 49, 57–60].

Such data is not available yet for CHF patients. Still, the use of TAP block as the primary anesthetic technique for PD catheter insertion should be considered in this patient group (authors' opinion).

7. Peritoneal ultrafiltration

7.1 Peritoneal membrane

The peritoneum is the most extensive serous membrane in the body, with a total surface of about 1.8 m^2. Human skin has a similar overall surface area. It helps to protect and separate the internal structures of the abdomen and pelvis.

The functions of the peritoneum:

a. Regulation of fluid for nutrient and mechanical purposes

b. Maintaining the position of organs by suspending them with ligaments

c. Prevention of friction while organs move

d. Conduction of vessels and nerves to the viscera

Peritonitis is inflammation of the peritoneum. Inflammation most often occurs as a result of a fungal or bacterial infection. Microorganisms can enter the abdomen due to an abdominal injury, some other condition such as perforation of a gastric ulcer, or during therapeutic procedures such as dialysis, esophagogastroduodenoscopy, gastrostomy. Inflammation of the peritoneum is a severe condition that requires urgent treatment. There are several types of peritonitis: acute and chronic by course, serous, fibrous, purulent, hemorrhagic by sort, diffuse, and circumscribed by localization. It can be divided into primary, secondary, and tertiary.

7.1.1 Structure of the peritoneal membrane

It consists of two layers: the parietal peritoneum (the outermost parietal layer), which surrounds the abdomen and pelvis, and the visceral peritoneum (inner visceral layer), which wraps around the abdominal organs. A potential space between the two layers contains small amounts of serous fluid (water, electrolytes, and immune cells). This fluid is a form of protection and acts as a lubricant between the layers. The parietal peritoneum covers the abdominal and pelvic walls and the diaphragm. The visceral peritoneum covers the intraperitoneal organs and forms various folds throughout the abdominal cavity. The greater omentum is a large fold of the visceral peritoneum and extends from the stomach downwards. Another fold of visceral peritoneum is the lesser omentum, which extends from the lesser curvature of the stomach to the liver. In addition to pain, the parietal peritoneum is sensitive to temperature, pressure, and laceration. The pain from the visceral peritoneum is poorly localized. It is only susceptible to extension and chemical irritation.

The visceral and parietal peritoneum has a similar histological structure: mesothelium, basal lamina, and submesothelial stroma. While mesothelium and basal lamina appear similarly throughout the abdomen, the submesothelial stroma may vary in thickness. Mesothelial cells are of mesodermal origin and, under specific conditions, can become even more similar to mesenchyme [61]. The mesothelial cells were considered inactive and contributed only to lubrication. It is known today that they play a crucial role in peritoneal homeostasis and produce a whole range of enzymes, cytokines, growth factors, and proteoglycans. They also provide the first line of defense against microorganisms and harmful chemical substances, which is why it is essential that the mesothelium can regenerate quickly and smoothly after injury.

At the basal surface, mesothelial cells are supported by the basal lamina. It consists of a layer of extracellular matrix less than 100 nm thick, composed of type IV collagen and laminin.

Connective tissue or stroma supports the mesothelial cells and the basal lamina. This supportive layer comprises collagen, mainly type I fibers, proteoglycans, fibronectin, (myo)fibroblasts, adipocytes, and blood and lymphatic vessels [62].

According to its structure, the peritoneum is a semipermeable membrane. Through its intercellular junctions and stomata, passive transport of liquids and dissolved substances takes place, as well as active transport through the formation of pinocytic vesicles. The transport of dissolved substances and small molecules through the peritoneum occurs quickly because the stroma, basal lamina, and mesothelium do not create resistance [63]. Transportation of large molecules is possible due to the network of collagen, fibronectin, elastin, and transcellular carriers in mesothelial cells [64]. The capacity of the peritoneum to transport fluids enables peritoneal UF/dialysis. Due to dialysate in the peritoneal cavity, UF and diffusion of water, salt, and uremic toxins through the membrane occur. Chronic exposure of the peritoneum to the dialysate evokes functional and morphological adaptions of the peritoneum. Chronic inflammation, progressive fibrosis, and angiogenesis thickening of the submesothelial stroma eventually lead to its loss of UF and blood purification capacity [65].

7.1.2 Aquaporins

The capillary endothelium, the interstitial space of the peritoneum, and the mesothelium represent a barrier to the exchange of soluble substances and water in the capillaries of the peritoneal cavity [66]. It should be emphasized that with this transport through the "pore" of the capillary walls, solutes larger than glucose are excessively lost, and the interstitium also modifies the transport of solutes *via* the barrier mentioned above [67]. The fluid exchange across the peritoneal membrane during PD is best explained with a "three-pore" model. The spaces between individual endothelial cells (inter endothelial clefts) represent the primary route for small-solute and fluid exchange. The radius of these clefts ("small pores") is cca. 40–50 Å. The small pores markedly impede the transit of albumin (36 Å) and ultimately prevent the passage of larger molecules, such as α_2-macroglobulin and immunoglobulins. The transendothelial pathways of the "large pores" (radius approx. 250 Å) are responsible for the penetration of large proteins into the interstitium and the peritoneal cavity [68]. Osmotic water transport occurs through ultra-small, water-only pores (radius approx. 2.5 Å), to which the capillary wall is highly susceptible.

Aquaporins (AQPs) are a family of integral plasma membrane proteins. Their discovery gave us insight into the molecular mechanisms for water transport through biological membranes. AQPs are usually specific for water permeability and exclude the passage of other solutes. All AQPs are impermeable to charged solutes, and water molecules traverse the AQP channel in a single file. It was assumed that water leaked through biological membranes, but the rapid movement of water across some cells remained unexplained. Although it had been predicted that water pores must exist in very leaky cells, it was not until 1992 that Peter Agre at Johns Hopkins University identified a specific transmembrane water pore later called aquaporin-1 (AQP1). AQP1 comprises a single peptide chain consisting of approximately 270 amino acids. It is distributed in the endothelium of capillaries, venules, and small veins of the peritoneum and is functionally identical to ultra-small pores [69].

An experimental mouse model showed that AQP1 is the most represented member of the AQP family in the peritoneum and is the only one found in the capillary endothelium. It was also experimentally shown that deletion of AQP1 does not affect the expression of other AQPs and the diameter or density of peritoneum capillaries. These data prove that AQP1 is important in peritoneal transport mechanisms [70].

Under non-PD conditions, approximately 60% of the net capillary UF occurs through small and 40% through large pores. Only 1–2% of total peritoneal transport occurs through ultra-small, water-only pores.

Under PD conditions, fluid removal is mainly reinforced by an osmotic agent in the peritoneal cavity. The osmosis mechanism is markedly affected by the type of osmotic agent used. For example, glycerol (radius approx. 3 Å) is a small osmotic agent with a weak effect on small pores and primarily on ultra-small, water-only pores. Unlike glycerol, glucose (radius approx. 3.7 Å) performs its ultrafiltration effect equally through ultra-small and small pores. Polyglucose (radius approx. 15–20 Å), a high-molecular-weight osmotic agent, ultrafilters liquid mainly through small pores. Polyglucose (radius approx. 15–20 Å), a high-molecular-weight osmotic agent, ultrafilters liquid mainly through small pores [71]. It is believed that AQP1 mediates 40–50% of osmotic-induced UF. A drop in dialysate sodium concentration is expected after 60 to 90 minutes of the dwell, as free water is transported through these pores, and this phenomenon is known as sodium sieving.

The relationship between AQPs, UF capacity, and sodium filtration is still debated in PD. On the other hand, understanding the molecular structure and role of ultra-small pores is vital for clinical practice regarding patient volume optimization.

7.1.3 Physiologic considerations

The final net UF in the peritoneal technique results from multiple transport mechanisms within the tissue surrounding the peritoneal cavity. Free water is transported through ultra-small pores, and an adequate volume of dialysate forces water and dissolved matter into the surrounding tissue. To achieve adequate UF from the capillaries of the peritoneum, it is necessary to maintain a high osmotic pressure in the peritoneal cavity. The osmotic pressure in the interstitium is lower than that in the peritoneal cavity. It is equal to the osmotic pressure in the plasma already in the first millimeter of tissue next to the peritoneum. Pure ultrafiltrate without dissolved substances results from the difference in osmotic pressure in the blood capillary and is produced by AQP1. If intraperitoneal pressure is too high, insufficient UF occurs. The most common reason for this is peritoneum inflammation when, due to capillary hyperpermeability, the osmotic agent quickly dissipates. Fibrosis of the peritoneum is the second possible reason because there is a reduced osmotic pressure near the blood supply, and there is no force to transport the fluid through the scar to the cavity. To solve problems in net UF, the key is to lower the volume and, secondary, the intraperitoneal pressure. Preventive measures are necessary to reduce chronic inflammation and peritonitis and preserve the peritoneal membrane and its transport characteristics.

The osmosis process is vital for transperitoneal water transport. Water moves from a low to high solute concentration area across a semipermeable membrane across all three pores. The effective surface area of the peritoneal membrane, the hydraulic conductance of the peritoneal membrane, the concentration and type of the osmotic agent used, and the influence of hydrostatic and oncotic pressure gradients across the peritoneal capillary are the factors that are responsible for the transcapillary water movement.

In the initial phase, the intraperitoneal volume is dominated by transcapillary UF. It is influenced by the crystalloid osmotic gradient created by glucose. On the other hand, it also governs relatively constant hydrostatic and oncotic pressure gradients (so-called "Starling forces") [72]. Intraperitoneal volume increases as the transcapillary UF rate exceeds lymphatic and tissue absorption [73]. The transcapillary UF rate decreases because of the steep decline in glucose concentration. A positive net UF occurs due to fluid transport imbalance because transcapillary UF exceeds lymphatic absorption. A state of balance in fluid transport that does not increase intraperitoneal volume is reached when the transcapillary UF rate drops to a value equal to the lymph flow rate. At that point, the intraperitoneal volume peak is reached. The negative net UF due to fluid absorption results from a difference between the decreasing transcapillary UF rate and the constant lymphatic tissue absorption, representing a new state of fluid transport imbalance.

A linear and stable decline is the second and last phase of intraperitoneal volume change. The peritoneal cavity's drainage time is responsible for the net clinical effect of peritoneal fluid movement. The drained volume may approach or even be less than the instilled volume if drainage is delayed until the end of the final phase.

Using glucose as an osmotic agent leads to the deterioration of the peritoneal membrane. Its well-known harmful effects on the peritoneum may lead to failure of the PD treatment in the mid-to-long term. With this in mind, an extensive effort has been made to find more biocompatible dialysis solutions, including icodextrin.

7.1.4 Advantages and safety considerations related to icodextrin solution

The icodextrin was launched in the mid-1990s, and its use has increased over time as more than 30,000 patients globally were receiving icodextrin treatment [74].

Different glucose concentrations in the PD solution are primarily used to meet the different UF needs. However, glucose has short-lived effects as an osmotic agent and degrades quickly in the peritoneum. Longer dwells of glucose solutions can often result in net fluid reabsorption from the dialysate into the patient rather than the expected outcome. Furthermore, glucose degradation products are formed, which harm the peritoneum, resulting in its damage in terms of fibrosis. These changes result in the peritoneum's functional inefficiency and the treatment method's viability [75]. Finally, these solutions lead to metabolic disorders such as hyperinsulinemia, hyperlipidemia., and hyperglycemia. Using icodextrin provides improved UF for long dwells compared to glucose solutions. It is also more efficient in volume status control. Further, Goossen et al.'s systematic review and meta-analysis demonstrated decreased mortality with icodextrin use [76]. Additional benefits from icodextrin are glucose-sparing properties, lipid status improvements, and echocardiographic parameters with reduced left ventricular mass.

The UF properties of icodextrin depend on the dwell time, whereby the maximum effect of icodextrin concerning glucose is achieved at a prolonged dwell time of 10–14 hours. Sometimes, full results are achieved as early as 10 hours of dwell, with minimal UF effect after that time. Compared to conventional glucose-based dialysates, icodextrin may offer improved peritoneal membrane biocompatibility by reducing glucose exposure, iso-osmolarity, and lesser carbonyl stress [77, 78]. Furthermore, the study of Posthum et al. showed that the concentrations of various peritoneal membrane markers (interleukin-8, CA125, amino-terminal propeptide of type III procollagen, and carboxyterminal propeptide of type III) did not differ between patients treated with glucose and icodextrin over 2 years [79]. Other clinical studies have confirmed that icodextrin is a safe and well-tolerated osmotic alternative solution to glucose [80]. The most significant side effect reported from using icodextrin is a skin hypersensitivity reaction [81]. Most likely, the hypersensitivity reaction is mediated by the immune complex. The peritonitis rate does not differ between patients treated with icodextrin and those treated with glucose solutions only, which has been confirmed in several randomized, controlled studies [82]. Long-term intraperitoneal use of icodextrin can permanently increase the plasma's maltose, maltotriose, and other oligosaccharides. This is significant because elevated maltose levels can interfere with specific glucose and amylase tests [83]. Therefore, one should be careful when interpreting the results of such tests when using icodextrin.

The most common antibiotics used to treat peritonitis (vancomycin, cephalosporins, and gentamicin) are compatible and stable with icodextrin [84]. Finally, the use of icodextrin has been associated with falls in serum sodium concentration and slight increases in serum osmolality, which are usually not clinically significant.

7.2 Rationale for peritoneal ultrafiltration in congestive heart failure

PUF is a treatment modality aimed at patients with diuretic-resistant CHF to control fluid retention adequately. While extracorporeal UF is more commonly used to treat acute decompensated HF, PUF has been proposed for long-term treatment of RCHF, especially in elderly patients, as a soothing therapeutic modality or as a bridge to definitive surgery or HTx. The potential benefits of this treatment modality include a quality-of-life improvement since it is a home-based therapy, better control of congestion and no need for central venous access (no problems associated with anticoagulation), and a reduction in hospitalization rates [85].

However, still unanswered questions show a need for future studies, starting with the patient inclusion criteria. According to Bertoli et al., an ideal candidate for PUF would be a patient with both CHF and CKD, on optimal medical therapy and at least three hospitalizations in the previous year. Secondly, it is still being determined if PUF would be suitable for patients with all HF types since, in most studies, patients had left ventricular systolic dysfunction [86].

7.3 Peritoneal ultrafiltration prescription in congestive heart failure

The global prevalence of HF is increasing due to aging populations, insufficiently controlled cardiovascular risk factors, and prolonged survival. Significant progress has been made in treating HF in recent decades due to new disease-modifying drugs and increasingly sophisticated devices [87]. However, the effectiveness of treatment is limited in some patients, and palliative care is the only option to improve the quality of life. Although progress has been made in the treatment of heart failure with improved survival, RCHF remains a growing health problem, already a significant cause of hospitalization, with associated costs [88]. CRS is dominated by a comprehensive pathophysiology in HF, regardless of EF. It is associated with poorer outcomes, more than 40% of all-cause mortality, and is a significant driver of repeat hospitalizations. Renal venous congestion and arterial insufficiency lead to "excretory renal failure" due to critical changes in intraglomerular filtration pressure. This results in inadequate volume control that causes recurrent cardiac decompensation [89]. Extracorporeal HD or UF is an alternative for treating congestion in case of diuretic resistance. HD is conventionally reserved for patients with concomitant ESRD, and UF is more commonly used in patients without ESRD [90]. There are conflicting results from clinical studies comparing UF with pharmacological therapy. In the UNLOAD study, patients treated with UF had better control of volume status and a lower frequency of hospitalization for HF than those treated with diuretics. However, in the CARESS-HF study, there was no difference in weight loss between patients treated with UF and those treated with higher doses of diuretics [3, 91]. More elevated serum creatinine values were observed in the group of patients treated with UF, which the authors assumed was due to a transient decrease in intravascular volume during this procedure.

More recently, there has been increased interest in UF via the peritoneal membrane with the updated terminology of PUF, reflecting the goal of fluid extraction across the peritoneal membrane [92]. PUF in RCHF reduces the incidence of decompensation episodes, which is particularly significant as each episode incrementally adds to mortality. Compared to extracorporeal therapies, this method offers potential advantages such as better preservation of residual renal function, tighter control of sodium balance, less neurohumoral activation, and the possibility of daily treatment in the home environment [93].

On the other hand, PUF offers excellent flexibility in a prescription best suited for a given patient. Success has been reported using a single-night time exchange with icodextrin. It is recommended to start the therapy with a smaller volume of the single-night icodextrin exchange and gradually increase it to the maximum tolerable level, which gives us an appropriate UF rate. The icodextrin exchange can be done twice daily in cases of greater hypervolemia. Such a prescription should be used for up to 2 weeks and then turn into one single-day exchange. An incremental therapeutic approach of the single-night exchange can be continued after achieving volume optimization of the patient, including regular outpatient monitoring. This implies pausing the therapy one or more days a week, according to the instructions of the supervising medical staff.

8. Conclusions

The presence of CKD is a poor prognostic factor in patients with CHF, and a number of these patients develop resistance to conventional medical therapy, primarily diuretics. PUF is a viable modality for both the short- and long-term managements of patients with RCHF. The role of PUF in short-term control is limited to situations where extracorporeal UF is not possible or available. However, for the long-term management of patients with RCHF, PUF should be the therapy of choice for ambulatory UF. It can be used as a bridge therapy for definitive interventions or palliative treatment for these patients. Using an intraperitoneal solution such as icodextrin promotes a slow and efficient PUF that better preserves residual renal function, is less invasive and is better tolerated by cardiac patients, improving clinical symptoms and quality of life.

Patients with CHF are usually fragile, with multiple comorbidities. The proper anesthesia technique and surgical approach for PD catheter placement in CHF patients must be based on the patient's characteristics (including comorbidities and previous operations), available equipment, and surgeon's experience. An open approach using a TAP block for PD catheter placement in patients with CHF is strongly recommended.

However, there is a need for controlled trials to define subgroups of patients with RCHF who are most likely to benefit from this treatment method. Non-randomized but more extensive observational studies should also be performed to provide more information and establish the best protocol for managing RCHF in patients without ESRD. Cost-benefit analyses and reimbursement policies should be implemented. All this may lead to a more widespread use of PUF with icodextrin in this group of patients.

Author details

Božidar Vujičić[1,2*], Koraljka Benko[2,3], Ana Petretić[2,3], Nenad Nemarnik[3], Matko Spicijarić[2,3], Dean Markić[2,4], Matej Bura[2,5], Fabio Kadum[3], Sanjin Rački[1,2] and Alen Ružić[2,3]

1 Department for Nephrology, Dialysis and Kidney Transplantation, Clinical Hospital Centre Rijeka, Rijeka, Croatia

2 School of Medicine, University of Rijeka, Rijeka, Croatia

3 Department for Cardiovascular Diseases, Clinical Hospital Centre Rijeka, Rijeka, Croatia

4 Department of Urology, Clinical Hospital Centre Rijeka, Rijeka, Croatia

5 Department of Anesthesiology, Reanimatology and Intensive Care Medicine, Clinical Hospital Centre Rijeka, Rijeka, Croatia

*Address all correspondence to: vujicic.bozidar@gmail.com

References

[1] Schneierson SJ. Continuous peritoneal irrigation in the treatment of intractable oedema of cardiac origin. The American Journal of the Medical Sciences. 1949;**218**(1):76-79

[2] Mailloux LU, Swartz CD, Onesti G, Heider C, Ramirez O, Brest AN. Peritoneal dialysis for refractory congestive heart failure. Journal of the American Medical Association. 1967;**199**(12):873-878

[3] Bart BA, Goldsmith SR, Lee KL, Givertz MM, O'Connor CM, Bull DA, et al. Ultrafiltration in decompensated heart failure with cardiorenal syndrome. The New England Journal of Medicine. 2012;**367**(24):2296-2304

[4] Gotloib L, Fudin R, Yakubovich M, Vienken J. Peritoneal dialysis in refractory end-stage congestive heart failure: A challenge facing a no-win situation. Nephrology, Dialysis, Transplantation. 2005;**20**:32-36

[5] McDonagh TA, Metra M, Adamo M, Gardner RS, Baumbach A, Böhm M, et al. ESC guidelines for the diagnosis and treatment of acute and chronic heart failure. European Heart Journal. 2021;**42**(36):3599-3726

[6] Bozkurt B, Coats AJS, Tsutsui H, Abdelhamid CM, Adamopoulos S, Albert N, et al. Universal definition and classification of heart failure: A report of the heart failure society of America, heart failure Association of the European Society of cardiology, Japanese heart failure society and writing committee of the universal definition of heart failure: Endorsed by the Canadian heart failure society, heart failure association of India, cardiac society of Australia and New Zealand, and Chinese heart failure association. European Journal of Heart Failure. 2021;**23**(3):352-380

[7] Mann DL, Chakinala M. Heart failure: Pathophysiology and diagnosis. In: Jameson J, Fauci AS, Kasper DL, Hauser SL, Longo DL, Loscalzo J, editors. Harrison's Principles of Internal Medicine, 20e. New York: McGraw Hill; 2018. pp. 1763-1764

[8] Figueroa MS, Peters JI. Congestive heart failure: Diagnosis, pathophysiology, therapy, and implications for respiratory care. Respiratory Care. 2006;**51**(4):403-412

[9] Stansfield WE, Ranek M, Pendse A, Schisler JC, Wang S, Pulinilkunnil T, et al. The pathophysiology of cardiac hypertrophy and heart failure. In: Willis M, Homeister JW, Stone JR, editors. Cellular and Molecular Pathobiology of Cardiovascular Disease. London: Elsevier, Inc; 2014. pp. 51-53

[10] Jones NR, Roalfe AK, Adoki I, Hobbs FDR, Taylor CJ. Survival of patients with chronic heart failure in the community: A systematic review and meta-analysis. European Journal of Heart Failure. 2019;**21**(11):1306-1325

[11] Coles AH, Tisminetzky M, Yarzebski J, Lessard D, Gore JM, Darling CE, et al. The magnitude of and prognostic factors associated with 1-year mortality after hospital discharge for acute decompensated heart failure based on ejection fraction findings. Journal of the American Heart Association. 2015;**4**(12)

[12] Godhiwala PP, Acharya S, Kumar S, Bagga C. Prognostic markers in advanced heart failure. Journal of Evolution of Medical and Dental Sciences. 2021;**10**(1):39-44

[13] Ledoux P. Les cardio-rénaux [Cardiorenal syndrome]. L'Avenir Médical. 1951;**48**(8):149-153

[14] Ronco C, McCullough P, Anker SD, Anand I, Aspromonte N, Bagshaw SM, et al. Cardio-renal syndromes: Report from the consensus conference of the acute dialysis quality initiative. European Heart Journal. 2010;**31**(6):703-711

[15] Uduman J. Epidemiology of cardiorenal syndrome. Advances in Chronic Kidney Disease. 2018;**25**(5):391-399

[16] Prothasis M, Varma A, Gaidhane S, Kumar S, Khatib N, Zahiruddin QS, et al. Prevalence, types, risk factors, and outcomes of cardiorenal syndrome in a rural population of Central India: A cross-sectional study. Journal of Family Medicine and Primary Care. 2020;**9**(8):4127-4133

[17] Matsushita K, Ballew SH, Wang AY, Kalyesubula R, Schaeffner E, Agarwal R. Epidemiology and risk of cardiovascular disease in populations with chronic kidney disease. Nature Reviews. Nephrology. 2022;**18**(11):696-707

[18] Iimori S, Naito S, Noda Y, Nishida H, Kihira H, Yui N, et al. Anaemia management and mortality risk in newly visiting patients with chronic kidney disease in Japan: The CKD-ROUTE study. Nephrology (Carlton, Vic.). 2015;**20**(9):601-608

[19] Ritchie J, Rainone F, Green D, Alderson H, Chiu D, Middleton R, et al. Extreme elevations in blood pressure and all-cause mortality in a referred CKD population: Results from the CRISIS study. International Journal of Hypertension. 2013;**2013**:1-8

[20] Tedeschi A, Agostoni P, Pezzuto B, Corra' U, Scrutinio D, La Gioia R, et al. Role of comorbidities in heart failure prognosis part 2: Chronic kidney disease, elevated serum uric acid. European Journal of Preventive Cardiology. 2020;**27**(Suppl. 2):35-45

[21] Forman DE, Butler J, Wang Y, Abraham WT, O'Connor CM, Gottlieb SS, et al. Incidence, predictors at admission, and impact of worsening renal function among patients hospitalised with heart failure. Journal of the American College of Cardiology. 2004;**43**(1):61-67

[22] Bubić I, Zaputović L, Rački S. Kardiorenalni sindrom. Medicina Fluminensis [Internet]. 2010;**46**(4): 391-402. Available from: https://urn.nsk.hr/urn:nbn:hr:184:388494 [Accessed: August 26, 2023]

[23] Ahmed A, Rich MW, Sanders PW, Perry GJ, Bakris GL, Zile MR, et al. Chronic kidney disease associated mortality in diastolic versus systolic heart failure: A propensity-matched study. The American Journal of Cardiology. 2007;**99**(3):393-398

[24] Khwaja A. KDIGO clinical practice guidelines for acute kidney injury. Nephron. Clinical Practice. 2012;**120**(4):c179-c184

[25] Ortega-Loubon C, Fernández-Molina M, Carrascal-Hinojal Y, Fulquet-Carreras E. Cardiac surgery-associated acute kidney injury. Annals of Cardiac Anaesthesia. 2016;**19**(4):687-698

[26] Stevens PE, Levin A. Evaluation and management of chronic kidney disease: Synopsis of the kidney disease: Improving global outcomes 2012 clinical practice guideline. Annals of Internal Medicine. 2013;**158**(11):825-830

[27] Peerapornratana S, Manrique-Caballero CL, Gómez H, Kellum JA. Acute kidney injury from sepsis: Current concepts, epidemiology, pathophysiology, prevention and treatment. Kidney International. 2019;**96**(5):1083-1099

[28] Murugan R, Karajala-Subramanyam V, Lee M, Yende S,

Kong L, Carter M, et al. Acute kidney injury in non-severe pneumonia is associated with an increased immune response and lower survival. Kidney International. 2010;**77**(6):527-535

[29] Liu J, Xie H, Ye Z, Li F, Wang L. Rates, predictors, and mortality of sepsis-associated acute kidney injury: A systematic review and meta-analysis. BMC Nephrology. 2020;**21**(1):318

[30] McMurray JJ, Packer M, Desai AS, Gong J, Lefkowitz MP, Rizkala AR, et al. Angiotensin-Neprilysin inhibition versus Enalapril in heart failure. The New England Journal of Medicine. 2014;**371**(11):993-1004

[31] Bardy GH, Lee KL, Mark DB, Poole JE, Packer DL, Boineau R, et al. Amiodarone or an implantable cardioverter-defibrillator for congestive heart failure. The New England Journal of Medicine. 2005;**352**(3):225-237. Erratum in: N Engl J Med. 2005 May 19;352(20):2146

[32] Solomon SD, McMurray JJV, Claggett B, de Boer RA, DeMets D, Hernandez AF, et al. Dapagliflozin in heart failure with mildly reduced or preserved ejection fraction. The New England Journal of Medicine. 2022;**387**(12):1089-1098

[33] Anker SD, Butler J, Filippatos G, Ferreira JP, Bocchi E, Böhm M, et al. Empagliflozin in heart failure with a preserved ejection fraction. The New England Journal of Medicine. 2021;**385**(16):1451-1461

[34] Nieminen MS, Fruhwald S, Heunks LM, Suominen PK, Gordon AC, Kivikko M, et al. Levosimendan: Current data, clinical use and future development. Heart Lung Vessel. 2013;**5**(4):227-245

[35] Verbrugge FH, Dupont M, Steels P, Grieten L, Swennen Q, Tang WHW, et al. The kidney in congestive heart failure: "Are natriuresis, sodium, and diuretics the good, the bad and the ugly?". European Journal of Heart Failure. 2014;**16**(2):133-142

[36] Braam B, Cupples WA, Joles JA, Gaillard C. Systemic arterial and venous determinants of renal hemodynamics in congestive heart failure. Heart Failure Reviews. 2012;**17**(2):161-175

[37] Singh D, Shrestha K, Testani JM, Verbrugge FH, Dupont M, Mullens W, et al. Insufficient natriuretic response to continuous intravenous furosemide is associated with poor long-term outcomes in acute decompensated heart failure. Journal of Cardiac Failure. 2014;**20**(6):392-399

[38] Ronco C, Ricci Z, Bellomo R, Bedogni F. Extracorporeal ultrafiltration for the treatment of overhydration and congestive heart failure. Cardiology. 2001;**96**(3-4):155-168

[39] Marenzi G, Lauri G, Grazi M, Assanelli E, Campodonico J, Agostoni P. Circulatory response to fluid overload removal by extracorporeal ultrafiltration in refractory congestive heart failure. Journal of the American College of Cardiology. 2001;**38**(4):963-968

[40] DiLeo M, Pacitti A, Bergerone S, Pozzi R, Tognarelli G, Segoloni G, et al. Ultrafiltration in the treatment of refractory heart failure. Clinical Cardiology. 1988;**11**(7):449-452

[41] Ronco C, Brendolan A, Bellomo R. Continuous versus intermittent renal replacement therapy in the treatment of acute renal failure. Nephrology, Dialysis, Transplantation. 1998;**13**:79-85

[42] Bellomo R, Ronco C, Mehta RL, Asfar P, Boisramé-Helms J, Darmon M,

et al. Acute kidney injury in the ICU: From damage to recovery: Reports from the 5th Paris International Conference. Annals of Intensive Care. 2017;**7**(1):49

[43] Mehta RL. Fluid management in CRRT. Contributions to Nephrology. 2001;**132**:335-348

[44] Eklund B, Honkanen E, Kyllönen L, Salmela K, Kala AR. Peritoneal dialysis access: Prospective randomised comparison of single-cuff and double-cuff straight Tenckhoff catheters. Nephrology, Dialysis, Transplantation. 1997;**12**(12):2664-2666

[45] Čala Z, Mimica Ž, Ljutić D, Janković N, Varlaj V, Čala S. Laparoscopic placement of the peritoneal dialysis catheter using specially designed trocar: A review of 84 patients. Dialysis & Transplantation. 2000;**29**(11):722-727

[46] Voss D, Hawkins S, Poole G, Marshall M. Radiological versus surgical implantation of the first catheter for peritoneal dialysis: A randomised non-inferiority trial. Nephrology, Dialysis, Transplantation. 2012;**27**(11):4196-4204

[47] Jain AK, Blake P, Cordy P, Garg AX. Global trends in rates of peritoneal dialysis. Journal of the American Society of Nephrology. 2012;**23**(3):533-544

[48] Markić D, Vujičić B, Ivanovski M, Krpina K, Gršković A, Živčić-Ćosić S, et al. Peritoneal dialysis catheter placement using an ultrasound-guided transversus abdominis plane block. Blood Purification. 2015;**39**(4):274-280

[49] Markić D, Vujičić B, Ivanovski M, Krpina K, Gršković A, Rahelić D, et al. Peritoneal dialysis catheter surgery using transversus abdominis plane block. Peritoneal Dialysis International. 2017;**37**(4):429-433

[50] Crabtree JH, Shrestha BM, Chow KM, Figueiredo AE, Povlsen JV, Wilkie M. Creating and maintaining optimal peritoneal dialysis access in the adult patient: 2019 update. Peritoneal Dialysis International. 2019;**39**(5):414-436

[51] Xie H, Zhang W, Cheng J, He Q. Laparoscopic versus open catheter placement in peritoneal dialysis patients: A systematic review and meta-analysis. BMC Nephrology. 2012;**13**:69

[52] Lancaster P, Chadwick M. Liver trauma secondary to ultrasound-guided transversus abdominis plane block. British Journal of Anaesthesia. 2010;**104**(4):509-510

[53] Jankovic Z, Ahmad N, Ravishankar N, Archer F. Transversus abdominis plane block: How safe is it? Anesthesia and Analgesia. 2008;**107**(5):1758-1759

[54] Eklund BH. Surgical implantation of CAPD catheters: Presentation of midline incision-lateral placement method and a review of 110 procedures. Nephrology, Dialysis, Transplantation. 1995;**10**(3):386-390

[55] Hagen SM, Lafranca JA, Steyerberg EW, Ijzermans JN, Dor FJ. Laparoscopic versus open peritoneal dialysis catheter insertion: A meta-analysis. PLoS One. 2013;**8**(2):e56351

[56] Abdijalil G, Shuijuan S. Laparoscopic versus open surgery catheter placement in peritoneal dialysis patients: A meta-analysis of outcomes. Indian Journal of Nephrology. 2022;**32**(5):406-413

[57] Varadarajan Y, Balasubramaniyam R. Ultrasound-guided rectus sheath and transversus abdominis plane block (TAP) for continuous ambulatory peritoneal dialysis (CAPD) catheterisation – Our

experience. Nephrology, Dialysis, Transplantation. 2012;**27**(2):ii464A

[58] Chatterjee S, Bain J, Christopher S, Gopal TV, Raju KP, Mathur P. Role of regional anaesthesia for the placement of peritoneal dialysis catheter under ultrasound guidance: Our experience with 52 end-stage renal disease patients. Saudi Journal of Anesthesia. 2015;**9**(2):132-135

[59] Henshaw DS, Baker ML, Weller RS, Reynolds JW, Jaffe JD. Transversus abdominis plane block is the primary anaesthetic for peritoneal dialysis catheter surgery. Journal of Clinical Anesthesia. 2016;**31**:182-188

[60] Jakšić A, Vujičić B, Deša D, Gršković A, Vukelić I, Španjol J, et al. Case report: Synchronous removal and implantation of peritoneal dialysis catheter using bilateral transversus abdominis plane block. Frontiers in Medicine (Lausanne). 2022;**9**:828930

[61] Sandoval P, Jiménez-Heffernan JA, Rynne-Vidal Á, Pérez-Lozano ML, Gilsanz Á, Ruiz-Carpio V, et al. Carcinoma-associated fibroblasts derive from mesothelial cells via mesothelial-to-mesenchymal transition in peritoneal metastasis. The Journal of Pathology. 2013;**231**(4):517-531

[62] Witz CA, Montoya-Rodriguez IA, Cho S, Centonze VE, Bonewald LF, Schenken RS. Composition of the extracellular matrix of the peritoneum. Journal of the Society for Gynecologic Investigation. 2001;**8**(5):299-304

[63] Flessner MF. Endothelial glycocalyx and the peritoneal barrier. Peritoneal Dialysis International. 2008;**28**(1):6-12

[64] De Vriese AS, White R, Granger DN, Lamiere NH. The peritoneal microcirculation in peritoneal dialysis. In: Khanna R, Krediet RT, editors. Nolph and Gokal's Textbook of Peritoneal Dialysis. 3rd ed. New York; Berlin: Springer; 2009. pp. 51-71

[65] Witowski J, Kawka E, Rudolf A, Jorres A. New developments in peritoneal fibroblast biology: Implications for inflammation and fibrosis in peritoneal dialysis. BioMed Research International. 2015;**2015**:1-7

[66] Rippe B, Rosengren BI, Venturoli D. The peritoneal microcirculation in peritoneal dialysis. Microcirculation. 2001;**8**(5):303-320

[67] Rippe B, Venturoli D. Simulations of osmotic ultrafiltration failure in CAPD using a serial three-pore membrane/fibre matrix model. American Journal of Physiology. Renal Physiology. 2007;**292**(3):F1035-F1043

[68] Rippe B, Haraldsson B. Transport of macromolecules across microvascular walls: The two-pore theory. Physiological Reviews. 1994;**74**(1):163-219

[69] Jung JS, Preston GM, Smith BL, Guggino WB, Agre P. Molecular structure of the water channel through aquaporin CHIP. The hourglass model. The Journal of Biological Chemistry. 1994;**269**(20):14648-14654

[70] Ni J, Verbavatz JM, Rippe A, Boisdé I, Moulin P, Rippe B, et al. Aquaporin-1 plays an essential role in water permeability and ultrafiltration during peritoneal dialysis. Kidney International. 2006;**69**(9):1518-1525

[71] Rippe B, Venturoli D, Simonsen O, de Arteaga J. Fluid and electrolyte transport across the peritoneal membrane during CAPD according to the three-pore model. Peritoneal Dialysis International. 2004;**24**(1):10-27

[72] Vonesh EF, Rippe B. Net fluid absorption under membrane transport models of peritoneal dialysis. Blood Purification. 1992;**10**(3-4):209-226

[73] Mactier RA, Khanna R, Twardowski Z, Moore H, Nolph KD. Contribution of lymphatic absorption to loss of ultrafiltration and solute clearances in continuous ambulatory peritoneal dialysis. The Journal of Clinical Investigation. 1987;**80**(5):1311-1316

[74] Silver SA, Harel Z, Perl J. Practical considerations when prescribing icodextrin: A narrative review. American Journal of Nephrology. 2014;**39**(6):515-527

[75] Ha H, Yu MR, Choi HN, Cha MK, Kang HS, Kim MH, et al. Effects of conventional and new peritoneal dialysis solutions on human peritoneal mesothelial cell viability and proliferation. Peritoneal Dialysis International. 2000;**20**(Suppl. 5): S10-S18

[76] Goossen K, Becker M, Marshall MR, Bühn S, Breuing J, Firanek CA, et al. Icodextrin versus glucose solutions for the once-daily long dwell in peritoneal dialysis: An enriched systematic review and meta-analysis of randomized controlled trials. American Journal of Kidney Diseases. 2020;**75**(6):830-846

[77] Posthuma N, Ter Wee P, Donker AJ, Dekker HA, Oe PL, Verbrugh HA. Peritoneal defense using icodextrin or glucose for daytime dwell in CCPD patients. Peritoneal Dialysis International. 1999;**19**(4):334-342

[78] Dawnay AB, Millar DJ. Glycation and advanced glycation end-product formation with icodextrin and dextrose. Peritoneal Dialysis International. 1997;**17**(1):52-58

[79] Posthuma N, Verbrugh HA, Donker AJ, van Dorp W, Dekker HA, Peers EM, et al. Peritoneal kinetics and mesothelial markers in CCPD using icodextrin for daytime dwell for two years. Peritoneal Dialysis International. 2000;**20**(2):174-180

[80] Posthuma N, Ter Wee PM, Donker AJ, Oe PL, Peers EM, Verbrugh HA. Assessment of the effectiveness, safety, and biocompatibility of icodextrin in automated peritoneal dialysis. The dextrin in APD in Amsterdam (DIANA) group. Peritoneal Dialysis International. 2000;**20**(Suppl. 2):S106-S113

[81] Queffeulou G, Bernard M, Vrtovsnik F, Skhiri H, Lebrun-Vigne B, Hufnagel G, et al. Severe cutaneous hypersensitivity requiring permanent icodextrin withdrawal in a CAPD patient. Clinical Nephrology. 1999;**51**(3):184-186

[82] Mistry CD, Gokal R, Peers E. A randomised multicenter clinical trial comparing isosmolar icodextrin with hyperosmolar glucose solutions in CAPD. MIDAS study group. Multicenter investigation of icodextrin in ambulatory peritoneal dialysis. Kidney International. 1994;**46**(2):496-503

[83] Janssen W, Harff G, Caers M, Schellekens A. Positive interference of icodextrin metabolites in some enzymatic glucose methods. Clinical Chemistry. 1998;**44**(11):2379-2380

[84] Choo CG, Titus AE, Zdarsky DM, Murphy GP, Kunzler JA, Scheithe JP. Compatibility of 7.5% polyglucose peritoneal dialysis solution with gentamicin, vancomycin, heparin and insulin. Peritoneal Dialysis International. 1997;**17**:S94

[85] Wańkowicz Z, Próchnicka A, Olszowska A, Baczyński D, Krzesiński P, Dziuk M. Extracorporeal

versus peritoneal ultrafiltration in diuretic-resistant congestive heart failure – A review. Medical Science Monitor. 2011;**17**(12):RA271-RA281

[86] Bertoli SV, Musetti C, Ciurlino D, Basile C, Galli E, Gambaro G, et al. Peritoneal ultrafiltration in refractory heart failure: A cohort study. Peritoneal Dialysis International. 2014;**34**(1):64-70

[87] Yancy CW, Jessup M, Bozkurt B, Butler J, Casey DE Jr, Colvin MM, et al. ACC/AHA/HFSA focused update of the 2013 ACCF/AHA guideline for the Management of Heart Failure: A report of the American College of Cardiology/American Heart Association task force on clinical practice guidelines and the Heart Failure Society of America. Circulation. 2017;**136**(6):e137-e161

[88] Virani SS, Alonso A, Aparicio HJ, Benjamin EJ, Bittencourt MS, Callaway CW, et al. Heart disease and stroke statistics-2021 update: A report from the American Heart Association. Circulation. 2021;**143**(8):e254-e743

[89] Bock JS, Gottlieb SS. Cardiorenal syndrome: New perspectives. Circulation. 2010;**121**(23):2592-2600

[90] Costanzo MR, Chawla LS, Tumlin JA, Herzog CA, McCullough PA, Kellum JA, et al. The role of early and sufficient isolated venovenous ultrafiltration in heart failure patients with pulmonary and systemic congestion. Reviews in Cardiovascular Medicine. 2013;**14**(2-4):e123-e133

[91] Costanzo MR, Guglin ME, Saltzberg MT, Jessup ML, Bart BA, Teerlink JR, et al. Ultrafiltration versus intravenous diuretics for patients hospitalised for acute decompensated heart failure. Journal of the American College of Cardiology. 2007;**49**(6):675-683

[92] Mehrotra R, Khanna R. Peritoneal ultrafiltration for chronic congestive heart failure: Rationale, evidence and future. Cardiology. 2001;**96**(3-4):177-182

[93] Puttagunta H, Holt SG. Peritoneal dialysis for heart failure. Peritoneal Dialysis International. 2015;**35**(6):645-649

Chapter 7

Medical Nutrition Therapy in Renal Replacement Therapy

Susan Atieno Onyango and Grace Nyawira Njuguna

Abstract

This chapter discusses Medical Nutrition Therapy in three modalities of renal replacement therapy (RRT), outlining the nutrient requirements for patients on maintenance hemodialysis, peritoneal dialysis, and kidney transplant in acute and chronic phases. The chapter takes note of the drastic impact of RRT on the patient's nutrition status and overall well-being, which puts them at high risk of morbidity and mortality, and thus emphasizes timely and regular comprehensive nutrition assessment to enable appropriate intervention. Recognizing that there are different modalities of RRT and that patients have different physiological characteristics as well as different laboratory test values, which may also vary for individual patients each time tests are run, nutrition therapy is individualized each time. The chapter takes a closer look at protein-energy wasting, a condition common among patients undergoing RRT, which is a predictor of mortality, discussing its prevention and treatment measures. Finally, the chapter takes a closer look at electrolytes, specifically potassium, sodium, calcium, and phosphorous, in relation to mineral bone disease.

Keywords: nutrition therapy, nutrient recommendations, nutrition assessment, protein energy wasting, mineral bone disease

1. Introduction

1.1 Medical nutrition therapy

Medical nutrition therapy (MNT) is an individualized nutrition evidence-based process that aims at treating and managing medical conditions. MNT comprises comprehensive nutrition assessment, diagnosis, specialized therapies, diet modifications, and nutrition counseling [1, 2].

A Renal Dietitian/Nutritionist, Registered Dietitian Nutritionist (RDN), a nutrition professional, or an international equivalent does the comprehensive nutrition assessment, including anthropometric measurements, nutrition-focused physical findings, monitoring and evaluating appetite, dietary intake, body weight changes, and biochemical data. This also assesses the effectiveness of MNT [3]. Renal replacement therapy significantly affects nutrition status, which in turn affects the well-being of the patients. Malnutrition is common among patients undergoing RRT, with more undernutrition leading towards those undergoing hemodialysis, while overnutrition may also be found among patients on peritoneal dialysis (PD) and post-transplant patient in the chronic phase. Malnutrition is common among patients with end-stage renal disease, with a prevalence ranging from 18 to 75% for patients on hemodialysis [4]. Patients often do not take adequate calories due to dietary restrictions, which is most common with hemodialysis, and reduced appetite caused by uremia. Other factors that cause malnutrition are loss of nutrients during RRT through dialysis membrane, metabolic acidosis, inflammation, as well as the catabolic effects of RRT [5].

1.2 Nutrition assessment

Comprehensive nutrition assessment, including but not limited to a history of dietary intake, appetite, body weight and body mass index (BMI), other anthropometric measurements, biochemical data, and nutrition-focused physical findings, is required. This should be done at least within the first 90 days of starting dialysis and monitored regularly. Nutrition assessment is the first step of the nutrition care process; therefore, doing it correctly will ensure appropriate intervention. A combination of screening tools and laboratory parameters is recommended [6].

For patients on maintenance hemodialysis (MHD) and PD, it is reasonable to measure body weight and composition at least monthly and at least quarterly for transplant patients to monitor for any changes. The routine anthropometric measurements include waist circumference, skin fold measurements, and creatinine kinetics. Although BMI should be used routinely for its usefulness in predicting mortality, it should not be used in isolation because it is not sufficient to diagnose Protein-energy wasting (PEW) unless it is less than 18 kg/m^2. Rather, percent change in the usual body may be more reliable for determining the risk of PEW [3].

The comprehensive nutrition assessment will inform the nutrition intervention prescribed. Based on the treatment plan, the renal nutritionist or international equivalent should therefore monitor key nutrition care outcomes, such as dietary nutrient intake, body composition, and serum biomarker levels, after which the plan will be re-assessed and adjusted accordingly to achieve the goals established. The Renal Dietitian will work with the multidisciplinary renal team throughout the nutrition care process. The patient and/or caregiver will be educated on dietary recommendations based on individual needs. Studies show that nutrition education effectively increases patients' compliance with dietary prescriptions [7].

The use of a combination of tools is recommended, including the global subjective tool (SGA) and malnutrition inflammation score (MIS).

When determining the energy requirements, the RDN should consider some factors, including but not limited to RRT modalities, level of physical activity, age, sex, weight status, disease-specific determinants, metabolic stressors, treatment goals, and the patient's overall health status. Studies suggest that diet therapy may aid in lowering dialysis doses to be used safely and effectively even as the glomerular filtration rate continues to decline [8].

2. Medical nutrition therapy in different renal replacement therapy modalities

This section discusses the different nutrient requirements for the different RRT modalities.

2.1 Nutrition therapy in maintenance hemodialysis

The goal of nutrition intervention in MHD patients is to optimize their nutritional status, control blood glucose and blood pressure and fluid overload, keep renal biochemistry within safe limits, and make dietary advice as practical as possible to assist in compliance. For this reason, all renal patients must have adequate renal-specific dietetic or nutritional support [9].

2.1.1 Energy requirements

Chronic Kidney Disease (CKD) impairs energy metabolism; therefore, it is prudent to maintain adequate energy intake, which is necessary to prevent PEW. To maintain a neutral nitrogen balance and nutrition status, studies suggest that energy intake should range between 30 and 35 kcal/kg/day [3].

2.1.2 Protein requirements

For metabolically stable patients, guidelines recommend a dietary protein intake of 1.0–1.2 g/kg body weight per day to maintain a stable nutritional status. However, higher dietary protein levels may need to be considered for patients at risk of hyperglycemia and/or hypoglycemia to maintain glycemic control. Dietary fat should not be restricted because they may be important sources of calories [10].

2.1.3 Potassium

Renal dieticians should focus on individualization, consistent checks on serum potassium levels, and clinical judgment, which would provoke the utilization of other interventions other than dietary restrictions to attain normal serum levels of potassium when appropriate. Studies suggest that dietary potassium restriction may limit heart-healthy diets and lead to the intake of more atherogenic diets [10].

It is important to note that there have not been any clinical trials done on how modifying diet can influence serum potassium levels in patients with CKD [3]. Several factors could influence the shift in serum potassium levels, including [11]: medications such as angiotensin-converting enzyme (ACE) inhibitors, thiazides, and loop diuretics; gastrointestinal problems (vomiting, diarrhea, constipation); acid–base balance; glycemic control; and catabolic state.

Individualized potassium recommendations can improve patient outcomes and quality of life. Moreover, pinpointing the root cause of hyperkalemia would be ideal to help with appropriate interventions. Lindsey suggests the following reflections to help in finding the root cause of hyperkalemia [12]: If the potassium level is consistent with the current trend; if it could be a laboratory error; if there are medications that would affect potassium levels/recent dose change; if there is constipation; the patient's carbon dioxide and blood sugar trend; recent muscle mass loss, reduced appetite, and recent food intake. The author further clarifies that restricting fruits and vegetable may not have a positive impact since most potassium in diets come from coffee, tea, savory foods, beer, animal protein, and dairy.

2.1.4 Phosphorous

Recent studies point out that restrictions on dietary phosphorous may lead to worse survival and poorer nutrition status [10]. The KDQOI guidelines recommend that to reach the decision of restricting dietary phosphorus, there needs to be the presence of progressively or persistently high serum phosphate levels, taking into consideration the trends rather than a single laboratory value and after paying attention to concomitant calcium and parathyroid hormone (PTH) levels [3].

In MHD patients, if the nutrition requirements cannot be met through the oral and enteral intake, intradialytic parenteral nutrition is recommended to improve and maintain nutritional status [3].

2.2 Nutrition therapy in peritoneal dialysis

Guidelines recommend comprehensive and regular nutrition assessment for patients with PD, including body measurements, patient appetite, nutrition-related laboratory markers, clinical status, and dietary intake. However, different factors influence dietary recommendations, and as such, dietary recommendations are not yet universal [13]. Energy requirements range from 30 to 35 kcal/kg/day, with patients below 60 years of age proposed to get 35 kcal/kg/day and those older than 60 years to get 30 kcal/kg/day incorporating the calories from the dialysate into the calculations, which are usually mostly the dextrose because absorption occurs into the patient's body [3].

Patients undergoing PD do quite a number of exchanges in a day; thus, they experience losses of essential elements and nutrients, including amino acids, peptides, vitamins, and trace elements. Dietary restrictions are, therefore, minimal compared to MHD patients. Guidelines suggest that dietary protein should range from 1.0 to 1.3 g/kg/day and even be higher up to 1.5 g/kg/day during peritonitis [3, 13]. Dietary potassium is generally not restricted, while sodium recommendation is <4 g based on serum levels. Phosphorous allowable is between 800 and 1000 mg/day, and phosphate binders with meals are recommended if serum levels are high. The fluid is adjusted based on the dextrose concentration of the dialysate.

2.3 Nutrition therapy in continuous renal replacement therapy

Continuous Renal Replacement Therapy (CRRT) is the modality of choice for critically ill patients. While it permits better control of fluids and is hemodynamically tolerated better than intermittent hemodialysis in critically ill patients, it has greater effects on nutrition [14–16]. The clearance of CCRT is not only specific to uremic toxins; it also clears low molecular substances, which are essential. Macronutrients and micronutrients are also cleared from the patient's blood into the waste [17–20]. Studies are limited on nutrition requirements, and as such, it is impossible to generalize given the different CCRT performance modalities, types of fluids, and different prescriptions [21]. However, some studies suggest that energy requirements range from 20 to 35 kcal/kg/day with a proportion of 60–70% being carbohydrates and 30–40 being lipids, respectively, considering the anabolic and catabolic phases while considering non-nutritional calories and being cautious about overfeeding [6, 19, 22]. Protein requirements range from 1.5 to 2.5 g/kg/IBW/day [23, 24]. There is no standard recommendation for the electrolytes, vitamins, and trace elements, but the medical team should continue monitoring the critically ill patients, checking the serum levels, and correcting/or adjusting the fluids/feeds as appropriate. The medical team should monitor serum levels of phosphorous, potassium, and calcium and adjust as appropriate.

2.4 Nutrition therapy in kidney transplant

Nutrition therapy is very crucial in the acute phase of the post-transplant period (up to eight weeks) to provide adequate nutrition. This would enable wound healing and prevent catabolism, prevent infections, correct clinically significant electrolyte and metabolic abnormalities caused by the immunosuppressive medications, and aid in restoring kidney function. In the chronic phase, nutrition helps to stabilize and prevent deterioration of kidney function and prevents the development of new-onset diabetes after transplant, hypertension, hyperglycemia, anemia, dyslipidemia, and bone disease [25, 26]. Adequate calories are recommended. Therefore, energy requirements should be between 30 and 35 kcal/kg/day and protein 1.2–2.0 g/kg/day in the early period post-transplant [26, 27]. After the first months, protein intake should be reduced to about 0.8 g/kg/day in patients with adequate graft function while adjusting both energy and protein intake for physical activity levels, gender, and age [28]. Some studies suggest that the protein recommendation for the chronic phase post-transplant for the recipients without diabetes should be 0.6–0.8 g/kg/day, while for those with diabetes, it should be 0.8–0.9 g/kg/day [29]. Dietary potassium in the acute phase ranges between 2 and 4 g if the patient has hyperkalemia and unrestricted in the chronic phase unless hyperkalemic. Fluids are generally unrestricted in both phases, and phosphorous should be given as the daily required intake and supplemented if the patient has hypophosphatemia in the acute phase. In the acute phase, sodium should be restricted if blood pressure and fluids dictate in the acute phase while in thechronic phase, sodium should range between 2 and 4 g if the patient has hypertension and/or edema.

Hypophosphatemia is often common in post-transplantation, especially in the first months, and often to lead osteodystrophy and osteomalacia; therefore, it is prudent to prescribe high-phosphorous intake through diet or supplements [3].

The nutrient requirements for each RRT modality are summarized in **Table 1**.

Nutrient requirements	Modality				
	Hemodialysis	PD	CRRT	Transplant	
				Acute phase	Chronic phase
Energy (kcal/kg/day)	30–35 [3] <age60 35 kcal >age60 30 kcal	30–35 [3] <age60 35 kcal >age60 30 kcal	Anabolic phase: 20–25 Catabolic phase: 25–35 [22]	25–35 [3] 30–35 [27] 30–35 [26]	Adjust to maintain body weight
Protein (g/kg/day)	1.0–1.2 [3]	1.0–1.2 [3] 1.2–1.3 [13] 1.3–1.5	1.5–1.7 [23] 1.7–2.0 [22] 2.0–2.5 [24]	1.2–2.0 [26–28]	0.8–1.0 limit with chronic graft dysfunction
Potassium (mg/day)	2300	Not restricted	Monitor serum levels and adjust/correct as appropriate	2000–4000 if hyperkalemic	Unrestricted unless hyperkalemic

Nutrient requirements	Modality				
	Hemodialysis	PD	CRRT	Transplant	
				Acute phase	Chronic phase
Sodium (mg/day)	<2400	3000–4000 Based on labs	Monitor serum levels and adjust/ correct as appropriate	Restrict if BP/ fluids dictate	2000–4000 with HTN and/ or edema
Phosphorous (mg/day)	800–1000	800–1000 Use phosphate binders	Monitor serum levels and adjust/ correct as appropriate	DRI Supplemented if serum levels are low	DRI
Calcium (mg/day)	<2000	<2000	Monitor serum levels and adjust/ correct as appropriate	1200–1500	1200–1500 [26]
Fluids (ml)	500–700 + urine output 1000 if anuric	Adjusted based on dextrose concentrations of dialysate	Individualized	Generally unrestricted	Generally unrestricted

DRI; Daily Recommended Intake.

Table 1.
Nutrient requirements in different RRT modalities.

3. Protein energy wasting

The International Society of Renal Nutrition and Metabolism (ISRNM) proposed the term protein-energy wasting (PEW) to characterize multiple metabolic alterations related to uremia, hypercatabolism, cachexia, and malnutrition associated with morbidity and mortality in kidney disease [2, 3, 30].

The major and most common cause of PEW is inadequate protein and energy intake, compounded by anorexia due to uremia, inflammation, dialysis procedure, and acidemia [31]. Insufficient nutrient intake may also result from glucose absorption from peritoneal dialysate and early satiety feeling, poor economic status, depression, and illness that affects gastrointestinal functions [32]. Nutrient loss during RRT, such as peptides, amino acids, vitamins, trace elements, and glucose, further put the patients at risk of PEW [33].

Studies suggest that adequate energy and protein intake, as recommended in **Table 1**, would help prevent PEW. Other strategies include dialysis adequacy, correcting metabolic acidosis, and treating inflammation and co-morbidities such as diabetes [34–36]. When standard preventive measures cannot reduce the loss of energy and protein stores, nutrition supplementation would suffice. A renal dietitian or equivalent can assess the patient for oral and enteral nutrition supplementation and further intradialytic parenteral nutrition [31].

4. Mineral bone disease

Many CKD patients are at an increased risk of developing CKD- Renal mineral bone disease (MBD). They develop bone lesions symptomatically showing up as pain, including back pain, tendon ruptures, pruritus, and an increased incidence of pathological fractures. Studies show that patients with renal mineral bone disorders are predisposed to calcification of the cardiovascular system and, consequently, increased morbidity and mortality.

This has led to a shift in the treatment of renal mineral bone diseases from just looking at a single biomarker, such as serum calcium levels, to further considering the disease's physiology, thus a look into serum phosphate and parathyroid hormone levels (PTH) [37].

Before the knowledge of fibroblast growth factor 23 (FGF23) and its influence on secondary hyperparathyroidism, phosphate retention was considered the main factor in the disorder occurring [38].

A series of physiological events are triggered by retained phosphate, including hyperphosphatemia, low vitamin D3, and reduced calcium levels, which stimulate parathyroid hormone secretion enhancing phosphate excretion and secondary hyperparathyroidism in end-stage renal disease [39].

There have been observations by authors that hyperphosphatemia and hypocalcemia were evidence of calcitriol deficiency, suggesting that it would be the main culprit to secondary hyperthyroidism noting the complexity of the disease because of the several elements in the pathophysiology [37].

Several studies have documented a strong relationship between serum Fibroblast growth factor 23 levels and creatinine clearance, noting that a decline in renal function had an increase in the FGF23 levels. Further, patients with End Stage renal disease would have up to a 1000-fold above the normal growth factor levels attributed to the reticence of phosphate and decline in renal clearance [40, 41].

The dire consequences associated with secondary hyperparathyroidism place an emphasis on the need to promptly manage CKD renal mineral bone diseases with a keen look and follow-up checks on markers such as serum calcium, phosphate, and parathyroid hormone and calcitriol levels. In light of this, the KDIGO guidelines recommend the onset of management dependent on serial trends of the markers [42].

Through proper nutrition education and counseling, there is a need to limit daily phosphate intake to less than 800 mg, and this is possible by educating the patients on how to read food labels to look out for high phosphate-containing foods and carbonated drinks as well as additives.

This should be done with close nutritional assessment and monitoring as most food sources that are protein in nature are rich in phosphorus. This, in turn, would help prevent protein-energy malnutrition in chronic kidney disease.

Individualized nutrition plans, as far as dietary sources of phosphates are concerned, should have the priority with consideration to intestinal absorption. Plant-based phosphate sources have lower intestinal absorption than those inorganic sources.

The use of phosphate binders has come a long way to help reduce intestinal absorption by allowing the formation of a non-absorbable complex with phosphorus in the food. Three classes of these binders are in use currently, that is, calcium-based binders, aluminum-based binders, and non-calcium-based binders. Caution should be taken with aluminum-based binders as their long-term use has been related to osteomalacia and encephalopathy.

The choice between calcium-based and non-calcium-based binder should, on the other hand, be guided by serum calcium, calcitriol levels, and parathyroid hormones Lest hypercalcemia occurs.

Low cholesterol levels, low uric acid levels, and anti-inflammatory effects have been attributed to using Savelamer, a non-calcium phosphate binder making it have some prominence, particularly where the serum calcium levels are normal. Dialysis is another efficient way of eliminating phosphorus from the bloodstream, yet this is possible with consideration of the type of dialysis, length of dialysis, and type of dialysate.

The most common length of hemodialysis is 4 hours with thrice-a-week sessions that eliminate up to 2600 mg of phosphate levels. However, this may be slightly lower for low resources settings where dialysis is done twice a week. Peritoneal dialysis will succeed at up to 220mmg of phosphate elimination when done four times a day with two-liter exchanges.

4.1 Emerging treatment options for CKD MBD

A new class of phosphate binders, sucroferric oxyhydroxide (PA21) and ferric citrate (JTT-751), are iron-based, calcium-free phosphate binders recently advanced into clinical practice. These have also been used to fix anemia in CKD and attenuate vascular calcification.

Klotho supplementation has also been suggested as a prophylactic or therapeutic therapy for averting secondary hyperparathyroidism. Equally, the usage of anti-FGF23 monoclonal antibodies (FGF23-Ab) to counteract the negative effects of high levels of FGF23 in animal models has been assessed. While counteraction of FGF23 has been characterized by improvement in secondary hyperparathyroidism, increased levels of serum phosphate, aortic calcification, and higher risk of mortality have been reported. Therefore, the therapeutic applicability of FGF23-Ab in humans is yet to be proven.

5. Conclusion

Renal replacement therapy has a great impact on the nutrition status and the overall well-being of renal patients. This chapter discussed medical nutrition therapy focusing on different modalities of renal replacement therapy. It delved into nutrition assessment. Its benefits, and nutrient requirements for each renal replacement therapy. It, finally, discussed the nutrition management of protein energy wasting and mineral bone disease, conditions which are very common among people with end-stage renal diseases.

Acknowledgements

We acknowledge the contribution of Dr. Francis Aila from the Department of Health, Homa Bay County, Kenya.

Conflict of interest

The authors declare no conflict of interest.

Author details

Susan Atieno Onyango[1*] and Grace Nyawira Njuguna[2]

1 Rachuonyo County Hospital, Homa Bay County, Kenya

2 Nanyuki County Teaching and Referral Hospital, Nanyuki, Kenya

*Address all correspondence to: susan.onyango1@gmail.com

References

[1] Sikand G, Handu D, Rozga M, de Waal D, Wong ND. Medical nutrition therapy provided by dietitians is effective and saves healthcare costs in the Management of Adults with Dyslipidemia. Current Atherosclerosis Reports. 2023;**25**(6):1-12. DOI: 10.1007/s11883-023-01096-0

[2] Lu M, Pilla SJ, Oh SH. Diabetes mellitus: Dietary management. In: Caballero B, editor. Encyclopedia of Human Nutrition. 4th ed. Oxford: Academic Press; 2023. pp. 234-251. DOI: 10.1016/B978-0-12-821848-8.00021-4

[3] Ikizler TA et al. KDOQI clinical practice guideline for nutrition in CKD: 2020 update. American Journal of Kidney Diseases. 2020;**76**(3):S1-S107. DOI: 10.1053/j.ajkd.2020.05.006

[4] As'habi A, Najafi I, Tabibi H, Hedayati M. Prevalence of protein energy wasting and its association with cardiovascular disease risk factors in Iranian peritoneal Dialysis patients. Iranian Journal of Kidney Diseases. 2019;**13**(1):8

[5] Visiedo L et al. The impact of nutritional status on health-related quality of life in hemodialysis patients. Scientific Reports. 2022;**12**(1):3029. DOI: 10.1038/s41598-022-07055-0

[6] Ostermann M, Lumlertgul N, Mehta R. Nutritional assessment and support during continuous renal replacement therapy. Seminars in Dialysis. 2021;**34**(6):449-456. DOI: 10.1111/sdi.12973

[7] Paes-Barreto JG et al. Can renal nutrition education improve adherence to a low-protein diet in patients with stages 3 to 5 chronic kidney disease? Journal of Renal Nutrition. 2013;**23**(3):164-171. DOI: 10.1053/j.jrn.2012.10.004

[8] Hanafusa N, Lodebo BT, Kopple JD. Current uses of dietary therapy for patients with far-advanced CKD. Clinical Journal of the American Society of Nephrology. 2017;**12**(7):1190-1195. DOI: 10.2215/CJN.09340916

[9] Rahman T et al. Provision of renal-specific nutrition knowledge for changing dietary practice in Bangladeshi hemodialysis patients. PEC Innovation. 2022;**1**:100028. DOI: 10.1016/j.pecinn.2022.100028

[10] Kalantar-Zadeh K et al. Dietary restrictions in Dialysis patients: Is there anything left to eat? Seminars in Dialysis. 2015;**28**(2):159-168. DOI: 10.1111/sdi.12348

[11] Udensi UK, Tchounwou PB. Potassium homeostasis, oxidative stress, and human disease. International Journal of Clinical and Experimental Physiology. 2017;**4**(3):111-122. DOI: 10.4103/ijcep.ijcep_43_17

[12] Zirker L. Updated Guidelines Challenge Current Standard for Potassium Intake in CKD. Florida, USA: Renal and Urology News; 2023. Available from: https://www. renalandurologynews.com/home/ departments/renal-nutrition-update/ diet-advice-for-blood-pressure-controlgoes-beyond-sodium-restriction/ [Accessed May 12, 2023]

[13] Kimball T, Holotka J, Habura I, Pawlaczyk K. Nutritional status in peritoneal Dialysis: Nutritional guidelines, adequacy and the Management of Malnutrition. Nutrients. 2020;**12**(6):1715. DOI: 10.3390/nu12061715

[14] Bonnassieux M et al. Renal replacement therapy modality in the ICU and renal recovery at hospital discharge. Critical Care Medicine. 2018;**46**(2):e102-e110

[15] Rabindranath KS, Adams J, MacLeod AM, Muirhead N. Intermittent versus continuous renal replacement therapy for acute renal failure in adults. Cochrane Database of Systematic Reviews. 2007;**18**(3):CD003773. DOI:10.1002/14651858.CD003773.pub3

[16] Symons JM et al. Demographic characteristics of pediatric continuous renal replacement therapy: A report of the prospective pediatric continuous renal replacement therapy registry. Clinical Journal of the American Society of Nephrology. 2007;**2**(4):732-738

[17] Fiaccadori E, Regolisti G, Maggiore U. Specialized nutritional support interventions in critically ill patients on renal replacement therapy. Current Opinion in Clinical Nutrition & Metabolic Care. 2013;**16**(2):217-224

[18] Frankenfield DC, Badellino MM, Reynolds HN, Wiles CE III, Siegel JH, Goodarzi S. Amino acid loss and plasma concentration during continuous hemodiafiltration. Journal of Parenteral and Enteral Nutrition. 1993;**17**(6):551-561

[19] Honoré PM et al. Nutritional and metabolic alterations during continuous renal replacement therapy. Blood Purification. 2013;**35**(4):279-284

[20] Bellomo R et al. High protein intake during continuous hemodiafiltration: Impact on amino acids and nitrogen balance. The International Journal of Artificial Organs. 2002;**25**(4):261-268

[21] Fishman G, Singer P. Metabolic and nutritional aspects in continuous renal replacement therapy. Journal of Intensive Medicine. 2023. DOI: 10.1016/j.jointm.2022.11.001

[22] Onichimowski D, Goraj R, Jalali R, Grabala J, Mayzner-Zawadzka E, Czuczwar M. Practical issues of nutrition during continuous renal replacement therapy. Anaesthesiology Intensive Therapy. 2017;**49**(4):309-316. DOI: 10.5603/AIT.a2017.0052

[23] Singer P et al. ESPEN guideline on clinical nutrition in the intensive care unit. Clinical Nutrition. 2019;**38**(1):48-79

[24] McClave SA et al. Guidelines for the provision and assessment of nutrition support therapy in the adult critically ill patient: Society of Critical Care Medicine (SCCM) and American Society for Parenteral and Enteral Nutrition (ASPEN). JPEN. Journal of Parenteral and Enteral Nutrition. 2016;**40**(2):159-211

[25] Veroux M et al. Nutrition in kidney transplantation. The International Journal of Artificial Organs. 2013;**36**(10):677-686

[26] Hong SH, Kim EM, Rha MY. Nutritional intervention process for a patient with kidney transplantation: A case report. Clinical Nutrition Research. 2019;**8**(1):74-78. DOI: 10.7762/cnr.2019.8.1.74

[27] Akbulut G, Gencer-Bingol F. Medical, nutritional therapy for renal transplantation in the COVID-19 pandemic. World Journal of Transplantation. 2021;**11**(6):212-219. DOI: 10.5500/wjt.v11.i6.212

[28] Losappio V et al. Nutrition-based Management of Inflammaging in CKD and renal replacement therapies. Nutrients. 2021;**13**(1):267. DOI: 10.3390/nu13010267

[29] Tiger NB. Owner's manual: Nutrition Care for Your Kidney Transplant. Journal of Renal Nutrition. 2019;**29**(3):249-255

[30] Carrero JJ et al. Etiology of the protein-energy wasting syndrome in chronic kidney disease: A consensus statement from the International Society of Renal Nutrition and Metabolism (ISRNM). Journal of Renal Nutrition. 2013;**23**(2):77-90. DOI: 10.1053/j.jrn.2013.01.001

[31] Alp Ikizler T et al. Prevention and treatment of protein energy wasting in chronic kidney disease patients: A consensus statement by the International Society of Renal Nutrition and Metabolism. Kidney International. 2013;**84**(6):1096-1107. DOI: 10.1038/ki.2013.147

[32] Wright M et al. Disturbed appetite patterns and nutrient intake in peritoneal dialysis patients. Peritoneal Dialysis International. 2003;**23**(6):550-556

[33] Ikizler TA, Flakoll PJ, Parker RA, Hakim RM. Amino acid and albumin losses during hemodialysis. Kidney International. 1994;**46**(3):830-837

[34] Schoenfeld P, Henry R, Laird N, Roxe D. Assessment of the nutritional status of the National Cooperative Dialysis Study population. Kidney International Supplement. 1983;**13**:S80-S88

[35] de Brito-Ashurst I, Varagunam M, Raftery MJ, Yaqoob MM. Bicarbonate supplementation slows progression of CKD and improves nutritional status. Journal of the American Society of Nephrology. 2009;**20**(9):2075-2084

[36] Goldstein SL, Ikizler TA, Zappitelli M, Silverstein DM, Ayus JC. Non-infected hemodialysis catheters are associated with increased inflammation compared to arteriovenous fistulas. Kidney International. 2009;**76**(10):1063-1069

[37] Moe SM, Drüeke T, Lameire N, Eknoyan G. Chronic kidney disease-mineral-bone disorder: A new paradigm. Advances in Chronic Kidney Disease. 2007;**14**(1):3-12. DOI: 10.1053/j.ackd.2006.10.005

[38] Isakova T et al. Fibroblast growth factor 23 is elevated before parathyroid hormone and phosphate in chronic kidney disease. Kidney International. 2011;**79**(12):1370-1378. DOI: 10.1038/ki.2011.47

[39] Habas ES, Eledrisi M, Khan F, Elzouki A-NY. Secondary hyperparathyroidism in chronic kidney disease: Pathophysiology and management. Cureus. 2021;**13**(7):e16388. DOI: 10.7759/cureus.16388

[40] Gutierrez O et al. Fibroblast growth factor-23 mitigates hyperphosphatemia but accentuates calcitriol deficiency in chronic kidney disease. Journal of the American Society of Nephrology. 2005;**16**(7):2205-2215. DOI: 10.1681/ASN.2005010052

[41] Damasiewicz MJ, Toussaint ND, Polkinghorne KR. Fibroblast growth factor 23 in chronic kidney disease: New insights and clinical implications. Nephrology (Carlton). 2011;**16**(3):261-268. DOI: 10.1111/j.1440-1797.2011.01443.x

[42] Kidney Disease: Improving Global Outcomes (KDIGO) CKD-MBD Update Work Group. KDIGO 2017 clinical practice guideline update for the diagnosis, evaluation, prevention, and treatment of chronic kidney disease-mineral and bone disorder (CKD-MBD). Kidney International Supplements (2011). 2017;**7**(1):1-59. DOI: 10.1016/j.kisu.2017.04.001

Chapter 8

Effect of Intra-Dialytic Physical Exercise on Depression in Hemodialysis Patients

Eman Abdelmohsen Sanad

Abstract

In hemodialysis (HD) patients, depression is linked to morbidity, mortality, a worse quality of life, a shorter life expectancy, and even suicidal thoughts. Intradialytic exercise is regarded as a crucial part of the clinical care management of HD patients because it enhances the effectiveness of HD, lowers systemic inflammation, increases exercise tolerance, lowers depressive symptoms, and improves quality of life.

Keywords: intradialytic exercise, depression, hemodialysis, quality of life, hemodialysis effectiveness, exercise tolerance, physical activity, Hamilton depression rating scale

1. Introduction

Hemodialysis (HD) is a common kind of renal replacement therapy for patients with end-stage renal disease (ESRD), which affects up to 90% of patients globally. Muscle wasting, decreased visceral protein storage, and physical function related to uremic myopathy and neuropathy all contribute to patients with ESRD having impaired physical function and activity [1].

Dialysis has a profound impact on how patients interact with their surroundings and how they may play social roles in their families and in society. The necessity of quitting their employment due to financial difficulties, acceptance of treatment schedules with set days and times, frequent hospital stays, and knowledge of their growing reliance on others [2].

The prevalence of depression among HD patients ranges from 20% to 60%, while the levels of worry and stress range from 21% to 48%. Physical activity among patients receiving HD is regarded as a safe and practical non-pharmacological method to lessen depression [3].

The physical and cognitive symptoms of depression include feelings of melancholy, worthlessness, difficulty sleeping, loss of appetite and sexual drive, as well as a lack of interest in routine tasks. When depressive symptoms last longer than 2 weeks, a clinical diagnosis of depression is made (**Figure 1**) [5].

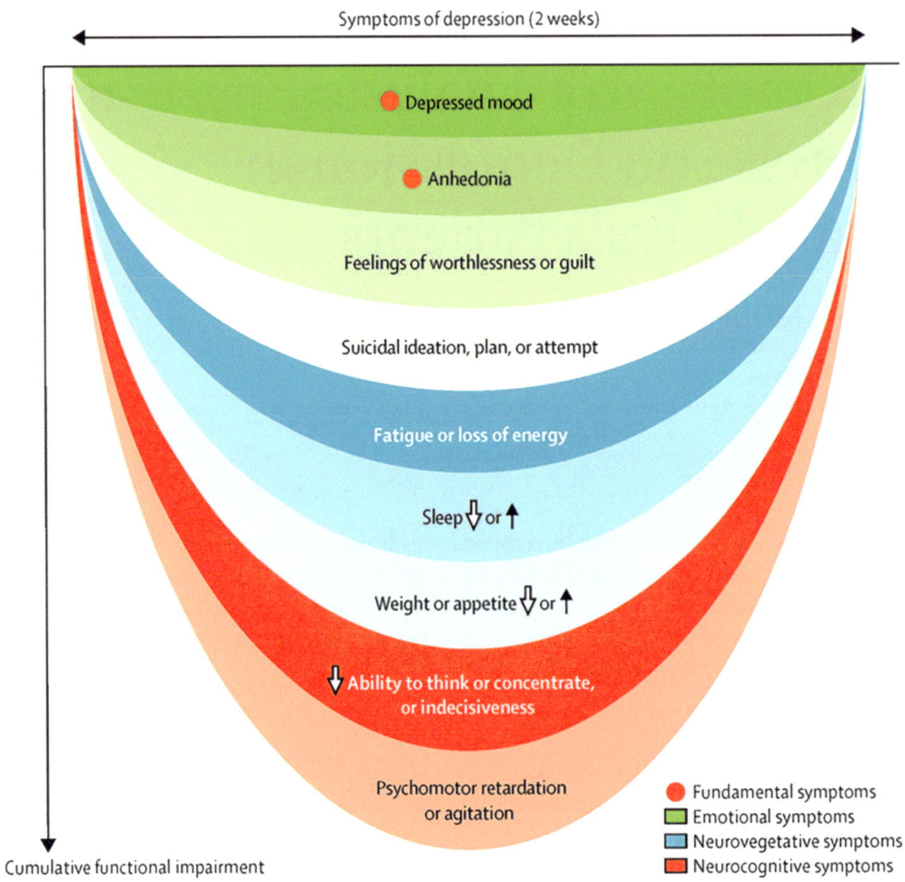

Figure 1.
Depression symptoms [4].

Chronic medical conditions advance significantly as a result of depression. Because depressed people are so hopeless, they are less likely to comply, which aggravates their medical condition. Additionally, nutritional shortages result from loss of appetite, which makes matters worse. A vicious loop would be created by physical health deterioration and depression. Patients on dialysis attempt suicide far more frequently than the overall population [6].

Patients on HD encounter a variety of changes and limits in their everyday life, such as hydration and nutrition restrictions, physical and cognitive impairment, and the inability to perform prior roles, responsibilities, or activities. Patients usually deal with severe psychological load, mostly anxiety and sadness, which has a detrimental impact on how the disease will progress. Death, illness, poor quality of life, limited lifespan, and, worst of all, suicidal thoughts are all associated with depression (**Figure 2**) [8].

Intradialytic exercise (IDE) is frequently advised to patients to promote their physical activity. IDE may be helpful in lowering the degree of exhaustion, improved sleep quality, increasing exercise tolerance, enhancing quality of life, and even improving psychological status, according to earlier studies. IDE can boost the effectiveness of dialysis, reducing inflammation and boosting nutrition and bone mineral density in the process [9].

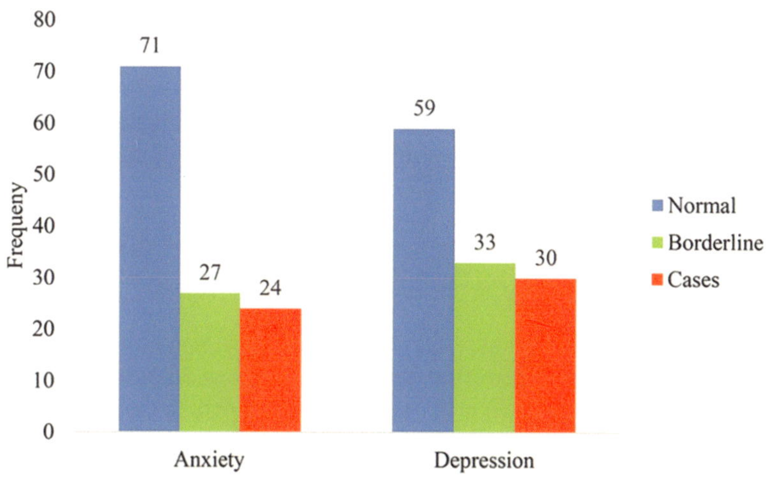

Figure 2.
Prevalence of anxiety and depression in chronic kidney disease patients undergoing HD [7].

The term "intradialytic exercise" refers to exercise training carried out during the HD session to improve the patient's strength and endurance, hence focusing on a variety of physiological and psychological characteristics. Different equipment is employed according to the type of exercise, ranging from stretching to weight training to aerobic activity. HD patients' general health and hospitalization rate have been shown to benefit via IDE [10].

Usually, the first 2 hours of HD therapy are spent engaging in intraadialytic activity. For HD patients, it is a practical non-pharmacological treatment. Placement of a cycle ergometer in front of the treatment chair or at the foot of a bed is the most typical example of IDE training (**Figure 3**) [12].

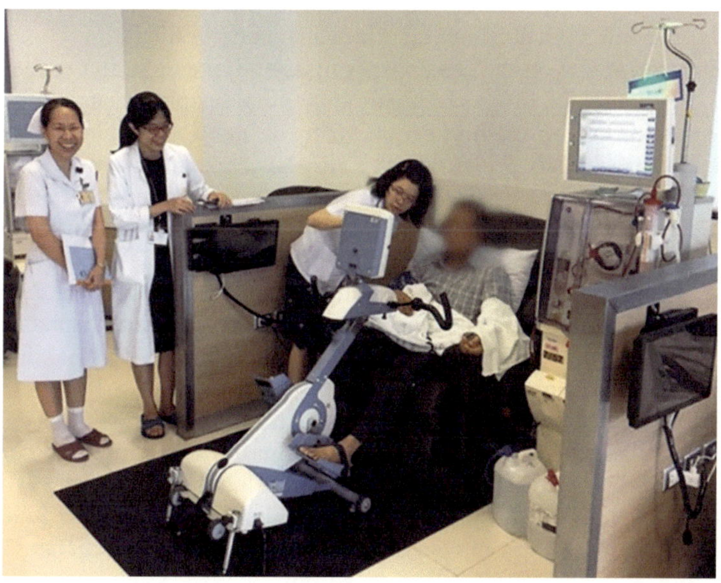

Figure 3.
Intradialytic cycling exercise training program [11].

These are some categories into which exercise may be divided: Aerobic exercise (AE), which works vast muscle groups, is rhythmic, continuous, and typically suggested to increase endurance. Strength training, also known as resistance exercise (RE), is known to enhance muscle growth and strength. Combination exercise (CE), which combines AE and RE, does the same. Every training plan has distinct fitness and health objectives [13].

2. Etiology of depression in HD patients

HD treatments alter the psychological well-being and personality of HD patients. These changes are a result of the continual stressful situations they are exposed to three times per week, as well as the many changes they must adapt to in their personal, social, and professional lives, the need to alter their lifestyle habits, their dependence on HD treatment and medical personnel, their loss of their jobs and social positions, their decreased financial situation, their dietary regimen, their sexual dysfunction, their access to dialysis-related issues, and their anxiety about mortality [14].

Dysphoria (depressed mood) and anhedonia (limited capacity for enjoyment) are characteristics of depression. It has a significant influence on people's social lives, including how interpersonal relationships are affected and how social roles are formed, as well as how neurocognitive abilities are affected. One of the primary emotional problems for which individuals seek treatment is depression. Additionally, depression is the primary cause of suicide fatalities [15].

Depression caused by dialysis has a complex etiology that is influenced by medical, psychological, and social processes. Increased cytokine levels and potential genetic susceptibility are two biological explanations. The loss of a job, sentiments of loss and lack of control, and disrupted family and social connections are examples of psychological and social variables. Fatigue is another factor that contributes to depression in HD patients. Fatigue is a subjective sensation that is defined by weakness, exhaustion, and lack of energy. On HD, between 60% and 97% of patients report feeling tired occasionally, and this has a detrimental effect on quality of life [16].

According to research on the behavioral causes of depression, increasing ESRD-related self-care demands, such as frequent doctor and hospital visits, dietary restrictions, more medication, and at-home monitoring of blood sugar, blood pressure, and weight, might cause despair. Patients with ESRD have been shown to isolate themselves from friends and family and experience financial hardships, both of which have been linked to depression. These patients typically encounter physical symptoms that are connected to uremia, dialysis, and medicines, and these symptoms have been linked to depression. It's still not known if these symptoms lead to depression or if sadness leads to somatic symptoms. Depression may increase the likelihood that people would engage in unhealthy risk-taking behaviors including smoking, staying inactive, and gaining weight [17].

A bidirectional relationship between inflammation and depression in chronic disease was substantiated by the biological mechanisms of depression. This connection is especially important for ESRD patients with high inflammatory markers. Depression has been linked to an increase in inflammation, which can hasten atherosclerosis and result in cardiovascular problems. Depression is also linked to changes in serotonin levels and autonomic nervous system activity, as well as an increase in platelet aggregation and changes in cortisol and norepinephrine production, all of which can result in stroke and cardiovascular events. The brain's ability to regulate mood may

DOI: http://dx.doi.org/10.5772/intechopen.113360

be directly impacted by cerebral vascular disease. For instance, certain post-stroke lesions in the frontal lobe, left anterior, and left basal ganglia have been linked to depression. By causing more inflammation, cerebral vascular disease may potentially indirectly alter mood. Depression has been linked to medication noncompliance, poor food choices, and missed dialysis in ESRD patients (**Figure 4**) [17].

In individuals with depression, several studies have discovered large increases in the levels of the pro-inflammatory cytokines IL-6 and tumor necrosis factor alpha (TNF-α) in the blood. Patients who received repeated injections of recombinant cytokines for the treatment of cancer, viral infections, or autoimmune illnesses showed depressive behaviors and mood changes, such as melancholy, depressed mood, and suicide thoughts. As a result, there seems to be a two-way interaction between depression and inflammation. In other words, both the inflammatory response and the onset of depressed symptoms have the potential to trigger inflammation [19].

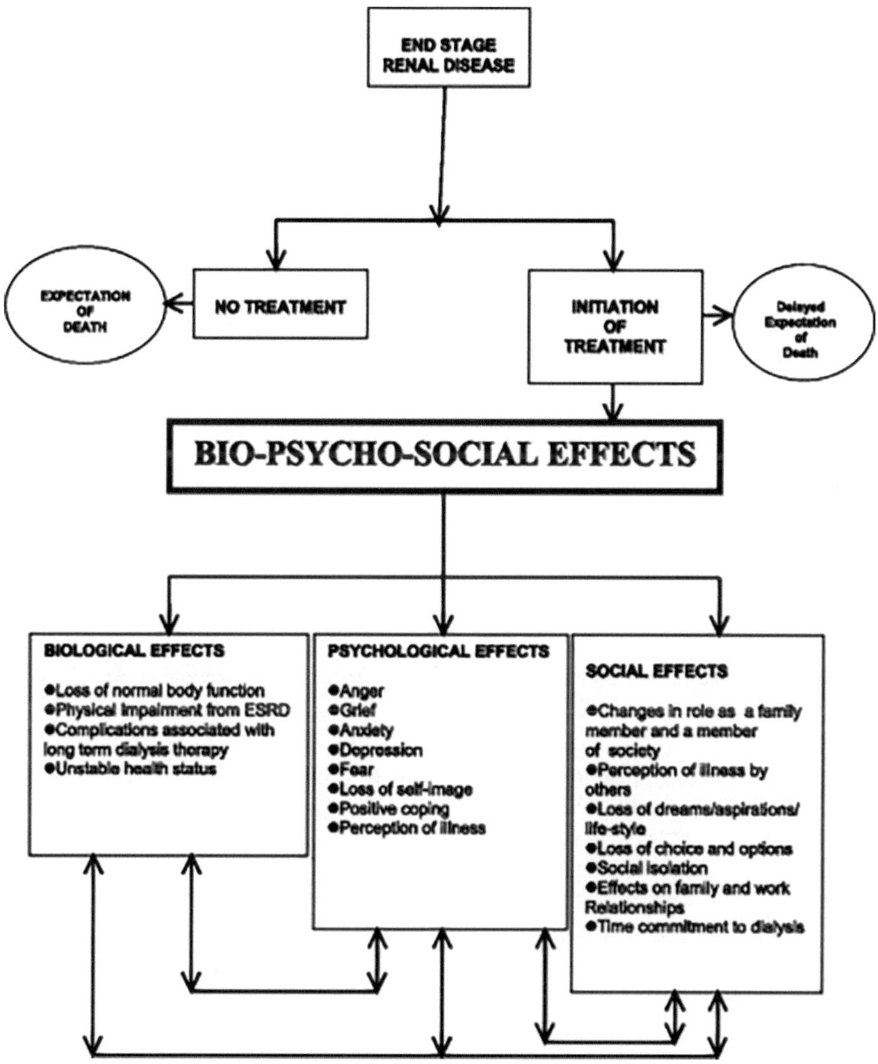

Figure 4.
A conceptual model of the bio-psychosocial links in ESRD [18].

According to the inflammatory theory of depression, cytokine production is dysregulated and immunological responses are too active. TNF-α, IL-1β, and IL-10 levels were all considerably greater in depressed patients, but IL-8 levels were significantly lower. The abnormal expression of inflammatory cytokines in depressed individuals implies that inflammation is triggered by depression. The pathophysiology of depression may be influenced by immunological disorders. Chronic stress has been linked to hypothalamic-pituitary-adrenal (HPA) axis dysfunction, which reduces serotonin synthesis [20].

The forms of vascular access were related to ESRD patients' survival after HD. Due to its decreased mortality and hospitalization rate, arteriovenous fistula (AVF), arteriovenous graft (AVG), and central venous catheter (CVC) are the most desired and suggested vascular access types. The use of CVC was linked to an increased risk of infection, which eventually led to a higher fatality rate. Despite this mounting evidence, CVC is still the method of choice for starting dialysis for more than half of incident HD patients. One of the modifiable variables for depression and health-related quality of life in dialysis patients appears to be the kind of vascular access [21].

In HD patients, uremic pruritus (UP) is a frequent and unsettling issue. Predialysis UP incidence ranges from 15% to 49%, whereas treatment-related UP incidence ranges from 50% to 90%. UP is assumed to have several factors, despite the fact that its pathogenesis is poorly understood. Recent theories contend that UP is caused by modifications to the immune and opioid systems. Increased blood urea nitrogen (BUN), calcium, phosphorus, and 2-microglobulin are risk factors for UP. Additional contributing variables include high ferritin levels, erythropoietin insufficiency, anemia, low transferrin, albumin levels, secondary hyperparathyroidism, elevated calcium, phosphate and magnesium levels, and an increase in chemicals produced by mast cells as histamine. The quality of life, sleep, emotional state, and social interactions of patients are all negatively impacted by UP [22].

Abnormal brain activity in numerous areas, including the prefrontal cortex, is associated with depression. Reduced prefrontal brain activity inhibits the ability to manage unpleasant emotions, which worsens the condition of one's mood [23]. The activity of the amygdala is also elevated during depression [24].

Depression is linked to high cortisol levels that increased during times of stress [25]. Depression is caused by cortisol, which makes the amygdala more active and the prefrontal cortex less active. According to cognitive theories of depression, depressive symptoms are brought on by unfavorable ideas, interpretations, self-evaluations, and expectancies [26].

Cognitive susceptibility and stressful life circumstances can also promote depression [27]. It has long been assumed that a stressful existence might lead to depression, and various studies have confirmed this [28]. Hopelessness theory is another cognitive theory of depression that proposes that a specific type of negative thinking leads to a sense of despair, which ultimately leads to depression [29].

Depression has the potential to negatively impact the medical outcome of ESRD patients through a variety of ways. In dialysis patients, depressive symptoms were linked to poor adherence. Depression has also been linked to changes in immune system function, notably lower cellular immunity and higher cytokine levels. Furthermore, depression has been associated to poor nutritional status and has been demonstrated to precede a decrease in blood albumin levels in ESRD patients (**Figure 5**) [30].

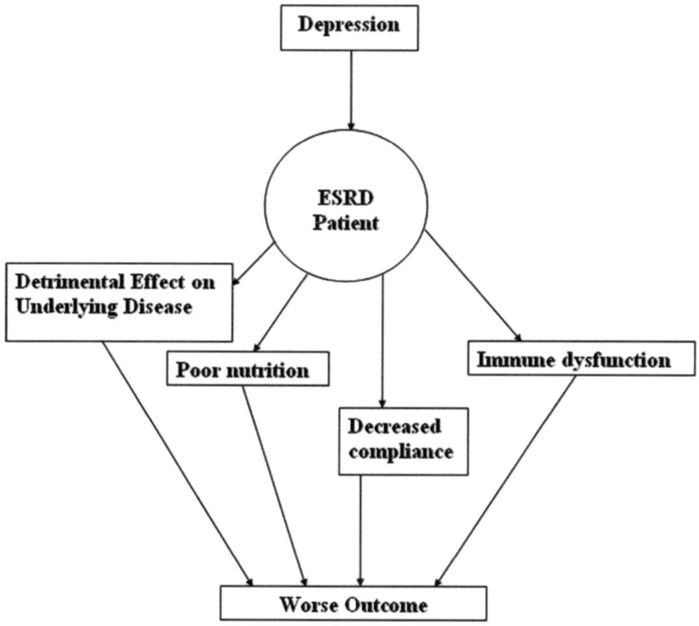

Figure 5.
The impact of depression on medical outcomes [30].

3. Epidemiology of depression in HD patients

Depression is more common among HD patients, with estimated rates ranging from 23% to 42% in the United States and Europe, and 45.9% in Taiwan. Furthermore, clinical depression and subthreshold depressed symptoms are closely linked to poor treatment adherence, increased mortality, and hospitalization rates [31].

ESRD is associated with high rates of both anxiety and depression, with 38% of kidney disease patients reporting anxiety and 27% reporting depression. Since these mood disorders are strongly associated with poor health-related quality of life and adverse outcomes including hospitalization, cardiovascular events, stopping dialysis, and death, it is crucial to detect patients with anxiety and/or depression in the setting of ESRD [32].

4. Depression diagnosis in HD patients

Due to the overlapping medical symptoms of uremia and depression, such as weariness, loss of appetite, disturbed sleep, and other symptoms, evaluating depression in ESRD patients can be challenging. These symptoms may also be influenced by other medical comorbidities, including as sleep apnea and vascular issues, which are common in ESRD [5].

Screening for depression in people with ESRD is critical. Several studies have been conducted to validate the more commonly used depression screening methods in chronic renal disease patients. The Beck Depression Inventory, the Hamilton Rating Scale for Depression, the Nine-Question Patient Health Questionnaire, and the

Center for Epidemiologic Studies Depression Scale are a few of the tests used to check for depression in patients with ESRD [30].

With a self-reported questionnaire, patients with uremic symptoms may test positive for depression. During a clinical interview, these uremic symptoms can be separated from depressed symptoms. As a result, the clinical interview remains the gold standard for detecting depression in ESRD patients [17].

For more than 40 years, the Hamilton depression scale has been the gold standard for assessing depression. It was created in the late 1950s to evaluate the efficacy of the first generation of antidepressants, and it was first published in 1960. The HDRS is the most often used clinician-administered depression scale. The original version has 17 items (HDRS17) referring to depressive symptoms encountered in the previous week. The rating is clinical, and the administration time is 20–30 minutes. The primary goal is to determine the intensity and change of depression symptoms. A score of 0–7 on the HDRS17 is considered normal (or in clinical remission), but a score of 20 or more (showing at least severe severity) is usually necessary for inclusion into a clinical trial [33].

5. Depression treatment in HD patients

Several research have recently examined the impact of antidepressants on cytokine levels and functions. Antidepressants appear to normalize blood levels of key inflammatory cytokines such as IL1 and IL6, as well as TNF. Antidepressants have been shown in certain clinical investigations to reduce the impact of proinflammatory cytokines by boosting the production of antiinflammatory cytokines. Antidepressants may have immune-modulatory effects by decreasing proinflammatory cytokines and increasing antiinflammatory cytokines [19].

Although evidence demonstrate that antidepressants are helpful and safe, side effects such as sleepiness, diarrhea, nausea, vomiting, ejaculatory dysfunctions, sleeplessness, and headache limited their use. As a result, it is critical to investigate non-pharmaceutical therapies. AE has been shown to be useful in the treatment of depression sufferers and has no negative side effects [34].

Physical exercise improves physical functionality, psychological status, and quality of life in ESRD patients, according to studies that have used it as part of their therapy regimen. Physical activity has been shown to significantly improve ESRD patients' levels of depression, quality of life, physical and mental health [35].

Many recent studies have emphasized the need of nonmedical therapies to address depression in HD patients rather than pharmacological therapy; some of these strategies include psychological, behavioral, modified regimens, supporting efforts by families, hypnotism, muscle relaxation, and meditation. Exercise and physical exercise are indicated as non-pharmacological treatments to treat or assist cure serious depression [36].

6. Physical exercise in HD patients

The participation of physical therapy professionals (physiotherapists and exercise physiologists) improved the efficacy and safety of individually recommended exercise regimens. The engagement of exercise professionals considerably contributes to increasing the "exercise culture" in HD units, which is the only way to build a sustainable excellent practice [37].

A nephrologist, a sports medicine doctor, a physiotherapist, nurses, an exercise physiologist, and even a renal nutritionist may establish an exercise dialysis team as a first step. For dialysis patients to successfully implement physical exercise, the following elements may be suggested:

- Involvement of fitness experts
- The dedication of the medical and dialysis personnel
- Thorough evaluation of the patient's physical capabilities
- Individualized workout program prescription for each patient
- Use of intra-dialysis exercise when practical
- Refraining from monotonous or boring workout routines
- Before beginning intra-dialysis exercise, fitness specialists should be present.
- Continual evaluation of the patient's physical capabilities
- Using a pedometer or diary recall to track regular daily exercise, provided you have the right tools [37].

A team of experts and professionals, including a cardiologist, physiotherapist, exercise physiologist, renal dietitian, and nurse, should be led by a nephrologist. Building an effective exercise team, establishing an exercise culture, and raising physical activity levels all contribute to more comprehensive and current clinical care treatment of ESRD patients [37].

The workout consists of the following phases: (a) Warm-up phase: 5 minutes of low-intensity cycling at a slow tempo. (b) Active phase: The patient cycled for 20–25 minutes at the speed obtained during the warm-up phase, after which the speed was increased in increments of nearly one cycle per second until the participant reached an intensity of stress with a fatigue score of 11–13 points, which corresponds to an exercise of (mild) intensity to (quite hard) on the Borg scale. (c) Cool down phase: Following the speed reduction to low speed, a 5-minute cooling down time followed, much like in the warming up phase. This type of training has the advantage that the quick burst of intense activity causes peripheral adaptations in the leg muscles without risking an overload in central mediation. In order to calculate an effort score between 11 and 13, or what would be considered (moderate) to (very hard) exercise on this scale, the bicycle load was maintained [38].

Patients with ESRD are constantly under oxidative stress due to an imbalance between reactive oxygen generation and inadequate endogenous antioxidant defense systems. As a result, oxidative stress encourages the activation of factors that trigger inflammatory processes in these individuals, resulting in a vicious cycle of oxidative stress and inflammation. This process is linked to an increased risk of developing cardiovascular disease (CVD). Physical workouts have been shown in recent research to lower oxidative stress indicators and boost the antioxidant defense system in HD patients; they may help diminish the inflammatory process in these individuals [39].

IDE has been shown to benefit HD patients. As they deal with the issues associated with ESRD, these people need to be less treated as "patients" and encouraged to take a more active role in their health. Obstacles must be overcome by medical and health professionals in order to encourage continued improvements in their patients' health and fitness. IDE programming that is well-planned and supervised can be both safe and efficient, with significant potential for enhanced quality of life [12].

Increasing physical activity should be a goal of clinical care management, however there are barriers that prevent physical exercise programs from being widely used in dialysis units. A HD exercise program may be maintained if three important characteristics are present: (a) participation of exercise specialists; (b) genuine commitment of nephrologists and dialysis professionals; and (c) unique patient customization of the exercise program [37].

Exercise training should be medically monitored and guided by an experienced exercise therapist (or physiotherapist) in HD patients. Physical examination, monitoring of heart rate, blood pressure, and rhythm before, during, and after exercise training should all be part of the supervision. A rigorous supervision allows for the verification of individual responses and tolerability, clinical stability, and the rapid identification of signs and symptoms suggesting the need for program adjustment or discontinuation [40].

However, there may be several exercise-related adverse effects such as fatigue, hypotensive episodes, musculoskeletal complications, and rare cardiovascular complications. The dialyzer experiences a significant flow of uremic toxins from the tissue to the vascular compartment during IDE. It results in increased capillary surface area and improved muscle blood flow. The IDE also showed increased compliance and lower drop-out rates in addition to enhanced adoption and adherence [41].

Exercise regimens must be adapted to each patient's physical capabilities and comorbidities. This is the primary method for implementing physical exercise in ESRD patients in a proper and safe manner. Dialysis nurses play an important role in encouraging and assisting patients during intravenous dialysis. This emphasizes the need of incorporating exercise specialists in a dialysis exercise team. To sum up, before suggesting an exercise program, either extra-dialysis or intra-dialysis, or both, a thorough evaluation of general condition, comorbidities, notably cardiovascular, nutritional state, and physical activity ability is essential. A multidisciplinary team of specialists and professionals, including a cardiologist, physiotherapist, exercise physiologists, renal dieticians, and nurses, should be led by nephrologists (**Figure 6**) [37].

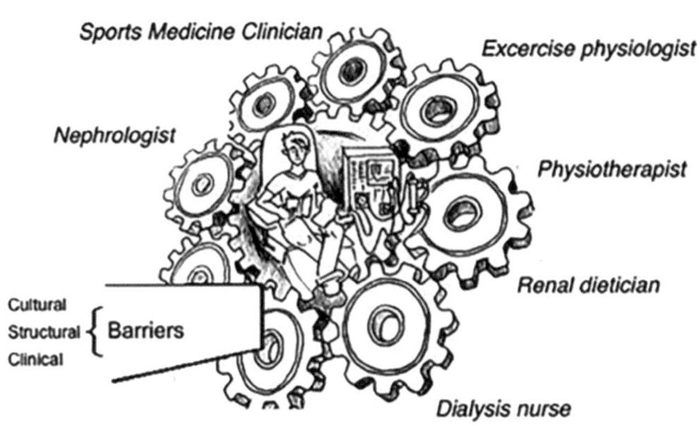

Figure 6.
The ideal exercise team [37].

7. Recommendations for safety and efficacy of exercise training in HD patients

Exercising should be done within the first hour of dialysis; do not exercise if you are hypertensive, cramping, or have a volume overload. Avoiding excessive weights on the vascular access limb; physicians in charge of a workout program Intradialytic or interdialytic exercise is preferable. Strength training is also impractical during dialysis [42].

Aerobic activities dominate intraadialytic exercise regimes. AE is performed with a cycle ergometer or bicycle training. There are several workout plans that use varied exercise frequency, intensities, and durations. It has been demonstrated that AE lasting from 8 weeks to 6 months improved peak VO_2 by around 17% in individuals with ESRD [43].

During dialysis, both endurance and RE training regimes have been routinely used. Most published research papers use intraadialytic cycling as the principal modality of endurance training. Patients bike on a cycle ergometer while receiving HD. Many research have employed intraadialytic resistance training as the predominant modality of exercise [44].

Whole body resistance training, in which muscles are progressively stressed by increasing weights or resistance over time, is the most effective way for enhancing muscular development, strength, and function. Unfortunately, patients confined to a dialysis chair or bed find it challenging to exercise, hence the majority of intradialytic resistance training regimens have relied on low- to moderate-intensity exercises employing ankle weights or elastic bands [45].

Because it affects intradialytic hemodynamic stress, exercise during dialysis session is best done within first 2 hours of dialysis. Exercise commonly raises blood pressure and results in post-exercise hypotension, as is widely recognized. The post-exercise hypotension is particularly alarming since it may raise the likelihood of harmful ischemia episodes, especially in the latter stages of HD when ultrafiltration is reducing the total blood volume [42].

Due to less limitations on the type, amount, and intensity of exercises that patients may conduct when they are not confined to a dialysis chair or bed, interdialytic exercise would appear to offer numerous advantages to intradialytic activities. IDE is supported primarily by the fact that it is highly time-effective for patients and that compliance can be thoroughly tracked [42].

Studies have shown that exercising while receiving dialysis treatments increases the effectiveness of the procedure. These studies' findings imply that intradialytic cycling can improve blood flow to the active leg muscles. This transfers the urea and other toxins that have been held in the muscle compartments to the blood stream for HD elimination. It has been proposed that an additional 20 minutes of dialysis might be equivalent to an hour of AE. Improvements in tiredness levels, sadness, quality of life, sleep, restless legs, inflammation, and hospitalization rates are also seen in the studies [12].

The following The Southern Alberta Renal Program (SARP) recommendations may aid in the delivery of IDE in HD units:

1. The physiotherapist should evaluate each patient's suitability for activity. ESRD comorbidities and etiology, all pertinent blood work, medications, cardiac history, bone health, symptoms (angina, shortness of breath, or pain), previous surgeries, injuries, hospitalizations, falls history, past/current exercise habits,

current living situation, ambulation aids, and ability to perform daily activities must all be covered in a thorough medical history.

2. Patients who have any of the following conditions should avoid exercising (or may need additional medical evaluation):

    - Unstable cardiac state (arrhythmias, severe arterio-venous stenosis, decompensated congestive heart failure, and angina pectoris)
    - Physical conditions that would make using the bike difficult
    - Ineffective blood glucose regulation
    - A current disease or infection
    - An ineffective CVC or AVF/AVG

3. A physiotherapist can do a daily assessment of the safety of activity. Prior to being allowed to exercise, the following prerequisites must be satisfied:

    - Aiming for an ultrafiltration rate (UFR) of less than 13 ml/h/kg
    - BP 180/100 or >100/50 mm Hg
    - Resting heart rate (BPM): 100
    - No illness or hospitalization in the previous week
    - AVF or AVG needing enough needling or a well working CVC
    - Absence of any unusual symptoms (headaches, nausea, dizziness, or the flu).
    - A minimum hemoglobin level of 9 g/dl is required; patients with more problematic cardiac histories may be put on hold until their hemoglobin levels rise.
    - Controlled blood sugar levels (between 126 and 252 mg/dl)
    - Without experiencing any symptoms, oxygen saturation levels should be over 90% at rest and above 88% during activity.

4. If a patient satisfies the safety requirements, the staff may place a pedal cycle in front of the patient's chair for them to use during the first 2 hours after starting dialysis. Patients get instruction on safety, progressive progression, and appropriate warm-up/cool-down techniques during the initial 5- to 10-min bike trial.

5. With the aim of getting at least 30 minutes of exercise during each dialysis treatment, patients self-progress their exercise time by 2–5 minutes every session. Pre-exercise, mid-exercise, and post-exercise vitals and oxygen saturation values are taken in all patients, and blood glucose levels are monitored pre-exercise and post-exercise in diabetics.

6. Special considerations:

    - Cardiac patients are sent for stress testing to ensure safety during exercise.
    - Because HD patients frequently use beta-blockers and may have changes in fluid gains, energy levels, and symptoms, the Borg scale is highly recommended for assessing exercise intensity.
    - No exercise is authorized if a patient misses their preceding HD treatment. Missed treatments might result in fluid overload and hyperkalemia symptoms.
    - Before beginning exercise, patients with a history of hyperkalemia may need at least 30 minutes of HD to reduce the risk associated with this condition.
    - IDE should be temporarily postponed until three consecutive successful HD sessions with double needles have been accomplished before establishing the needling of a new AVF or AVG.
    - HD patients who experience thirst can be advised to chew on ice cubes to help slake their thirst as a way to reduce water intake due to fluid limitations.
    - Patients with intradialytic hypotension could need longer cool-downs. In addition, as soon as activity is stopped, all patients' feet should be raised on the footrest of the chair.
    - Due to the improved blood flow to the leg muscles and peripheral areas, patients may enjoy relief from cramps [12].

The Renal Association Clinical Practice Guideline on Hemodialysis indicated that once patients get accustomed to exercising during dialysis, they be encouraged to do it on non-dialysis days [46].

8. Conclusions

1. In HD patients, a simple AE program provides a supplementary, safe, and successful therapeutic therapy strategy.

2. IDE may alleviate depression by enhancing inflammation, physical performance, and dialysis adequacy.

3. IDE can improve physical performance of ESRD patients

4. It is probable that correctly screening, diagnosing, and treating depression in these people will result in an increase in quality of life.

5. Future research for the development of patient exercise systems must continue to focus on high-quality data and expand the number of plans for varied patient situations. Furthermore, investigations examining the potential negative effects of exercise on HD patients are advised in order to give more thorough data for establishing effective exercise programs.

Abbreviations

HPA	hypothalamic-pituitary-adrenal
HD	hemodialysis
ESRD	end-stage renal disease
IDE	intradialytic exercise
HDRS	Hamilton depression rating scale
TNF-α	tumor necrosis factor alpha
6MWT	six-minute walk test
RAPA	rapid assessment of physical activity
peak VO_2	peak volume of oxygen consumption
PTH	parathyroid hormone
ECG	electro-cardiogram
6MWD	six-minute walk distance
URR	urea reduction ratio
Ca	calcium
PO_4	phosphorus
HB	hemoglobin
ELISA	enzyme linked immune-sorbent assay
T. Sat	transferrin saturation
TSH	thyroid stimulating hormone
IQR	inter quartile range
CVC	central venous catheter
AVF	arterio-venous fistula
AVG	arterio-venous graft

Author details

Eman Abdelmohsen Sanad
Faculty of Medicine, Department of Nephrology and Internal Medicine,
Ain Shams University, Cairo, Egypt

*Address all correspondence to: emysanad90@gmail.com

References

[1] Chung YC, Yeh ML, Liu YM. Effects of intradialytic exercise on the physical function, depression and quality of life for haemodialysis patients: A systematic review and meta-analysis of randomised controlled trials. Journal of Clinical Nursing. 2017;**26**(13-14):1801-1813

[2] Dziubek W, Kowalska J, Kusztal M, Rogowski Ł, Gołębiowski T, Nikifur M, et al. The level of anxiety and depression in dialysis patients undertaking regular physical exercise training-a preliminary study. Kidney and Blood Pressure Research. 2016;**41**(1):86-98

[3] Alradaydeh MF, Khalil AA. The effectiveness of physical exercise on psychological status, and sleep quality among jordanian patients undergoing hemodialysis: Literature review. Open Journal of Nursing. 2019;**9**(12):1267

[4] Malhi GS, Mann JJ. Depression. The Lancet. 2018;**392**(10161):2299-2312

[5] Xing L, Chen R, Diao Y, Qian J, You C, Jiang X. Do psychological interventions reduce depression in hemodialysis patients? A meta-analysis of randomized controlled trials following PRISMA. Medicine. 2016;**95**(34):e4675

[6] Anees M, Barki H, Masood M, Ibrahim M, Mumtaz A. Depression in hemodialysis patients. Pakistan Journal of Medical Sciences. 2008;**24**(4):560-565

[7] Mosleh H, Alenezi M. Prevalence and factors of anxiety and depression in chronic kidney disease patients undergoing hemodialysis: A cross-sectional single-center study in Saudi Arabia. Cureus. 2020;**12**(1):1-8

[8] Lilympaki I, Makri A, Vlantousi K, Koutelekos I, Babatsikou F, Polikandrioti M. Effect of perceived social support on the levels of anxiety and depression of hemodialysis patients. Materia Socio-Medica. 2016;**28**(5):361

[9] Pu J, Jiang Z, Wu W, Li L, Zhang L, Li Y, et al. Efficacy and safety of intradialytic exercise in haemodialysis patients: A systematic review and meta-analysis. BMJ Open. 2019;**9**(1):e020633

[10] Salhab N, Karavetian M, Kooman J, Fiaccadori E, El Khoury CF. Effects of intradialytic aerobic exercise on hemodialysis patients: A systematic review and meta-analysis. Journal of Nephrology. 2019;**32**:549-66

[11] Assawasaksakul N, Sirichana W, Joosri W, Kulaputana O, Eksakulkla S, Ketanun C, et al. Effects of intradialytic cycling exercise on daily physical activity, physical fitness, body composition, and clinical parameters in high-volume online hemodiafiltration patients: A pilot randomized-controlled trial. International Urology and Nephrology. 2021;**53**(2):359-371

[12] Parker K. Intradialytic exercise is medicine for hemodialysis patients. Current Sports Medicine Reports. 2016;**15**(4):269-275

[13] Cho JH, Lee JY, Lee S, Park H, Choi SW, Kim JC. Effect of intradialytic exercise on daily physical activity and sleep quality in maintenance hemodialysis patients. International Urology and Nephrology. 2018;**50**(4):745-754

[14] Čengič B, Resic H. Depression in hemodialysis patients. Bosnian Journal of Basic Medical Sciences. 2010;**10**(Suppl. 1):S73

[15] Tavares AC, Lima RF, Tokumaru RS. Evolutionary theories of depression:

Overview and perspectives. Psicologia USP. 2021;**32**:1-10

[16] Armaly Z, Farah J, Jabbour A, Bisharat B, Abd-El Qader A, Saba S, et al. Major depressive disorders in chronic hemodialysis patients in Nazareth: Identification and assessment. Neuropsychiatric Disease and Treatment. 2012;**8**:329

[17] Shirazian S, Grant CD, Aina O, Mattana J, Khorassani F, Ricardo AC. Depression in chronic kidney disease and end-stage renal disease: Similarities and differences in diagnosis, epidemiology, and management. Kidney International Reports. 2017;**2**(1):94-107

[18] White Y, Grenyer BF. The biopsychosocial impact of end-stage renal disease: The experience of dialysis patients and their partners. Journal of Advanced Nursing. 1999;**30**(6):1312-1320

[19] Taraz M, Taraz S, Dashti-Khavidaki S. Association between depression and inflammatory/anti-inflammatory cytokines in chronic kidney disease and end-stage renal disease patients: A review of literature. Hemodialysis International. 2015;**19**(1):11-22

[20] Zou W, Feng R, Yang Y. Changes in the serum levels of inflammatory cytokines in antidepressant drug-naïve patients with major depression. PLoS One. 2018;**13**(6):e0197267

[21] Kim DH, Park JI, Lee JP, Kim YL, Kang SW, Yang CW, et al. The effects of vascular access types on the survival and quality of life and depression in the incident hemodialysis patients. Renal Failure. 2020;**42**(1):30-39

[22] Ozen N, Cinar FI, Askin D, Mut D. Uremic pruritus and associated factors in hemodialysis patients: A multi-center study. Kidney Research and Clinical Practice. 2018;**37**(2):138

[23] Fitzgerald PB, Laird AR, Maller J, Daskalakis ZJ. A meta-analytic study of changes in brain activation in depression. Human Brain Mapping. 2008;**29**(6):683-695

[24] Drevets WC, Bogers W, Raichle ME. Functional anatomical correlates of antidepressant drug treatment assessed using PET measures of regional glucose metabolism. European Neuropsychopharmacology. 2002;**12**(6):527-544

[25] Halligan SL, Herbert J, Goodyer I, Murray L. Disturbances in morning cortisol secretion in association with maternal postnatal depression predict subsequent depressive symptomatology in adolescents. Biological Psychiatry. 2007;**62**(1):40-46

[26] McDouall J, editor. Mood disorders. In: Introduction to Psychology. Southern Alberta Open Education; 2021. Available from: https://openeducationalberta.ca/saitintropsychology/chapter/mood-disorders/

[27] Gotlib IH, Joormann J. Cognition and depression: Current status and future directions. Annual Review of Clinical Psychology. 2010;**6**:285

[28] Mazure CM. Life stressors as risk factors in depression. Clinical Psychology: Science and Practice. 1998;**5**(3):291

[29] Abramson LY, Metalsky GI, Alloy LB. Hopelessness depression: A theory-based subtype of depression. Psychological Review. 1989;**96**(2):358

[30] Cohen SD, Norris L, Acquaviva K, Peterson RA, Kimmel PL. Screening, diagnosis, and treatment of depression in patients with end-stage renal disease. Clinical Journal of the American Society of Nephrology. 2007;**2**(6):1332-1342

[31] Liu X, Yang X, Yao L, Zhang Q, Sun D, Zhu X, et al. Prevalence and

related factors of depressive symptoms in hemodialysis patients in northern China. BMC Psychiatry. 2017;**17**(1):1-7

[32] Collister D, Rodrigues JC, Mazzetti A, Salisbury K, Morosin L, Rabbat C, et al. Single questions for the screening of anxiety and depression in hemodialysis. Canadian Journal of Kidney Health and Disease. 2019;**6**:2054358118825441

[33] Hamilton M. A rating scale for depression. Journal of Neurology, Neurosurgery, and Psychiatry. 1960;**23**(1):56

[34] Zhao C, Ma H, Yang L, Xiao Y. Long-term bicycle riding ameliorates the depression of the patients undergoing hemodialysis by affecting the levels of interleukin-6 and interleukin-18. Neuropsychiatric Disease and Treatment. 2017;**13**:91

[35] Rajan EJ, Subramanian S. The effect of depression and anxiety on the performance status of end-stage renal disease patients undergoing hemodialysis. Saudi Journal of Kidney Diseases and Transplantation. 2016;**27**(2):331

[36] Rezaei J, Abdi A, Rezaei M, Heydarnezhadian J, Jalali R. Effect of regular exercise program on depression in hemodialysis patients. International Scholarly Research Notices. 2015;**2015**:1-6

[37] Capitanini A, Lange S, D'Alessandro C, Salotti E, Tavolaro A, Baronti ME, et al. Dialysis exercise team: The way to sustain exercise programs in hemodialysis patients. Kidney and Blood Pressure Research. 2014;**39**(2-3):129-133

[38] Henrique DM, Reboredo MD, Chaoubah A, Paula RB. Aerobic exercise improves physical capacity in patients under chronic hemodialysis. Arquivos brasileiros de cardiologia. 2010;**94**:823-828

[39] Esgalhado M, Stockler-Pinto MB, de França Cardozo LF, Costa C, Barboza JE, Mafra D. Effect of acute intradialytic strength physical exercise on oxidative stress and inflammatory responses in hemodialysis patients. Kidney Research and Clinical Practice. 2015;**34**(1):35-40

[40] Liao MT. Intradialytic aerobic cycling exercise alleviates inflammation and improves endothelial progenitor cell count and bone density in hemodialysis patients. Medicine. 2016;**95**(27):e4134

[41] Rhee SY, Song JK, Hong SC, Choi JW, Jeon HJ, Shin DH, et al. Intradialytic exercise improves physical function and reduces intradialytic hypotension and depression in hemodialysis patients. The Korean Journal of Internal Medicine. 2019;**34**(3):588

[42] Wilund KR, Jeong JH, Greenwood SA. Addressing myths about exercise in hemodialysis patients. Seminars in Dialysis. 2019;**32**(4):297-302

[43] Johansen KL. Exercise in the end-stage renal disease population. Journal of the American Society of Nephrology. 2007;**18**:1845-1854

[44] Fang HY, Burrows BT, King AC, Wilund KR. A comparison of intradialytic versus out-of-clinic exercise training programs for hemodialysis patients. Blood Purification. 2020;**49**(1-2):151-157

[45] Piercy KL, Troiano RP, Ballard RM, et al. The Physical Activity Guidelines for Americans. JAMA. 2018;**320**(19):2020-2028

[46] Baker LA, March DS, Wilkinson TJ, Billany RE, Bishop NC, Castle EM, et al. Clinical practice guideline exercise and lifestyle in chronic kidney disease. BMC Nephrology. 2022;**23**(1):1-36

Chapter 9

Psychological Interventions for End-Stage Renal Disease Patients' Receiving Hemodialysis

Haseeba Shouket

Abstract

Hemodialysis is the lifesaving treatment for End-Stage Renal Disease (ESRD) patients; however, the treatment's nature impacts the patient's quality of life and mental health. Focusing on the mental health of patients receiving hemodialysis, the chapter draws attention to the psychological interventions that can improve patient's quality of life. The mental health of ESRD patients receiving hemodialysis can be improved with cognitive-behavioral therapy, psychoeducation, relaxation techniques, peer support groups, spiritual therapy, and technology-based psychological interventions.

Keywords: hemodialysis, mental health, quality of life, psychological interventions, end-stage renal disease

1. Introduction

Globally, hemodialysis is one of the most common forms of renal replacement therapy for End-Stage Renal Disease (ESRD) patients. Around 69% of all kidney replacement therapies and 89% of all dialysis treatments are performed *via* hemodialysis (HD) [1, 2]. HD is performed in the center; hence, the procedure requires frequent visits to the hospital or HD centers, often three times a week for three to four hours, as a result, patients' normal living patterns are substantially altered [3, 4]. Moreover, HD treatment leads to weakness and fatigue along with the limitations of fluid and diet [5, 6]. In addition to these limitations, HD patients face social and financial challenges [7]. Hence, the logical implications of HD influence the patients' life overall and impact their quality of life [8–10].

HD patients are not the only ones affected by the magnitude of change, but also their families, as they depend largely on their families to care for them and provide them with financial support [11–14]. Even though HD treatment improved health maintenance and life extension, the quality of life of the patients is compromised by their survival treatment [15]. In a study [16], untreated depression in high prevalence among HD patients was reported and one of the main reason was the reluctance of patients toward psychotherapy.

A high proportion of patients receiving HD experience a compromised quality of life [17] and report mental health challenges due to adaptive difficulties during

 IntechOpen

disease management [15, 18, 19]. Mental and emotional distress is associated with HD due to restrictions in lifestyle, the constant threat of death, and other physical symptoms that can discourage self-management among patients [20]. According to an estimation, one in five HD patients experience depression [21, 22]. Other commonly reported symptoms are stress, anxiety, fatigue, lowered self-esteem, and social isolation [23–25]. HD patients experience anxiety, depression, and poor quality of life [26]. These mental health problems impact the response of HD patients to their treatment [27]; hence, needs attention.

2. Psychological interventions

Psychological interventions are set of strategies that can be used to change behavior, cognition, or emotions [28]. It refers to relationships designed to increase an individual's ability to adapt to a situation and optimize his or her personal resources in relation to autonomy, self-knowledge, and self-help [29]. Psychological interventions not only have the potential to reduce depression and anxiety among patients receiving hemodialysis [30] but also improves their quality of life [31, 32]. In other words, psychological interventions can promote mental health that can prevent the occurrence of psychological disorders, for example, depression. It is extremely important to understand that mental health is more than just the absence of mental disorders [33]. According to World Health Organization, mental health is described as:

> *"Mental health is a state of mental well-being that enables people to cope with the stresses of life, realize their abilities, learn well and work well, and contribute to their community. It is an integral component of health and well-being that underpins our individual and collective abilities to make decisions, build relationships and shape the world we live in" [33].*

Therefore, it is important to improve the quality of life even in the absence of any mental health problem by fostering healthy thoughts and behaviors [34], which can be possible by incorporating psychological interventions in health care of HD patients. Hence, the use of psychological intervention with ESRD patients on maintenance HD is extremely important.

3. Psychological interventions for ESRD patients receiving HD

Psychological interventions can be effectively improving the mental health of ESRD patients receiving HD. These interventions are delivered either individually [35], in groups [36, 37], or by guided self-help [38, 39]. Cognitive-behavioral therapy (CBT), psychoeducation/educational interventions, relaxation techniques, peer support groups, spiritual therapy, technology-based psychological interventions, and other psychotherapeutic techniques are effective in improving the mental health of ESRD patients receiving HD (**Figure 1**) [40, 41].

3.1 Cognitive-behavioral therapy (CBT)

CBT is the widely used psychological intervention for HD patients [32]. It aims to develop a positive attitude toward hemodialysis by countering negative thoughts and

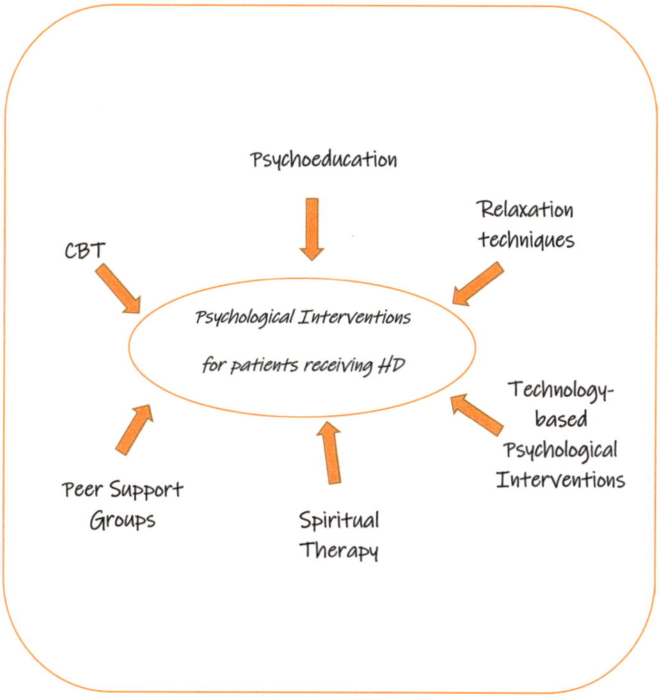

Figure 1.
Psychological interventions for ESRD patients receiving HD.

improving the patients' acceptance and understanding of their disease and HD [42]. Moreover, CBT helps to internalize HD patients' locus of control [43]. Therefore, reduce depression [44, 45] and anxiety and improves quality of life of the patients undergoing HD [46, 47]. CBT is effective in increasing hope among ESRD patients receiving HD and dealing with their death anxiety [48].

The benefits of CBT extend into physical health as well. For instance, HD patients can benefit from CBT techniques, including sleep hygiene, to reduce their sleep disturbances [49, 50]. Furthermore, fluid control, which is integral to HD [51], can be achieved by using techniques such as reinforcement, self-monitoring, self-contracting, and other CBT techniques [52, 53]. Moreover, mindfulness meditation improves the biological markers of ESRD patients receiving HD [54]. BReF is specially designed CBT to reduce fatigue among ESRD patients receiving HD by creating consistent activity and rest routines throughout the day [55].

In a systematic review [56], it was concluded that the most promising psychological interventions were thought to be those that have cognitive and behavioral components. These findings highlight the importance of CBT for ESRD patients receiving HD. However, despite the evidence from the literature for the effectiveness of CBT in improving the quality of life and self-management among patients receiving HD patients, it is not being incorporated into practice [57].

3.2 Psychoeducation

Psychoeducation educates patients about the nature of their illness and how to manage the problems associated with illness [58]. These education-based psychological interventions for ESRD patients receiving HD are aimed to surge their capability of goal setting and health literacy [32]. ESRD patients receiving HD were when psycho-educated, it changed their understanding and some beliefs about their survival treatment; hence, improves adherence behavior toward treatment [59]. In the case of HD, psychoeducation is beneficial at any stage of HD, but when used either before starting HD or in the initial stage exhibits significant advantages [60]. Psychoeducation can be used to address anxiety and depression among hemodialysis [61]. Al saraireh, Aloush [62] preferred psychoeducation over CBT for depression among patients receiving HD. Family-based psychoeducation program is beneficial for HD patients and their families [63]. In most studies [61, 62, 64, 65], ESRD patients undergoing HD were educated about normal kidney function and renal failure, demonstration of the dialysis procedure, diet and fluid, hygiene, essential needed care, and renal replacement options. However, only a few studies included information about potential problem-solving skills, individual stress management, adaptive responses, such as muscle relaxation [61, 62] and emotion-focused coping strategies [64].

3.3 Relaxation techniques

Patients with ESRD who receive HD can benefit from relaxation techniques. Psychological interventions based on relaxation promote self-regulation, emotional, cognitive, and behavioral flexibility among ESRD patients receiving HD [32]. Moreover, literature illustrates that relaxation technique can improve sleep quality [66–68], activity level [69], adherence to HD and other biomedical markers [70] and reduces pain [71, 72], fatigue [73], depression [74], and anxiety [75] among patients' receiving HD.

Relaxation techniques, including Benson's relaxation technique [66, 67, 69, 70, 72, 74], progressive muscle relaxation [71, 75, 76], and music relaxation therapy [77], can help ESRD patients undergoing HD. These techniques can be used in combination with other relaxation techniques, for instance, Benson relaxation with progressive muscle relaxation [78] and music therapy [79]. Aerobic exercise with relaxation techniques can improve the psychological health of ESRD patients undergoing HD [80]. However, relaxation techniques were suggested to use consistently for longer time, for example, one month among hemodialysis patients [81]. Relaxation techniques can effectively reduce psychological symptoms and improve the quality of life among elderly ESRD patients receiving HD. Hence, it is recommended to use these relaxation techniques in hospitals or HD centers [67].

3.4 Peer support

Peer-to-peer support improves the quality of life [82], self-management [83], hope [84], and mental health [85, 86] of the HD patients undergoing. Moreover, physical outcomes among HD patients receiving were also reported due to peer support [87]. Patient's "real knowledge" can be more beneficial to other patients undergoing hemodialysis if they share it with other fellow patients [83].

Peer to support benefits both; mentors and mentees in terms of knowledge, self-efficacy, and social support [88]. However, mentors should be trained prior to peer-to-peer mentoring about kidney disease, active listening, communication skills, privacy, and confidentiality [88]. Peer support sessions can also be moderators with the help of facilitators [84]. Generally, patients' can be benefited from informational, spiritual, instrumental, and emotional support from their fellow patients undergoing maintenance hemodialysis [84]. Moreover, peer support groups promoting self-transcendence were found to improve physical health status and quality of life among HD patients [37].

Peer support for ESRD patients undergoing HD can be done face-to-face or remote. However, HD patients prefer face-to-face peer support instead of remote telephonic peer support [89]. Online peer support was found effective for adolescents [90] and pediatric HD patients [91]. In a study [83], peer support programs were suggested to introduced in the early phase of HD to ESRD patients. Early support from their peers can help them manage their problems and themselves. Although peer support is found effective in improving physical health and psychological well-being, it is not taken advantage of this psychological intervention [92].

3.5 Spiritual practices

ESRD undergoing HD who use their religious beliefs and practices to cope with their lifelong survival treatment are less likely to experience psychological problems [23, 93, 94]. Spiritual therapy was effectively used with patients' receiving HD to improve their well-being [95], lifestyle [96], hope [97], resilience [98], and reducing their stress, anxiety, depression [99, 100].

In cases of HD, spiritual therapy proved especially effective since HD patients' lifestyle changes have affected their quality of life and researchers found that spirituality improves quality of life [101, 102]. In this context, spiritual interventions became increasingly important for HD patients [103]. Through religious practices, reading religious books, listening to spiritual music, and changing perspectives, spiritual therapy promotes optimism, hope, gratitude, contemplation, patience, raising awareness, and addressing problems through religious beliefs [91, 95, 99, 104, 105]. Further, Hosseini, Naseri-Salahshour [106] found that HD-related fear of death can be addressed through religious counseling. Therefore, spiritual therapy should be utilized as a complement to health care to increase treatment effectiveness [99].

3.6 Tech-based psychological intervention

Digital technologies (e.g., websites, applications, VR, and telephone) have been increasingly incorporated to optimize HD patients' quality of life. The use of technology-based psychological interventions is accepted, feasible, and needs minimum additional resources to address the mental health of patients on maintenance HD [107]. With the help of technology, it is possible to manage depression, anxiety, fatigue, self-efficacy, and self-management among patients receiving HD [108].

Psychological interventions with the help of digital technologies were tested in various forms with ESRD patients undergoing HD. The use of internet-based positive psychological interventions is an effective therapeutic option for HD patients with depression [109]. Internet-delivered CBT can reduce depression and anxiety among HD patients [110]. Further, therapist-guided Internet-based cognitive-behavioral therapy interventions address the problems associated with HD patients' experience [111]. Video-based ACT can also help HD patients to cope with the challenges associated with HD [112]. App-based self-management intervention can potentially improve the self-efficacy and basic psychological needs of elderly HD patients [113]. Additionally, immersed virtual reality during HD proved to be an active detraction and has the potential to address dialysis-related problems [114].

On the other hand, in tablet-based educational and motivational interviewing interventions when used with patients during HD, certain problems were reported in the user interface [115]. Similarly, HD patients with depression seem not to benefit from guided internet-based self-help problem-solving therapy [116]. In a systematic review, Marin and Redolat [108], the majority of the tech-based psychological intervention studies focused on psychological symptoms associated with HD, and there is a scarcity of literature aiming to target the cognitive functioning of patients' receiving HD. Hence, there is a need to carefully design the content and approachability of the psychological intervention of HD patients.

4. Conclusion

Psychological intervention in several forms also positively changes the HD experience for ESRD patients. Social activity, for instance, participating in theater play reduces depression and improves self-esteem among HD patients [117]. Motivational interviewing can improve the well-being of ESRD patients undergoing HD [32]. Counseling of ESRD patients undergoing HD can improve their quality of life [118]. Guided imagery has the potential to influence the psychological and physical health of hemodialysis patients [119]. These non-pharmacological psychological interventions are extremely important and should be part of the health care for ESRD patients undergoing HD [15] because HD is not merely a treatment procedure for ESRD it actually leads to the major lifestyle change that challenges patients' mental health [19].

Author details

Haseeba Shouket
Edith Cowan University, Perth, Australia

*Address all correspondence to: hshouket@our.ecu.edu.au; haseebashoukat@gmail.com

References

[1] Bello AK, Okpechi IG, Osman MA, Cho Y, Htay H, Jha V, et al. Epidemiology of haemodialysis outcomes. Nature Reviews Nephrology. 2022;**18**(6):378-395

[2] Liyanage T, Ninomiya T, Jha V, Neal B, Patrice HM, Okpechi I, et al. Worldwide access to treatment for end-stage kidney disease: A systematic review. The Lancet. 2015;**385**(9981):1975-1982

[3] Avramovic M, Stefanovic V. Health-related quality of life in different stages of renal failure. Artificial Organs. 2012;**36**(7):581-589

[4] Gerasimoula K, Lefkothea L, Maria L, Victoria A, Paraskevi T, Maria P. Quality of life in hemodialysis patients. Materials Sociomedicine. 2015;**27**(5):305-309

[5] Hatthakit U. Lived experiences of patients on hemodialysis: A meta-synthesis. Nephrology Nursing Journal. 2012;**39**(4)

[6] Chiaranai C. The lived experience of patients receiving hemodialysis treatment for end-stage renal disease: A qualitative study. Journal of Nursing Research. 2016;**24**(2):101-108

[7] Al-Ghabeesh S, Suleiman K. The lived experience of patients' with end stage renal disease on hemodialysis: A phenomenological study. International Journal of Medicine and Medical Sciences. 2014;**47**(1):1423-1429

[8] Chuasuwan A, Pooripussarakul S, Thakkinstian A, Ingsathit A, Pattanaprateep O. Comparisons of quality of life between patients underwent peritoneal dialysis and hemodialysis: A systematic review and meta-analysis. Health and Quality of Life Outcomes. 2020;**18**(1):191

[9] Lim KH, Kwon GS. Factors affecting quality of life in Hemodialysis patients. Journal of Korean Academic Fundamental Nursing. 2023;**30**(1):1-12

[10] El-Habashi AF, El-Agroudy AE, Jaradat A, Alnasser ZH, Almajrafi HH, Alharbi RH, et al. Quality of life and its determinants among Hemodialysis patients: A single-Center study. Saudi Journal of Kidney Diseases and Transplantation. 2020;**31**(2):460-472

[11] Abebe A, Arba A, Paulos K, Abera W, Sidamo T, Shiferaw S, et al. The lived experience of primary family caregivers of patients on Hemodialysis treatment in southern Ethiopia: A phenomenological study. International Journal of Nephrology and Renovascular Disease. 2022;**15**:41-52

[12] Beard MP. The impact of hemodialysis and transplantation on the family. Critical Care Nursing Quarterly. 1978;**1**(2):87

[13] Ebadi A, Sajadi SA, Moradian ST, Akbari R. Psychological consequences for family caregivers of patients receiving hemodialysis: Threat or opportunity? BMC Psychology. 2021;**9**(1):154

[14] Farzi S, Farzi S, Moladoost A, Ehsani M, Shahriari M, Moieni M. Caring burden and quality of life of family caregivers in patients undergoing Hemodialysis: A descriptive-analytic study. International Journal of Community Based Nursing Midwifery. 2019;**7**(2):88-96

[15] Schmidt DB. Quality of life and mental health in hemodialysis patients: A challenge for multiprofessional practices. SciELO Brasil. 2019;**2019**:10-11

[16] Johnson S, Dwyer A. Patient perceived barriers to treatment of depression and anxiety in hemodialysis patients. Clinical Nephrology. 2008;**69**(3):201-206

[17] Elhadad AA, Ragab AZEA, Atia SAA. Psychiatric comorbidity and quality of life in patients undergoing hemodialysis. Middle East Current Psychiatry. 2020;**27**(1):9

[18] Ginieri-Coccossis M, Theofilou P, Synodinou C, Tomaras V, Soldatos C. Quality of life, mental health and health beliefs in haemodialysis and peritoneal dialysis patients: Investigating differences in early and later years of current treatment. BMC Nephrology. 2008;**9**(1):14

[19] Goyal E, Chaudhury S, Saldanha D. Psychiatric comorbidity in patients undergoing hemodialysis. Industrial Psychiatry Journal. 2018;**27**(2):206-212

[20] Nataatmadja M, Evangelidis N, Manera KE, Cho Y, Johnson DW, Craig JC, et al. Perspectives on mental health among patients receiving dialysis. Nephrology Dialysis Transplantation. 2020;**36**(7):1317-1325

[21] Amira O. Prevalence of symptoms of depression among patients with chronic kidney disease. Nigerian Journal of Clinical Practice. 2011;**14**(4):460-463

[22] Mosleh H, Alenezi M, Al Johani S, Alsani A, Fairaq G, Bedaiwi R. Prevalence and factors of anxiety and depression in chronic kidney disease patients undergoing Hemodialysis: A cross-sectional single-Center study in Saudi Arabia. Cureus. 2020;**12**(1):e6668

[23] Senmar M, Razaghpoor A, Mousavi AS, Zarrinkolah F, Esmaeili F, Rafiei H. Psychological symptoms in patients on Dialysis and their relationship with spiritual well-being. Florence Nightingale Journal of Nursing. 2020;**28**(3):243-249

[24] Alkhaqani A. Psychological impact of chronic kidney disease and Hemodialysis: Narrative review. Psychosometric Medical Research. 2022;**4**(2):1-5

[25] Marthoenis M, Syukri M, Abdullah A, Tandi TMR, Putra N, Laura H, et al. Quality of life, depression, and anxiety of patients undergoing hemodialysis: Significant role of acceptance of the illness. The International Journal of Psychiatry in Medicine. 2021;**56**(1):40-50

[26] Daniel SC, Azuero A, Gutierrez OM, Heaton K. Examining the relationship between nutrition, quality of life, and depression in hemodialysis patients. Quality of Life Research. 2021;**30**:759-768

[27] Anjomshoa F, Esmaeili-Abdar M, Rafiei H, Arjmand-Kermani M, Hassanarabi F, Hasani A, et al. Depression among hemodialysis patients: A cross-sectional study in southeast of Iran. International Journal of Epidemiological Research. 2014;**1**(1):24-28

[28] Antonio Sandu AF, Unguru E. Ethics in Research Practice and Innovation. Hershey, PA, USA: IGI Global; 2018

[29] Horvath AO, Del Re A, Flückiger C, Symonds D. Alliance in individual psychotherapy. Psychotherapy. 2011;**48**(1):9

[30] Bargiel-Matusiewicz K, Łyś A, Stelmachowska P. The positive influence of psychological intervention on the level of anxiety and depression in dialysis patients: A pilot study. The International Journal of Artificial Organs. 2019;**42**(4):167-174

[31] Lerma A, Perez-Grovas H, Bermudez L, Peralta-Pedrero ML, Robles-García R, Lerma C. Brief cognitive behavioural intervention for depression and anxiety symptoms improves quality of life in chronic haemodialysis patients. Psychology and Psychotherapy: Theory, Research and Practice. 2017;**90**(1):105-123

[32] Barello S, Anderson G, Acampora M, Bosio C, Guida E, Irace V, et al. The effect of psychosocial interventions on depression, anxiety, and quality of life in hemodialysis patients: A systematic review and a meta-analysis. International Urology and Nephrology. 2023;**55**(4):897-912

[33] Mental Health [Internet]. 2022. Available from: https://www.who.int/news-room/fact-sheets/detail/mental-health-strengthening-our-response

[34] Feldman DB, Dreher DE. Can hope be changed in 90 minutes? Testing the efficacy of a single-session goal-pursuit intervention for college students. Journal of Happiness Studies. 2012;**13**(4):745-759

[35] Anson HM, Byrd MR, Koch EI. Cognitive behavioral treatment to improve adherence to hemodialysis fluid restrictions: A case report. Case Reports in Medicine. 2009;**2009**:835262. DOI: 10.1155/2009/835262

[36] Sharp J, Wild MR, Gumley AI, Deighan CJ. A cognitive behavioral group approach to enhance adherence to hemodialysis fluid restrictions: A randomized controlled trial. American Journal of Kidney Diseases. 2005;**45**(6):1046-1057

[37] Milani MJ, Amiri P, Vejdani M, Salehiniya H, Malek-Khahi A. The effect of peer support group on self-transcendence in patients undergoing haemodialysis. Biomedical Research and Therapy. 2017;**4**(03):1198-1209

[38] Nadort E, Schouten RW, Dekker FW, Honig A, van Oppen P, Siegert CE. The (cost) effectiveness of guided internet-based self-help CBT for dialysis patients with symptoms of depression: Study protocol of a randomised controlled trial. BMC Psychiatry. 2019;**19**:1-9

[39] Vogt W. Acceptance and Commitment Therapy Self-Help Intervention for Depression in Haemodialysis Patients: a Feasibility Randomised Controlled Trial. Lincoln, England: University of Lincoln; 2016

[40] Xing L, Chen R, Diao Y, Qian J, You C, Jiang X. Do psychological interventions reduce depression in hemodialysis patients?: A meta-analysis of randomized controlled trials following PRISMA. Medicine (Baltimore). 2016;**95**(34):e4675

[41] Natale P, Palmer SC, Ruospo M, Saglimbene VM, Rabindranath KS, Strippoli GFM. Psychosocial interventions for preventing and treating depression in dialysis patients. Cochrane Database of Systematic Reviews. 2019;**12**(12):CD004542. DOI: 10.1002/14651858.CD004542.pub3

[42] Ng CZ, Tang SC, Chan M, Tran BX, Ho CS, Tam WW, et al. A systematic review and meta-analysis of randomized controlled trials of cognitive behavioral therapy for hemodialysis patients with depression. Journal of Psychosomatic Research. 2019;**126**:109834

[43] Mehrtak M, Habibzadeh S, Farzaneh E, Rjaei-Khiavi A. Effectiveness of teaching cognitive-behavioral techniques on locus of control in hemodialysis patients. Electronic Physician. 2017;**9**(10):5631-5637

[44] Marvi A, Bayazi MH, Rahmani M, Deloei AK. Studying the effect of cognitive Behavioral group training on depression in Hemodialysis patients. Procedia – Social and Behavioral Sciences. 2011;**30**:1831-1836

[45] Daniel Cukor PD. Use of CBT to treat depression among patients on Hemodialysis. Psychiatric Services. 2007;**58**(5):711-712

[46] Duarte PS, Miyazaki MC, Blay SL, Sesso R. Cognitive–behavioral group therapy is an effective treatment for major depression in hemodialysis patients. Kidney International. 2009;**76**(4):414-421

[47] Rouhi M, Manzari Tavakoli A, Tajrobehkar M. The effectiveness of cognitive Behavioral therapy on coherent self- knowledge, emotion regulation, and quality of life of Hemodialysis patients: A quasi-experimental study. Journal of Rafsanjan University of Medical Sciences. 2023;**21**(10):1055-1070

[48] Saki M, Khoshnood S, Mohammadipour F, Ebrahimzadeh F, Rezaei F. The effect of cognitive–behavioral intervention on hope and death anxiety level in patients undergoing hemodialysis. The Journal of Mental Health Training, Education and Practice. 2022;**17**(3):181-190

[49] Chen H-Y, Cheng IC, Pan Y-J, Chiu Y-L, Hsu S-P, Pai M-F, et al. Cognitive-behavioral therapy for sleep disturbance decreases inflammatory cytokines and oxidative stress in hemodialysis patients. Kidney International. 2011;**80**(4):415-422

[50] Hou Y, Hu P, Liang Y, Mo Z. Effects of cognitive behavioral therapy on insomnia of maintenance hemodialysis patients. Cell Biochemistry and Biophysics. 2014;**69**(3):531-537

[51] Canaud B, Chazot C, Koomans J, Collins A. Fluid and hemodynamic management in hemodialysis patients: Challenges and opportunities. Jornal Brasileiro de Nefrologia. 2019;**41**(4):550-559

[52] Sagawa M, Oka M, Chaboyer W, Satoh W, Yamaguchi M. Cognitive behavioral therapy for fluid control in hemodialysis patients. Nephrology Nursing Journal. 2001;**2001**:37

[53] Sharp J, Wild MR, Gumley AI. A systematic review of psychological interventions for the treatment of nonadherence to fluid-intake restrictions in people receiving hemodialysis. American Journal of Kidney Diseases. 2005;**45**(1):15-27

[54] Sohn BK, Oh YK, Choi JS, Song J, Lim A, Lee JP, et al. Effectiveness of group cognitive behavioral therapy with mindfulness in end-stage renal disease hemodialysis patients. Kidney Research Clinical Practise. 2018;**37**(1):77-84

[55] Picariello F, Moss-Morris R, Norton S, Macdougall IC, Da Silva-Gane M, Farrington K, et al. Feasibility trial of cognitive behavioral therapy for fatigue in Hemodialysis (BReF intervention). Journal of Pain and Symptom Management. 2021;**61**(6):1234-46.e5

[56] Matteson ML, Russell C. Interventions to improve hemodialysis adherence: A systematic review of randomized-controlled trials. Hemodialysis International. 2010;**14**(4):370-382

[57] Shirazian S, Smaldone A, Rao MK, Silberzweig J, Jacobson AM, Fazzari M, et al. A protocol for a pilot randomized controlled trial to assess the feasibility and effect of a cognitive behavioral

intervention on quality of life for patients on hemodialysis. Contemporary Clinical Trials. 2018;**73**:51-60

[58] Taylor S. 11.11 - pandemics and clinical psychology. In: Asmundson GJG, editor. Comprehensive Clinical Psychology. Second ed. Oxford: Elsevier; 2022. pp. 151-166

[59] Karamanidou C, Weinman J, Horne R. Improving haemodialysis patients' understanding of phosphate-binding medication: A pilot study of a psycho-educational intervention designed to change patients' perceptions of the problem and treatment. British Journal of Health Psychology. 2008;**13**(2):205-214

[60] Devins GM, Hollomby DJ, Barré PE, Mandin H, Taub K, Paul LC, et al. Long-term knowledge retention following Predialysis psychoeducational intervention. Nephron. 2000;**86**(2): 129-134

[61] Espahbodi F, Hosseini H, Mirzade MM, Shafaat AB. Effect of psycho education on depression and anxiety symptoms in patients on Hemodialysis. Iran Journal of Psychiatry Behavioural Science. 2015;**9**(1):e227

[62] Al Saraireh FA, Aloush SM, Al Azzam M, Al Bashtawy M. The effectiveness of cognitive behavioral therapy versus psychoeducation in the management of depression among patients undergoing haemodialysis. Issues in Mental Health Nursing. 2018;**39**(6):514-518

[63] Sousa H, Ribeiro O, Paúl C, Costa E, Frontini R, Miranda V, et al. "Together we stand": A pilot study exploring the feasibility, acceptability, and preliminary effects of a family-based psychoeducational intervention for patients on Hemodialysis and their family caregivers. Healthcare. 2021;**9**(11):1585

[64] Bakarman MA, Felimban MK, Atta MM, Butt NS. The effect of an educational program on quality of life in patients undergoing hemodialysis in western Saudi Arabia. Saudi Medical Journal. 2019;**40**(1):66

[65] Hudson JL, Moss-Morris R, Game D, Carroll A, McCrone P, Hotopf M, et al. Improving distress in dialysis (iDiD): A feasibility two-arm parallel randomised controlled trial of an online cognitive behavioural therapy intervention with and without therapist-led telephone support for psychological distress in patients undergoing haemodialysis. BMJ Open. 2016;**6**(4):e011286

[66] Rambod M, Pourali-Mohammadi N, Pasyar N, Rafii F, Sharif F. The effect of Benson's relaxation technique on the quality of sleep of Iranian hemodialysis patients: A randomized trial. Complementary Therapies in Medicine. 2013;**21**(6):577-584

[67] El-Gilany A-H. The effect of Benson's relaxation technique on anxiety, depression and sleep quality of elderly patients undergoing Hemodialysis. International Journal of Nursing Didactics. 2019;**9**:23

[68] Sayed Ahmed S. The effect of relaxation techniques on quality of sleep for patients with end-stage renal failure undergoing hemodialysis. SESAGA Younis International Journal of Innovative and Applied Research. 2014;**2**(7):83-94

[69] Rambod M, Pasyar N, Sharif F, Rafii F, Pourali MN. The effect of relaxation technique on physical activity of Hemodialysis patients. Iran Journal of Nursing. 2014;**27**(90):22-32

[70] Pasyar N, Rambod M, Sharif F, Rafii F, Pourali-Mohammadi N. Improving adherence and biomedical markers in hemodialysis patients: The effects of relaxation therapy. Complementary Therapies in Medicine. 2015;**23**(1):38-45

[71] Al Hasbi H, Chayati N, Makiyah S. Progressive muscle relaxation to reduces chronic pain in hemodialysis patient. Medisains. 2020;**17**:62-66

[72] Rambod M, Sharif F, Pourali-Mohammadi N, Pasyar N, Rafii F. Evaluation of the effect of Benson's relaxation technique on pain and quality of life of haemodialysis patients: A randomized controlled trial. International Journal of Nursing Studies. 2014;**51**(7):964-973

[73] Sutinah S, Azhari R. The effects of relaxation breathing on fatigue in patients with chronic kidney disease undergoing hemodialysis. Malahayati International Journal of Nursing and Health Science. 2020;**3**(1):15-21

[74] Heshmatifar N, Sadeghi H, Mahdavi A, Shegarf Nahaee M, Rakhshani M. The effect of Benson relaxation technique on depression in patients undergoing Hemodialysis. Journal of Babol University of Medical Sciences. 2015;**17**(8):34-40

[75] Alarcon RD, Jenkins CS, Heestand DE, Scott LK, Cantor L. The effectiveness of progressive relaxation in chronic hemodialysis patients. Journal of Chronic Diseases. 1982;**35**(10):797-802

[76] Saeedi M, Torab T, Saatchi K, Zayeri F, Akbari S. The effect of progressive muscle relaxation on sleep quality of patients undergoing hemodialysis. IJCCN. 2012;**5**:23-28

[77] Damayanti S, Fadlilah S, Yoshima Nekada CD, Tanda SU, Nugroho A, Mindarsih E. Music relaxation therapy effectively reduces fatigue in patients under hemodialysis. International Medical Journal. 2023;**30**(1):44-47

[78] Purba TUP, Dharmajaya R, Siregar CT. The effectiveness of progressive muscle relaxation with Benson relaxation on the sleep quality in hemodialysis patients. Indian Journal of Public Health Research & Development. 2020;**11**(1):1392-1396

[79] Eroglu H, Gok MZ. Benson relaxation technique combined with music therapy for fatigue, anxiety, and depression in Hemodialysis patients : A randomized controlled trial. Holistic Nursing Practice. 2022;**36**(3):139-148

[80] Amini E, Goudarzi I, Masoudi R, Ahmadi A, Momeni A. Effect of progressive muscle relaxation and aerobic exercise on anxiety, sleep quality, and fatigue in patients with chronic renal failure undergoing hemodialysis. International Journal of Pharmaceutical and Clinical Research. 2016;**8**(12):1634-1639

[81] Abu Maloh HIA, Soh KL, Chong SC, Ismail SIF, Soh KG, Abu Maloh DI, et al. The effectiveness of Benson's relaxation technique on pain and perceived stress among patients undergoing Hemodialysis: A double-blind, cluster-randomized, active control clinical trial. Clinical Nursing Research. 2022;**32**(2):288-297

[82] Lilia Cervantes MC, Hasnain-Wynia R, Steiner JF, Havranek E, Hull M, Rice J, et al. Peer navigator intervention for Latinos on Hemodialysis: A single-arm clinical trial. Journal of Palliative Medicine. 2019;**22**(7):838-843

[83] Husain A, Kusuma H, Johan A. Effects of peer support program on self-management in patients with end-stage

renal disease undergoing hemodialysis. Nurse Media Journal of Nursing. 2020;**10**(2):171-181. DOI: 10.14710/nmjn.v10i2.26502

[84] Pasyar N, Rambod M, Jowkar M. The effect of peer support on hope among patients under hemodialysis. International Journal of Nephrology and Renovascular Disease. 2020;**13**:37-44

[85] Malek Khahi A, Jadid Milani M, Amiri P. The effect of peer support groups on sexual function in patients treated with haemodialysis. Journal of Sabzevar University of Medical Sciences. 2016;**23**(2):304-312

[86] Malek Khahi A, Jadid Milani M, Amiri P. The effects of peer support groups on mental health of Hemodialysis patients. Iran Journal of Nursing. 2015;**28**(96):40-49

[87] Jadid Milani M, Malek Khahi A, Jafarzadeh M, Rakhshani M. The effect of peer support groups on physical health status in patients treated with hemodialysis. Journal of Sabzevar University of Medical Sciences. 1970;**21**(6):993-1000

[88] Russell J, Southerland S, Huff ED, Thomson M, Meyer KB, Lynch JR. A peer-to-peer mentoring program for In-Center Hemodialysis: A patient-Centered quality improvement program. Nephrology Nursing Journal. 2017;**44**(6):481-496

[89] Bennett PN, Hussein WF, Argentina M, Damron KC, Atwal J, Schiller B. The feasibility of remote patient peer mentoring in hemodialysis. Kidney Medicine. 2022;**4**(10):100529

[90] Nicholas DB, Picone G, Vigneux A, McCormick K, Mantulak A, McClure M, et al. Evaluation of an online peer support network for adolescents with chronic kidney disease. Journal of Technology in Human Services. 2009;**27**(1):23-33

[91] Mathews A, Swain R, White M, Lehmann H, Furth S. Evaluating the use of an online gaming community in a pediatric hemodialysis center. American Medical Informatics Association Annual Symposium Proceedings. 2005;**2005**:1046

[92] Longley RM, Harnedy LE, Ghanime PM, Arroyo-Ariza D, Deary EC, Daskalakis E, et al. Peer support interventions in patients with kidney failure: A systematic review. Journal of Psychosomatic Research. 2023;**171**:111379

[93] Musa AS, Pevalin DJ, Al Khalaileh MAA. Spiritual well-being, depression, and stress among Hemodialysis patients in Jordan. Journal of Holistic Nursing. 2017;**36**(4):354-365

[94] Li C-Y, Hsieh C-J, Shih Y-L, Lin Y-T. Spiritual well-being of patients with chronic renal failure: A cross-sectional study. Nursing Open. 2021;**8**(5):2461-2469

[95] Darvishi A, Otaghi M, Mami S. The effectiveness of spiritual therapy on spiritual well-being, self-esteem and self-efficacy in patients on Hemodialysis. Journal of Religion and Health. 2020;**59**(1):277-288

[96] Salahinezhad M, Kia B, Mahmoodi M, Fereidouni Sarigeh P. The effect of spiritual therapy on the life style of Hemodialysis patients. Military Caring Sciences. 2021;**8**(2):193-201

[97] Oshvandi K, Amini S, Moghimbeigi A, Sadeghian E. The effect of a spiritual care on Hope in patients

undergoing Hemodialysis: A randomized controlled trial. Current Psychiatry Research and Reviews. 2020;**16**

[98] Sarijeh P, Kia B, Mahmoodi M, Nejad M. The effect of spiritual therapy on resiliency of Hemodialysis patients. Avicenna Journal of Nursing and Midwifery Care. 2021;**29**:264-272

[99] Durmuş M, Ekinci M. The effect of spiritual care on anxiety and depression level in patients receiving Hemodialysis treatment: A randomized controlled trial. Journal of Religion and Health. 2022;**61**(3):2041-2055

[100] Moodi V, Arian A, Moodi JR, Dastjerdi R. Effectiveness of spiritual therapy on depression, anxiety, and stress in Hemodialysis patients. Modern Care Journal. 2020;**17**(4):e108879

[101] Dewi DSE, Hamzah HB. The relationship between spirituality, quality of life, and resilience. In: 6th International Conference on Community Development (ICCD 2019). Dordrecht, Netherlands: Atlantis Press; 2019

[102] Lima S, Teixeira L, Esteves R, Ribeiro F, Pereira F, Teixeira A, et al. Spirituality and quality of life in older adults: A path analysis model. BMC Geriatrics. 2020;**20**:1-8

[103] Finkelstein FO, West W, Gobin J, Finkelstein SH, Wuerth D. Spirituality, quality of life and the dialysis patient. Nephrology Dialysis Transplantation. 2007;**22**(9):2432-2434

[104] Dalal K, Sankhe A, Zope J. A prospective, controlled study to assess effect of spiritual therapy in patient undergoing hemodialysis at Bhaktivedanta hospital. Saudi Journal of Kidney Diseases and Transplantation. 2021;**32**(6):1570-1576. DOI: 10.4103/1319-2442.352417

[105] Eloia SMC, Ximenes MAM, Eloia SC, Galindo Neto NM, Barros LM, Caetano JÁ. Religious coping and hope in chronic kidney disease: A randomized controlled trial. Revista da Escola de Enfermagem da USP. 2021;**55**:e20200368. DOI: 10.1590/1980-220X-REE USP-2020-0368

[106] Hosseini SM, Naseri-Salahshour V, Farsi Z, Esmaeili M, Sajadi M, Maddah Z, et al. The effect of spirituality-oriented psychological counseling on the fear of death among patients undergoing chronic hemodialysis: A randomized controlled trial. European Journal of Integrative Medicine. 2022;**49**:102103

[107] Jakubowski KP, Jhamb M, Yabes J, Gujral S, Oberlin LE, Bender FH, et al. Technology-assisted cognitive-behavioral therapy intervention for end-stage renal disease. Translational Behavioral Medicine. 2019;**10**(3):657-663

[108] Marin A-E, Redolat R, Gil-Gómez J-A, Mesa-Gresa P. Addressing cognitive function and psychological well-being in chronic kidney disease: A systematic review on the use of technology-based interventions. International Journal of Environmental Research and Public Health. 2023;**20**(4):3342

[109] Hernandez R, Burrows B, Wilund K, Cohn M, Xu S, Moskowitz JT. Feasibility of an internet-based positive psychological intervention for hemodialysis patients with symptoms of depression. Social Work in Health Care. 2018;**57**(10):864-879

[110] Chan R, Dear BF, Titov N, Chow J, Suranyi M. Examining internet-delivered cognitive behaviour therapy for patients with chronic kidney disease on haemodialysis: A feasibility open trial. Journal of Psychosomatic Research. 2016;**89**:78-84

[111] Tommel J, Evers AWM, van Hamersvelt HW, van Dijk S, Chavannes NH, Wirken L, et al. E-health treatment in long-term dialysis (E-HELD): Study protocol for a multicenter randomized controlled trial evaluating personalized internet-based cognitive-behavioral therapy in dialysis patients. Trials. 2022;**23**(1):477

[112] Elander J, Kapadi R, Coyne E, Taal MW, Selby NM, Stalker C, et al. Using patient feedback to adapt intervention materials based on acceptance and commitment therapy for people receiving renal dialysis. BMC Urology. 2021;**21**(1):157

[113] Min Y, Park M. Effects of a Mobile-app-based self-management support program for elderly hemodialysis patients. Healthcare Information Research. 2020;**26**(2):93-103

[114] Hernandez R, Burrows B, Browning M, Solai K, Fast D, Litbarg NO, et al. Mindfulness-based virtual reality intervention in Hemodialysis patients: A pilot study on end-user perceptions and safety. Kidney360. 2021;**2**(3):435-444

[115] Willis M, Brand Hein L, Hu Z, Saran R, Argentina M, Bragg-Gresham J, et al. Usability evaluation of a tablet-based intervention to prevent intradialytic hypotension in Dialysis patients during In-clinic Dialysis: Mixed methods study. JMIR Human Factors. 2021;**8**(2):e26012

[116] Nadort E, Schouten RW, Boeschoten RE, Smets Y, Chandie Shaw P, Vleming LJ, et al. Internet-based treatment for depressive symptoms in hemodialysis patients: A cluster randomized controlled trial. General Hospital Psychiatry. 2022;**75**:46-53

[117] Sertoz OO, Ascı G, Toz F, Duman S, Elbi H, Ok E. Planning a social activity to improve psychological well-being and quality of life of hemodialysis patients: A pilot study. Therapeutic Apheresis and Dialysis. 2009;**13**(4):366-372

[118] Abraham S, Venu A, Ramachandran A, Chandran PM, Raman S. Assessment of quality of life in patients on hemodialysis and the impact of counseling. Saudi Journal of Kidney Diseases and Transplantation. 2012;**23**(5):953-957

[119] Beizaee Y, Rejeh N, Heravi-Karimooi M, Tadrisi SD, Griffiths P, Vaismoradi M. The effect of guided imagery on anxiety, depression and vital signs in patients on hemodialysis. Complementary Therapies in Clinical Practice. 2018;**33**:184-190

Chapter 10

Shared Decision-Making for Choosing Renal Replacement Therapy

Mansour Ghafourifard

Abstract

Chronic kidney disease is common worldwide, and the number of patients with end-stage kidney disease (ESKD) is expected to rise over the next decade. These patients must select one of the three main treatments available to them: conservative care, dialysis (hemodialysis or peritoneal dialysis), and kidney transplantation. Hemodialysis can occur in a dialysis center (in-center dialysis) or in a person's home (home dialysis). The international guidelines support the approach of shared decision-making (SDM) for selecting renal replacement therapy. In this approach, patients and healthcare providers collaborate to make medical decisions that incorporate the patient's values and preferences in conjunction with the best evidence. However, in some clinical practice, patients feel that they do not receive the full knowledge of all available options or that the selection of certain treatment is not well reasoned. In this chapter, the application of SDM for the selection of renal replacement therapies will be discussed in detail.

Keywords: end-stage kidney disease (ESKD), chronic kidney disease (CKD), renal replacement therapy, shared decision-making, dialysis, kidney replacement

1. Introduction

Chronic kidney disease as a long-term condition is a common chronic disease characterized by progressive and irreversible damage and loss of the function of kidneys and often leads to end-stage kidney disease (ESKD) [1, 2]. The prevalence of ESKD continues to increase globally [3, 4]. In 2010, there were 2.62 million patients with ESKD worldwide receiving renal replacement therapies, and the number of people needed for dialysis was projected to double by 2030 [5]. Moreover, it has been predicted that chronic kidney disease will be the fifth leading cause of mortality by 2040 [6]. Chronic kidney disease has a major global economic impact and influence on global health and quality of life of patients and their family [7].

2. Shared decision-making

When there are numerous treatment options in the healthcare systems, healthcare professionals should involve patients and their families in the process of decision-making on their care so that they can select care that meets their preferences and value needs and reflects what is important to them. This process is called shared decision-making [8]. Shared decision-making (SDM) is defined as a process in which patients, their family, and healthcare professionals try to collaborate with each other to choose the best treatment option for patients [9]. SDM engage patients and their families in the process of decision-making about diagnosis, treatment, or follow-up when more than one medically reasonable option is available [10, 11]. In fact, SDM is made by knowing and understanding the best available evidence on the benefits, harms, risks, and effectiveness of all available options; considering the patient's personal preferences and values; and mutually agreeing upon the course of care [8].

SDM is based on the notion that healthcare professionals are the expert persons on the evidence of medical and patients are the experts on what matters most to them [12].

In a systematic review by Makoul & Clayman [13], 161 definitions were found for SDM. They summarized the main elements of SDM in an integrative model of SDM. The model showed nine crucial elements and features that can be used in a variety of healthcare settings. Healthcare professionals could use these SDM-related specific behaviors during consultations with patients and families:

- Explain and define the patient's diagnosis, treatment, or follow-up process
- Present all available options
- Discuss the pros and cons of all available options (risks, benefits, costs)
- Identify patient preferences and values
- Discuss patient skills, abilities, and self-efficacy
- Provide full knowledge of what is known and provide the necessary recommendations
- Clarify and evaluate the patient's understanding
- Make a decision or defer decision-making
- Organize the follow-up.

In many healthcare encounters, the notion that only healthcare providers could access evidence is no longer accepted. As a substitute, shared decision-making assumes that both the healthcare professional and patient require access to information about the evidence for providing a decision. Thus, considering and respecting both the healthcare professional's recommendations and the patient's preferences is necessary for providing an effective SDM [8].

2.1 Outcomes of shared decision-making

Shared decision-making (SDM) has many positive outcomes for patients and families. A systematic review showed that SDM was most likely related to affective-cognitive patient outcomes (54%), compared with 25% of health outcomes and 37% of behavioral outcomes [14].

Shared decision-making (SDM) is considered an essential factor of safe and effective healthcare when there are available options to patients. Moreover, SDM is in line with the notion of "No decision about me without me" and supports patient-centered healthcare [15].

2.2 The steps of shared decision-making

Although there are some models for SDM, the following simple steps proposed by Stiggelbout et al. [10] could be understood easily:

Step 1. The healthcare professional should inform the patients and their families that a decision is to be made, and it is important to consider the patient's view.

Step 2. All the available choices should be explained by healthcare professionals. Moreover, they should clarify the pros and cons of each option.

Step 3. Both the patient and healthcare professional discuss the patient's values and preferences; the professional try to support the patient in the discussion.

Step 4. Both the patient and healthcare professional discuss the patient's decisional role preference, make the decision or defer it, and discuss possible follow-up plans.

3. Conservative care

Conservative care for kidney disease means that the healthcare professionals continue the care without performing dialysis or kidney transplantation. The aim of conservative care is to improve the patient's quality of life, manage the symptoms, and preserve kidney function for as long as possible [1, 16].

4. Renal replacement therapies (RRTs)

Equity of access to renal replacement therapy (RRT) varies between countries based on rationing and finance. Renal replacement therapy (RRT) is a therapy for patients with kidney failure that replaces kidney function (i.e., blood filtration, electrolyte homeostasis, fluid regulation, toxin removal/secretion, and filtrate transport and drainage). Currently available RRT approaches include dialysis and kidney transplantation.

4.1 Dialysis

Dialysis options include hemodialysis (HD), which can either be done at home (HHD) or in-center (ICHD), or peritoneal dialysis (PD). There are two types of PD including Continuous Ambulatory Peritoneal Dialysis (CAPD) or Automated Peritoneal Dialysis (APD). In CAPD method, the schedule of dialysis fluid exchanges is done by hand. However, in the APD method, a machine called "cycler" is used to empty and fill the peritoneal cavity three to five times during the night [3, 16, 17].

4.2 Kidney transplantation

Kidney transplantation is the most effective and preferred form of renal replacement therapy which has a significant survival benefit compared with other renal replacement therapies. Using a kidney transplantation procedure, a new healthy donor kidney is placed in the patient's body. It can offer a longer and more active life for patients with kidney failure. Moreover, there are fewer limitations on diet and fluid intake. However, patients should take immunosuppressant or anti-rejection medicines as long as the new kidney works to keep the immune system less active [18].

5. Shared decision-making in patients with chronic kidney disease

SDM in nephrology settings is a challenging issue because of the complexity of chronic kidney disease and the preference-sensitive choice to be made [19]. When chronic kidney disease progresses toward end-stage kidney disease (ESKD), patients need to make decisions for different renal replacement therapies to be survived [1]. They must continue receiving one of the RRT treatments for the rest of their lives. Therefore, it is important for patients to select the treatment option that is the most suitable and acceptable treatment based on the preference and values of patients [20].

To help patients for making timely treatment modality decisions, international guidelines in nephrology suggest shared decision-making (SDM), where the treatment is selected based on patient's values and preferences [21]. SDM in nephrology engage the patients in decisions that best suit patients' preferences and their living and medical situations [22]. In the SDM process for renal replacement therapies, both healthcare providers and patients choose the best treatment option together after assessing the evidence and discussing the pros and cons of all available options (including kidney transplantation, hemodialysis, and peritoneal dialysis), individual preferences, and the circumstances of the patient. During the SDM process, outcomes from weighing the clinical guidelines are weighed against personal beliefs and preferences [22].

5.1 Shared decision-making for the selection of renal replacement therapies

Patients suffering from advanced chronic kidney disease should make complex decisions for selection of all possible renal replacement therapies [1]. Each option of RRT could impact their everyday life. The selection of RRT is a usual situation for 'informed shared decision-making' (iSDM). Van Dulmen et al. [23] proposed four essential elements for iSDM in RRT: (a) at least two persons are engaged in decisions, (b) both share information according to the evidence-based care, and (c) building an agreement on the preferred choice, and where (d) a consensus is made on the treatment option with joint responsibility.

5.2 Time of shared decision-making for selection of RRT

Because kidney function of patients with chronic kidney disease usually declines progressively, the healthcare providers especially the nephrologists and nurses have multiple opportunities to discuss all available options of renal replacement therapy.

There are when shared decision-making for a patient with CKD is important at least three times: when the patient enters stage 4 (estimated glomerular filtration rate [eGFR] < 30 ml/min/1.73 m^2), when the patient is going to start RRT in the near time (eGFR <15 ml/min/1.73 m^2), or when the healthcare provider find no evidence that further treatment will prolong life (age ≥ 75 years and multiple comorbidities, or eGFR <5 ml/min/1.73 m^2). In this stage, a nephrologist should discuss all available options for renal replacement therapy with the patient and family and support the patient in the selection of a suitable lifesaving treatment based on the patient's preferences and the best evidence [24].

6. Outcomes of shared decision-making for selection of RRT

According to the literature review, SDM is considered an important factor for positive patient-centered outcomes. Successful SDM could increase patients' adherence and compliance, their satisfaction, as well as the promotion of awareness about the disease. Moreover, SDM can decrease the cost of treatments and reduce the symptoms [25].

A study in Germany conducted by Robinski et al. showed that successful shared decision-making is one of the main factors increasing the satisfaction of dialysis patients on long-term treatment [26].

Patients with ESKD need to be assisted and encouraged to choose the most suitable renal replacement therapy in an active manner proactively rather than being passive and relying on healthcare professionals' decisions. Patients' participation in the decisions could improve the patients' empowerment and autonomy in making treatment decisions [27].

During the SDM process, healthcare professionals provide information and evidence regarding different types of treatments, whereas the patients express their own preferences and opinions. The exchange of this information could help to ensure that patients and their families understand the appropriate information, thereby it reduces decision conflicts [28]. Moreover, receiving support during the effective SDM increases patients' self-efficacy [20]. Moreover, it has also been reported that SDM can optimize decisional outcomes, improve treatment compliance, reduce anxiety, and lower demand for healthcare resources [29].

7. Strategies for improving SDM in the choice of renal replacement therapy

Patients with CKD have numerous sources of information which could help them to make an informed decision. The nephrologists, due to their medical competence, could play a main role in providing medical advice. Moreover, Nurses can play a crucial role in explaining the available choices of RRT in and in providing emotional support for them. Patient's family members could be engaged in decoctions and providing support [23].

In a recent study, Stoye et al. [23] conducted a study to explore nurses' and nephrologists' perceptions of their participation in shared decision-making for selecting renal replacement therapy. The results showed that due to the high disease burden on patient's life, shared decision-making for the selection of renal replacement therapy is mostly difficult issue. Providing full education and training for patients and the consistent participation of nursing staff and peer education facilitated the SDM process [23].

Although nephrologists and nursing professionals are professional experts, family members of patients and peers are considered experts by virtue of their experience [30]. Structured peer mentoring programs or peer counseling could help patients to select a desired option.

Shifting the paradigm of medicine from a predominant biomedical and technical orientation to a person-centered orientation of SDM might improve decision-making practices [31].

8. Conclusion

Collaboration of healthcare providers and patients with kidney disease as a team in the shared decision-making process increases the patient's capacity to develop person-centered care and effective life plan that not only improves patients' survival but also prepares them for end-of-life care. This collaborative approach can improve the quality of care for all patients who suffer from CKD. However, a shared decision-making process should be developed in each country based on the heath care policies, resources, and facilities to engage patients and their families in the decision for the selection of kidney replacement therapies (KRTs).

Acknowledgements

I would like to thank all the healthcare professionals who support the idea of shared decision-making in patients with CKD.

Conflict of interest

The authors declare no conflict of interest.

Author details

Mansour Ghafourifard
Tabriz University of Medical Sciences, Tabriz, Iran

*Address all correspondence to: m.ghafori@yahoo.com

References

[1] Hamroun A, Speyer E, Ayav C, Combe C, Fouque D, Jacquelinet C, et al. Barriers to conservative care from patients' and nephrologists' perspectives: The CKD-REIN study. Nephrology Dialysis Transplantation. 2022;**37**(12):2438-2448

[2] Ghodsian S, Ghafourifard M, Ghahramanian A. Comparison of shared decision making in patients undergoing hemodialysis and peritoneal dialysis for choosing a dialysis modality. BMC Nephrology. 2021;**22**(1):1-9

[3] Yu X, Nakayama M, Wu M-S, Kim Y-L, Mushahar L, Szeto CC, et al. Shared decision-making for a dialysis modality. Kidney International Reports. 2022;**7**(1):15-27

[4] Ghafourifard M, Mehrizade B, Hassankhani H, Heidari M. Hemodialysis patients perceived exercise benefits and barriers: The association with health-related quality of life. BMC Nephrology. 2021;**22**:1-9

[5] Liyanage T, Ninomiya T, Jha V, Neal B, Patrice HM, Okpechi I, et al. Worldwide access to treatment for end-stage kidney disease: A systematic review. The Lancet. 2015;**385**(9981):1975-1982

[6] Foreman KJ, Marquez N, Dolgert A, Fukutaki K, Fullman N, McGaughey M, et al. Forecasting life expectancy, years of life lost, and all-cause and cause-specific mortality for 250 causes of death: Reference and alternative scenarios for 2016-40 for 195 countries and territories. The Lancet. 2018;**392**(10159):2052-2090

[7] van Eck van der Sluijs A, Vonk S, Bonenkamp AA, Prantl K, Riemann AT, Van Jaarsveld BC, et al. Value of patient decision aids for shared decision-making in kidney failure. Journal of Renal Care. 2023:1-9

[8] Légaré F, Stacey D, Turcotte S, Cossi MJ, Kryworuchko J, Graham ID, et al. Interventions for improving the adoption of shared decision making by healthcare professionals. Cochrane Database of Systematic Reviews. 2014;(9)

[9] Elwyn G, Frosch D, Thomson R, Joseph-Williams N, Lloyd A, Kinnersley P, et al. Shared decision making: A model for clinical practice. Journal of General Internal Medicine. 2012;**27**:1361-1367

[10] Stiggelbout AM, Pieterse AH. De Haes JCJPe, counseling. Shared Decision Making: Concepts, Evidence, and Practice. 2015;**98**(10):1172-1179

[11] Schrager S, Phillips G, Burnside E. Shared decision making in cancer screening. Family Practice Management. 2017;**24**(3):5

[12] Bomhof-Roordink H, Gärtner FR, Stiggelbout AM, Pieterse AH. Key components of shared decision making models: A systematic review. BMJ Open. 2019;**9**(12):e031763

[13] Makoul G, Clayman ML. An integrative model of shared decision making in medical encounters. Patient Education Counseling. 2006;**60**(3):301-312

[14] Shay LA, Lafata JE. Where is the evidence? A systematic review of shared decision making and patient outcomes. Medical Decision Making. 2015;**35**(1):114-131

[15] Joseph-Williams N, Elwyn G, Edwards A. Knowledge is not power

for patients: A systematic review and thematic synthesis of patient-reported barriers and facilitators to shared decision making. Patient education counseling. 2014;**94**(3):291-309

[16] Murtagh FE, Burns A, Moranne O, Morton RL, Naicker S. Supportive care: Comprehensive conservative care in end-stage kidney disease. Clinical Journal of the American Society of Nephrology. 2016;**11**(10):1909-1914

[17] Hamidi M, Roshangar F, Khosroshahi HT, Hassankhani H, Ghafourifard M, Sarbakhsh P. Comparison of the effect of linear and step-wise sodium and ultrafiltration profiling on dialysis adequacy in patients undergoing hemodialysis. Saudi Journal of Kidney Diseases and Transplantation. 2020;**31**(1):44-52

[18] Gordon E, Butt Z, Jensen S, Lehr AL-M, Franklin J, Becker Y, et al. Opportunities for shared decision making in kidney transplantation. American Journal of Transplantation. 2013;**13**(5):1149-1158

[19] Firanek CA, Garza S, Gellens ME, Lattrel K, Mancini A, Robar A, et al. Contrasting perceptions of home dialysis therapies among in-center and home dialysis staff. Nephrology Nursing Journal. 2016;**43**(3):195-205

[20] Ya-Fang H, Yu-Chi C, Huang C-C, Wen-Yu H, Kuan-Chia L. The effects of shared decision making on different renal replacement therapy decisions in patients with chronic kidney disease. Journal of Nursing Research. 2020;**28**(4):e109

[21] Engels N, de Graav G, van der Nat P, van den Dorpel M, Bos WJ, Stiggelbout AM. Shared decision-making in advanced kidney disease: A scoping review protocol. BMJ Open. 2020;**10**(2):e034142

[22] van Dulmen S, Roodbeen R, Schulze L, Prantl K, Rookmaaker M, van Jaarsveld B, et al. Practices and perspectives of patients and healthcare professionals on shared decision-making in nephrology. BMC Nephrology. 2022;**23**(1):1-13

[23] Stoye A, Zimmer JM, Girndt M, Mau W. The role of different nephrology experts in informed shared decision-making for renal replacement therapy. Journal of Renal Care. 2022;**48**(3):177-184

[24] Tuso P. Choosing wisely and beyond: Shared decision making and chronic kidney disease. The Permanente Journal. 2013;**17**(4):75

[25] Oshima Lee E, Emanuel E. Shared decision making to improve care and reduce costs. New England Journal of Medicine. 2013;**368**(1):6-8

[26] Robinski M, Mau W, Wienke A, Girndt M, counseling. Shared decision-making in chronic kidney disease: A retrospection of recently initiated dialysis patients in Germany. Patient education counseling. 2016;**99**(4):562-570

[27] Obeidat RF. Shared decision making among individuals with cancer in non-Western cultures: A literature review. Number 5/September. 2013;**40**(5):454-463

[28] Gionfriddo MR, Leppin AL, Brito JP, LeBlanc A, Boehmer KR, Morris MA, et al. A systematic review of shared decision making interventions in chronic conditions: A review protocol. Systematic Reviews. 2014;**3**(1):1-7

[29] Frazier R, Levine S, Porteny T, Tighiouart H, Wong JB, Isakova T, et al. Shared decision making among older adults with advanced CKD.

American Journal of Kidney Diseases. 2022;**80**(5):599-609

[30] Cordier J-F. The expert patient: Towards a novel definition. European Respiratory Journal. 2014;**44**(4):853-857

[31] Verberne WR, Stiggelbout AM, Bos WJW, van Delden JJM. Asking the right questions: Towards a person-centered conception of shared decision-making regarding treatment of advanced chronic kidney disease in older patients. BMC Medical Ethics. 2022;**23**(1):47

Chapter 11

Health Economics of Renal Replacement Therapy

Tomoyuki Takura, Naotsugu Ichimaru and Atushi Aikawa

Abstract

The medical treatment of renal failure is increasingly being discussed in terms of medical economics against the background of disease mechanisms, treatment techniques, and related systems. Particularly, renal replacement therapy requires considerable medical resources and results in high medical costs; therefore, the interest in medical economics is increasing worldwide. This article discusses the cost-effectiveness of renal replacement therapy using macro- and micro-analyses. Based on the macroscopic analysis of international comparisons of renal replacement therapy systems based on medical expenses per patient with end-stage renal disease and a one-year mortality rate, Japan performed better than other developed countries. A clinical economic study of renal replacement therapy is significant because it quantitatively demonstrates the socioeconomic value of life-saving and health benefits (Hemodialysis: approximately 6.5 million JPY/Qaly). In other words, even with high annual medical expenses and a heavy financial burden, the level of medical fees is appropriate from the perspective of the public's value judgment. A micro-analysis comparing the cost-effectiveness of marginal and standard donors revealed no statistically significant difference in their cumulative medical costs per long-term life expectancy. Thus, evidence and decision-making related to medical economics are required for the sustainable development of the medical system for end-stage renal disease.

Keywords: health economy, medical innovation, cost-effectiveness analysis, renal replacement therapy, kidney transplantation, marginal donor, universal health coverage, international comparison

1. Introduction

The estimated worldwide prevalence of chronic kidney disease (CKD) in 2017 was 9.1%, an increase of 29.3% since 1990 [1]. In Japan, the number of patients with CKD is increasing annually, with one in eight adults estimated to have CKD. Under these circumstances, the medical economics of renal replacement therapy for patients with end-stage renal disease (ESRD) are attracting global attention against the backdrop of medical system sustainability. Based on these trends, this paper discusses the medical economics of renal replacement therapy by combining theories of medical value assessment and clinical economic studies. These findings are presumed to contribute to the further development of CKD treatment.

2. Socio-economy and medical innovation

In general, since economic trends and the rate of the aging population affect the balance of social security payments that support medical care, recent circumstances have increased the severity of socioeconomic trends surrounding medical care, leading to discussions on increasing the national burden and improving productivity [2]. For example, medical expenditures in the areas of coronary and kidney diseases are growing faster than the gross domestic product (GDP) in Japan [3]. Against this background, the insurance premiums borne by beneficiaries cover only approximately half of the financial structure of the universal health insurance system, and public funds (compensation from general revenue sources with a debt of approximately 30%), which are widely borne by the public, account for nearly 40%.

When discussing health policy as a system, this situation (social income-expenditure imbalance) is regarded as one of the uncertainties concerning a stable supply of medical services in the future.

In other words, social security debt is problematic because whether it can be regarded as an "investment" that can be expected to increase social added value (return) is unclear. However, since the field of pediatric medicine targets the group that will become the working population in the future, it is relatively easy to discuss "investment and recovery" based on the above-mentioned perspective. Additionally, in the field of medical care for older adults, the socioeconomic added value can be discussed while creating new medical innovations and building social models that are beneficial for everyone. We hope that these perspectives will be discussed further in the future.

In recent years, themes related to the sustainability of systems and social harmony in the medical field have been emphasized, and concepts such as Sustainable Development Goals (SDGs) and Appropriate Use Criteria (AUC) have been introduced. Hence, even with the further development of artificial organs and transplantation medicine, socioeconomic perspectives are becoming increasingly significant. Therefore, it is important to realize the economic added value of these medical treatments and share them with the stakeholders. Particularly, it should be reaffirmed that a robust universal health insurance system is necessary to encourage related research and development [4].

For example, an analysis aimed at clarifying the preliminary interactions between Universal Health Coverage (UHC) and medical innovations regarding the security and continued progress of medical services showed that UHC levels and medical innovations (drug discovery) were positively correlated ($r = 0.629$, $R^2 = 0.395$, $p < 0.05$; **Figure 1**) through the health economic mechanism (value chain).

This study conducted a correlation analysis using statistical data from 11 countries (World Bank and the Japanese government) on the relationship between UHC indicators and medical innovations. The UHC index was converted into an integral value of the UHC index (0–100 score) and the total population (in millions) while considering the contribution of each level to the population. Focusing on drug discovery as a major aspect of medical innovation, we selected the share of the top 100 ethical drugs worldwide according to the country of origin. Pearson's correlation coefficient was used for the correlation analysis. The statistical significance level was set at 5%. Notably, this figure is represented by a logarithmic transformation.

A country's UHC level is generally affected by its real economy (e.g., GDP) (**Table 1**) [5]. Particularly, the impact of fluctuations in public medical costs is significant. Additionally, the ratio of medical expenses per capita is considered to

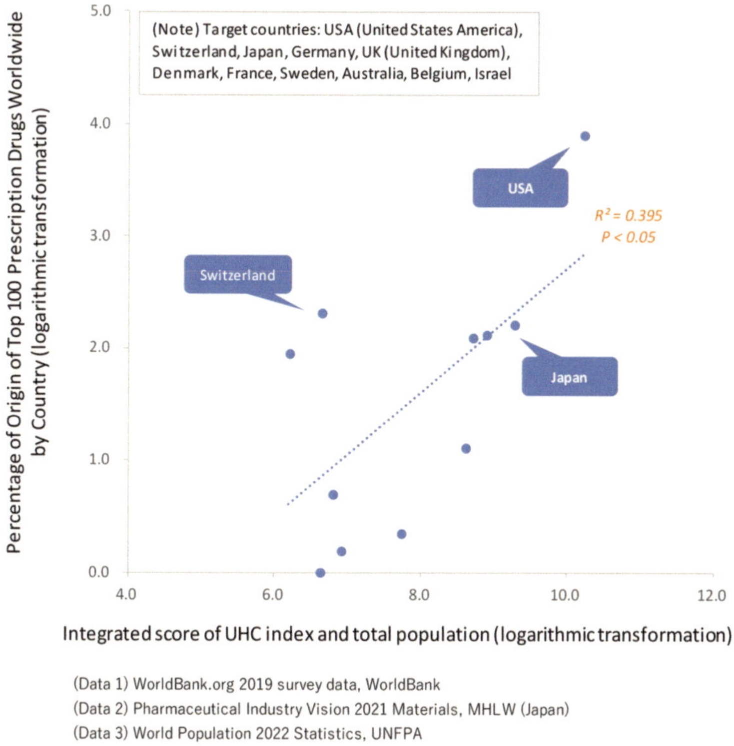

Figure 1.
An international comparison of correlations between medical innovation (drug discovery ability) and UHC levels.

UHC Index of Service Coverage (SCI)	Partial Regression Coefficient	Standardized Partial Regression Coefficient	S.E.	*p*-value	95% CI
Population (total: million people)	0.0049	0.1921	0.0012	0.0001	0.0025–0.0074
GDP per capita (current USD)	0.0017	1.6129	0.0002	<0.001	0.0013–0.0021
Health expenditure (% of GDP)	2.3481	0.4116	1.5748	0.136	−0.7386–5.4347
Government health expenditures (% of general government expenditures)	1.4511	0.6575	0.2804	<0.001	0.9015–2.0006
Unemployment rate (%: ratio of unemployed persons)	−1.4764	−0.2253	0.7105	0.0377	−2.8689–−0.0838
Poverty rate (%: poverty gap)	−1.6736	−0.2303	0.4674	0.0003	−2.5897–−0.7575

Model: $R^2 = 0.991$, F test: $p < 0.001$.
GDP, gross domestic product; UHC, universal health coverage; SCI, service coverage index; S.E., standard error; CI, confidence interval.

Table 1.
Panel data analysis of the impact of the economic level (GDP, health expenditure, unemployment, and poverty) on the UHC level (SCI). (source: Ref. [5]).

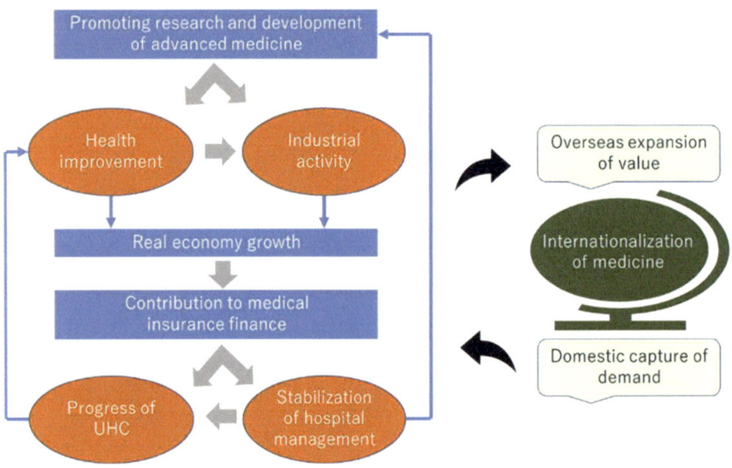

Figure 2.
Progress mechanisms of healthcare and socioeconomic factors associated with medical innovation: Value chain, including UHC. (source: Ref. [4]).

affect the spread of innovative medical technologies that have been developed [5]. Thus, economic growth is important for promoting medical innovation. Therefore, sustainable and equitable capital investment in medical care (i.e., the improvement of UHC) is crucial. Furthermore, the active expansion of public medical resources is essential to enhance the synergistic effect between medical innovation and UHC. In future, these factors should be systematically discussed as value chains (**Figure 2**).

3. Life-saving value and cost-effectiveness

In the discussion on medical value that advocates the real-world economy, it is generally possible, albeit limited, to evaluate the value of medical services by applying cost-effectiveness analysis and marginal utility theory. The main theories are outlined below. Usually, in microeconomics, the efficiency of service provision is maximized through price convergence based on the supply and demand equilibrium, backed by the fundamental utility theory [6]. Additionally, the prices at which the supply and demand are in equilibrium represent this value.

On the other hand, in the medical field that has a high public interest, the perspective of equity (balance of well-being) is considered along with efficiency. It is necessary to discuss the value of public interest while considering the harmony between the patient's medical care requests (preferences and willingness to pay) and the government's medical finances (income redistribution and fiscal balance). Therefore, the value of medical care should be examined in terms of the balance between utility (health outcomes) and costs (resource consumption) per health program unit, while interweaving the relationship between individuals and society against the background of welfare economics (**Figure 3**) [7].

Consequently, when utility is maximized within a certain budget range, the higher the performance, the greater the utility of the group as a whole and the higher the "value" of stakeholders. Compared with other conceptual discussions, this approach to value assessment in medical care is relatively consistent with the values of the real

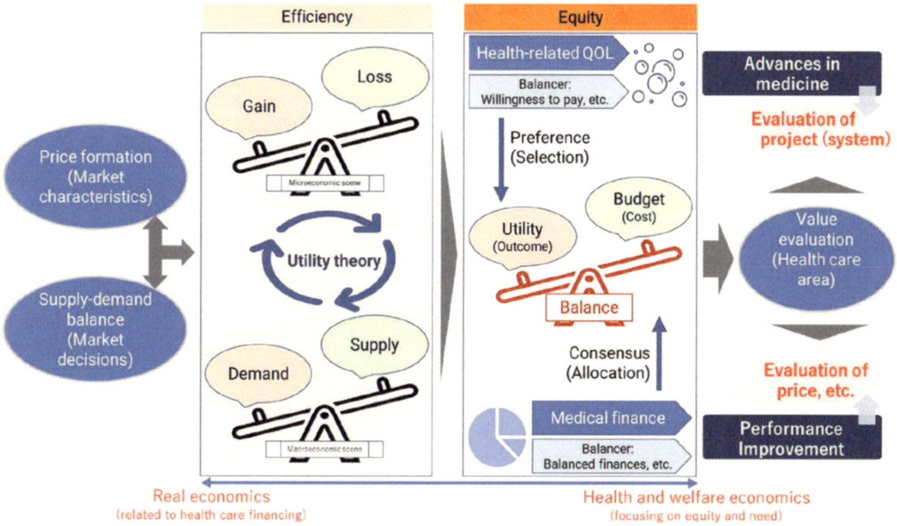

Figure 3.
The concept of medical valuation (application of the utility theory and cost-effectiveness). (source: Ref. [7]).

economy and daily life (national consensus) (e.g., approximately 6 million yen per quality-adjusted life year [Qaly]). Therefore, it is suitable to examine the value of medical services in the public sector [8].

For example, a Japanese report assessed the value of renal replacement therapy (hemodialysis, HD) for ESRD, whose annual medical expenses are approximately 5 million JPY and the financial burden is approximately 1.6 trillion JPY (**Figure 4**) [9, 10]. This study is significant because it quantitatively demonstrates the socioeconomic value of life-saving and health (HD: approximately 6.5 million JPY/Qaly). In other words, even with high annual medical expenses and a heavy financial burden, the level of medical fees is appropriate from the perspective of the public's value judgment. This is further supported by the macro analysis based on the international comparison shown below.

In the previous section, it was stated that an increase in public medical expenses is necessary to promote innovative treatment technologies and improve treatment outcomes. The next point of contention is whether the amount of medical resource consumption is appropriate to improve medical outcomes. Part of the answer to this question derives from cost-effectiveness. For example, ESRD treatment costs and public healthcare budget were positively correlated (**Figure 5**). Based on this, when a macro cost-effectiveness analysis was performed on the annual total medical expenses and one-year life prognosis of ESRD, Japan had the best performance compared to other countries (**Figure 6**). Thus, renal replacement therapy in Japan is highly valuable to the general public.

Since the medical insurance system that advocates UHC includes a stable supply as one part of the system, its sustainable development is considered as the most significant medical value to the public. Although there may be variations in the national culture and disease characteristics, it can be inferred that saving lives is the most common value. It is essential to remember that lifesaving not only results in opportunities for other medical interventions (opportunities for disease improvement) but also provides assurance of the quality of life (QOL) in the long run, which

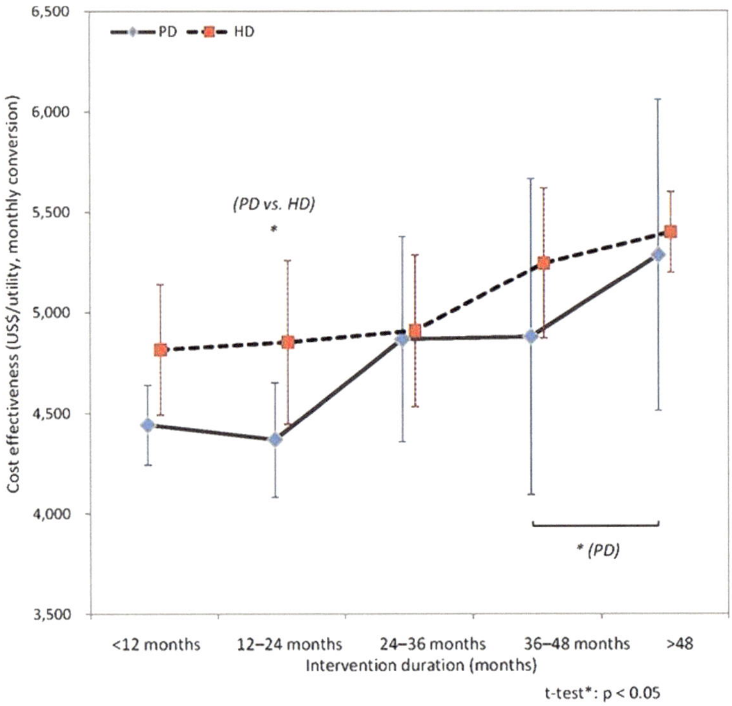

Figure 4.
Cost-effectiveness of dialysis intervention (artificial kidney): Hemodialysis versus peritoneal dialysis. (source: Ref. [9]).

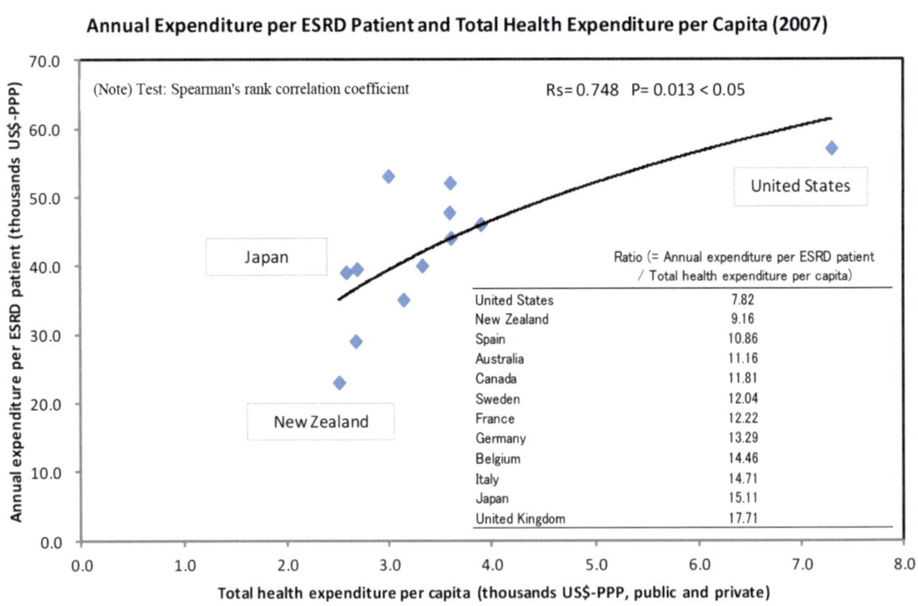

Figure 5.
The relationship between patients' medical expenses in the field of end-stage renal disease (ESRD) and medical expenses per capita. Data source: Refs. [11, 12].

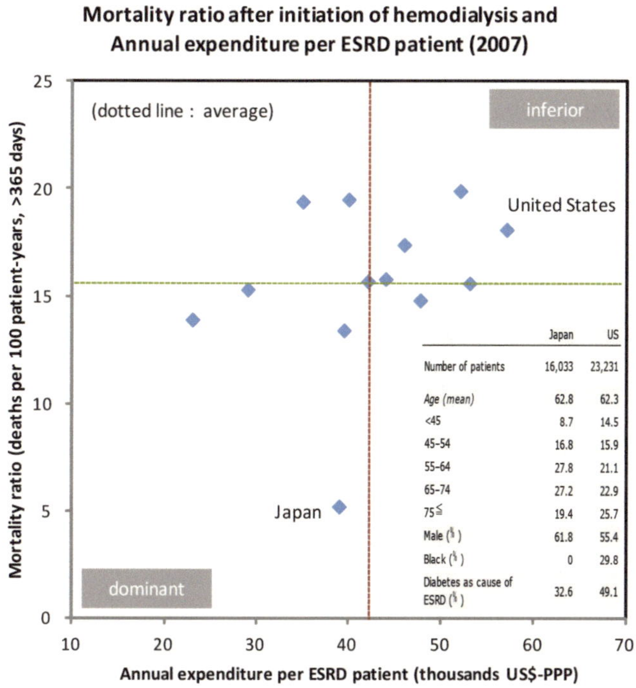

Figure 6.
An international comparison of the cost-effectiveness of the clinical system for end-stage renal disease (ESRD). (note) U.S., United States. Data source: Refs. [11, 13].

is of considerable significance in due course. Therefore, the potential value of renal replacement therapy (HD) is significant.

However, the assessment of medical value involves stakeholders' interests and is affected by the application of subjective outcomes and the macro real economy. Therefore, there are some restrictions on its use, along with difficulties in data analysis and direct recognition. However, against the background of tight medical finances and progress in innovation, cost-effectiveness analysis, which is a part of health technology assessment (HTA), is being actively introduced globally. Based on this trend, medical value assessments are expected to increase.

4. Cost-effectiveness of renal replacement therapy

Although the disease and economic burden associated with kidney diseases are increasing worldwide, there have been few international reports evaluating the cost-effectiveness of renal replacement therapy in recent years. Several recent reports have systematically reviewed the cost-effectiveness of dialysis. This section briefly introduces the contents of this study and discusses a research report on the cost-effectiveness evaluation of renal replacement therapy in Japan.

The main report [14] conducted a systematic review of the costs and health outcomes of dialysis modalities between January 2000 and December 2017. The survey sources included the MEDLINE, National Health Service Economic Evaluation

Database, Health Technology Assessment Database from the Center of Reviews and Dissemination, Cochrane Library, and Econlit. They identified 16 health economic evaluation reports that compared dialysis modalities from both high- and low-income countries. Two similar review papers have also been published [15, 16].

These studies examined the cost and health outcomes of multiple dialysis modalities and reported average cost-effectiveness rather than incremental cost-effectiveness (ICER). Nearly all evaluations suggest that home dialysis is less costly and provides similar or better health outcomes than institutional dialysis, which is the

Author (year)	ICER/main results	Authors' conclusions
Moradpour et al. (2020)	PD was dominant over HD; ICER for KT vs. PD: $1446/Qaly.	KT is cost-effective compared with PD at a WTP threshold of $12,400, and HD was dominated.
Rosselli et al. (2015)	KT was a cost-effective alternative from the second year and became the dominant alternative after the fourth year.	KT improves the overall survival rates and quality of life and is a cost-saving alternative compared with dialysis.
Jensen et al. (2014)	KT holds a dominant position over dialysis with both lower costs (810,516 DKK versus 1,032,934 DKK) and higher effects (4.4 Qaly versus 1.7 Qaly).	KT was the dominant treatment when compared with dialysis.
Shimizu et al. (2012)	Base scenario (current composition of KRT) was dominated by Scenario 2 (likelihood of a preemptive LT increased by 2.4 times), Scenario 3 (likelihood of a LT increased by 2.4 times), and Scenario 4 (likelihood of a DT increased by 22 times).	Increased rate of KT and PD can reduce costs and improve health outcomes.
	The ICER of Scenario 1 (likelihood of starting with PD increased by 2.3 times) over Base scenario was $5458/Qaly.	
Villa et al. (2012)	Scenario 1 (57% of scheduled incident patients on any RRT modality) was dominated by all the proposed scenarios: Scenario 2 (increased proportion of overall scheduled incident patient to 75% from 57%), Scenario 3 (increased proportion of scheduled patients on PD to 30% from 10%) and Scenario 4 (combined scenarios 2 and 3)	An increase in the overall scheduled incidence of KRT on PD should be promoted.
Haller et al. (2011)	Scenario 1 (current policy of assigning 90.6% of incident ESKD patients to HD, 7.2% to PD, 0.1% to LT, and 2.1% to DT) was dominated by Scenario 2 (increasing PD to 20%), and Scenario 3 (increasing PD to 20% and increasing KT to 10%)	KT and PD are more cost-effective than HD.

NR, not reported; QALY, quality-adjusted life year; ESKD, end-stage kidney disease; KRT, kidney replacement therapy; HD, hemodialysis; PD, peritoneal dialysis; CAPD, continuous ambulatory peritoneal dialysis; KT, kidney transplantation; LT, living-donor transplantation; DT, deceased-donor transplantation; ICER, incremental cost-effectiveness ratio; SA, sensitivity analysis; PAS, probabilistic sensitivity analysis; WTP, willingness-to-pay.

Table 2.
Example of the cost-effectiveness of renal replacement therapy: A systematic review. (source: Ref. [14]).

mainstay intervention. Therefore, home dialysis, which includes both hemodialysis (HD) and peritoneal dialysis (PD), is generally more cost-effective than institutional dialysis (**Table 2**). However, there are few reports with high-quality study designs.

In Japan, some studies have preliminarily evaluated the cost-effectiveness of HD, PD, and kidney transplantation (KT) for renal replacement therapy. The results are summarized in **Table 3**. Although both reports were observational studies, and the level of evidence was not high, it is possible to estimate the level of performance of renal replacement therapy in Japan. Particularly, the analytical approach was unified using a cost-utility analysis, which is suitable for mutual comparison of the medical economics of each modality.

The most cost-effective renal replacement therapy has been PD [9]. The reason for this is a good quality of life in home care, as found in a previous study. However, the PD selection rate in Japan is approximately 9%, which is lower than that of other countries. There are several reasons for this, but the previous paper has discussed the

Renal replacement therapy	**Kidney transplant**	**Peritoneal dialysis**	**Hemodialysis**	**Hemodialysis (Online-HD)**
Publication year	2017	2019	2015	2013
Research design	Prospective observational study, Multicenter study (Added: Model calculation for 3 years)	Prospective observational study, Multicenter study	Prospective observational study, Multicenter study	Prospective observational study, Multicenter study
Number of patients (n)	25	179	29	24
Observation period (months)	12	36	437 dialysis sessions (average: 15 months)	4
Evaluation index	Health-related QOL, Life year, Medical fee claim (Including donor medical expenses)	Health-related QOL, Life year, Medical fee claim	Health-related QOL, Life year, Medical fee claim	Health-related QOL, Life year, Medical fee claim
Result of the analysis				
ICUR (Kidney death as nonintervention)	66,000 (USD/Qaly; 12 months), 51,600 (USD/Qaly; Model calculation for 3 years)	55,019 (USD/Qaly)	68,800 (USD/Qaly)	65,700 (USD/Qaly)
ICUR (Other control therapy)		126,034 (USD/Qaly; APD vs. CAPD)		
Reference number	14	9	10	15

(Note) Exchange rates were averages for the publication year or observation period. ICUR, incremental cost-utility ratio.

Table 3.
Japanese report on the cost-effectiveness of renal replacement therapy.

socioeconomic significance of "PD first for older adults" based on the characteristics of bacterial peritonitis, which is one of the reasons for limiting the duration of PD. Thus, there is a perspective on the sustainability of the medical system in the selection of renal replacement therapy.

KT is approximately at the same level as PD and tends to be more cost-effective [17]. Particularly, KT has the best incremental cost-utility ratio (ICUR) for renal death at 51,600 (USD/Qaly) when converted to medical costs using the exchange rate of the year of publication. Furthermore, it should be noted that the results of this study did not reflect the superiority of the treatment mechanism or the cumulative cost of transplantation medicine because of a short observation period (analysis period) of 3 years. Thus, it can be inferred that KT outperforms other modalities in terms of long-term clinical and economic performance.

HD, which accounts for the majority of renal replacement therapy in Japan, has almost the same results as the cost-effectiveness judgment criteria in the medical insurance system set by the government authorities, and as described in the previous section, its socioeconomic usefulness is significant [10]. Additionally, online HD with improved dialysate quality significantly improves the QOL and function [18]. In Japan, HD is advantageous in terms of facility access and medical management. Therefore, it is essential to select a therapy suitable for the condition and lifestyle of each patient to further develop a treatment system for ESRD.

5. Health economics evaluation of marginal donors

As discussed in the previous section, KT, as a therapy for ESRD, is generally considered economically superior. Therefore, although the widespread use of KT is desired, a solution to the limitations of therapy selection (e.g., securing a donor) has long been expected. As the burden of renal failure increases in Japan, the use of marginal donors in kidney transplantation medicine is expanding. Therefore, based on the definition of a marginal donor developed in a research project, we introduce a preliminary report that verifies its medical economic usefulness through a cost-effectiveness analysis.

This study [19] utilized renal transplant registry data from the Japan Society for Transplantation and Tokyo University Health Economy Big Data (TheBD). The evaluation group included marginal donors, while the control group included standard donors. The eGFR cut-off of 70 mL/min/1.73 m^2 was used to separate the two. Clinical results (engraftment rate, mortality rate, etc.) were analyzed from the renal transplant registry data, and the cost elements (hospitalization and outpatients by disease) of the medical economic big data were extrapolated to the obtained results. In the cost-effectiveness analysis, total medical costs (kidney transplantation medical costs and related disease treatment costs) were used as cost indicators and life-years (LYs) were used as effect indicators. Survival analysis was performed using the Kaplan-Meier method and Wilcoxon rank-sum test.

There were 3336 marginal donors and 7960 standard donors (**Table 4**). There was no significant difference ($p = 0.681$) in survival between the two groups (**Figure 7**). Regarding cost-effectiveness, the standard donor group tended to be slightly better in each observation period, but there was no statistically significant difference between the two (overall:2.59 million JPY/LY/year vs. 2.48 million JPY/LY/year, $p = 0.849$). Multiple regression analysis revealed that donor eGFR at transplantation, recipient age at transplantation, and dialysis duration were statistically significant factors

Item	(parameter)	Unit	Standard donor			Marginal donor			p-value
Number of samples	Whole population	N	7960			3336			
Observation period		year	4.1	±	2.4	3.8	±	2.3	NS
Donor type		%							
	Living donor		100.0			100.0			
	Deceased donor		0.0			0.0			
Sex		Male ratio (%)							
	Recipient		63.6			62.3			
	Donor		36.0			38.3			
Age		year							
	Recipient		44.7	±	16.0	47.3	±	14.7	NS
	Donor		54.9	±	11.2	61.8	±	8.7	NS
Primary disease	(top 50%)	%							
	IgA nephropathy		16.2			15.6			
	Diabetic Nephropathy (NIDDM)		15.0			14.3			
	Not clear		17.8			21.5			
Dialysis history	(recipient prior treatment)								
	Hemo/ Peritoneal/ Combination	%	80.1			78.9			
	Introduction period	year	3.4	±	4.7	3.4	±	5.0	NS
Recipient comorbidity	(at the time of transplantation: overlap)	%							
	Cardiovascular complications		83.8			82.7			
	Diabetic complications		12.5			23.2			
Donor test value									
	BMI	kg/m^2	22.8	±	9.8	23.2	±	9.0	NS
	Blood pressure (systolic)	mmHg	123.2	±	14.7	125.6	±	15.1	NS
	Serum creatinine	mg/dL	0.64	±	0.12	0.82	±	0.15	< 0.05
	eGFR	$mL/min/1.73m^2$	85.9	±	12.9	62.2	±	6.7	< 0.05
Donor history		%							
	Diabetes		4.8			3.9			
	Heart disease		1.5			2.2			

(Note) NIDDM, non-insulin-dependent diabetes mellitus. (Source: Ref. [19])

Table 4.
Composition of the target population.

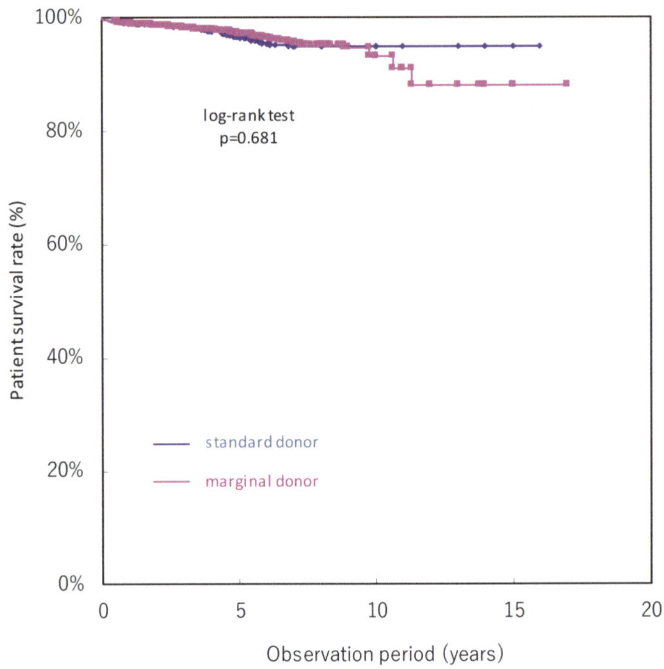

Figure 7.
Comparison of survival rates between marginal and standard donor groups (Kaplan-Meier curve).

influencing cost-effectiveness (**Table 5**). No statistically significant difference was observed in the analysis in which the conditions for setting the standard donor group were stricter and the age at transplantation and dialysis history were the same for both groups (**Table 6**).

Item	Standard partial regression coefficient	F-value	p-value	Standard error	VIF
d_eGFR at transplantation	−0.033	6.164	< 0.05	0.181	1.02
d_Postoperative hospital stay	0.003	0.044	NS	0.559	1.02
d_BMI value	0.002	0.026	NS	0.916	1.05
d_Systolic blood pressure	0.014	1.145	NS	0.189	1.06
d_Diabetes	0.011	0.654	NS	5.288	1.01
r_Age at transplantation	0.031	5.134	< 0.05	0.199	1.08
r_Duration of dialysis	0.054	16.375	< 0.01	0.587	1.05
r_Diabetes	0.007	0.270	NS	5.976	1.13
r_Cardiovascular disease	0.020	2.220	NS	3.380	1.06
Constant term		0.131	NS	43.281	

Model: $p < 0.01$.
(Note) d_, donor; r_, recipient.

Table 5.
Factors affecting cost-effectiveness (multiple regression analysis).

Item	Standard donor	Marginal donor	p-value
Standard donor's conditions (cut-off) and patient's background conditions (age, dialysis)	Donor eGFR>80	Donor eGFR<70	
	Donor age<70	Recipient age: adjusted	
	Donor complications: None	History of dialysis introduction: adjustment	
	Donor BMI<25	Pediatric exclusion	
Recipient age (years)	44.4 ± 16.5	44.3 ± 12.7	NS
History of dialysis introduction (years)	3.6 ± 4.9	3.3 ± 4.7	NS
Donor eGFR (mL/min/1.73m^2)	88.4 ± 14.2	62.2 ± 6.8	< 0.05
Cost-effectiveness (10,000 JPY/LY/year)	199.7 ± 191.1	215.7 ± 453.5	NS

(Note) Units in the table are eGFR: mL/min/1.73m^2, age: years old, and BMI: kg/m^2.
Supplement: SD notation.

Table 6.
Cost-effectiveness analysis with more detailed conditions for standard donors. (source: Ref. [19]).

The results of this study showed that the survival and cost-effectiveness in the marginal donor group were not significantly lower than those in the standard donor group. These results are generally valid in the clinical settings in Japan, where the practice of marginal donors is expanding while maintaining the clinical results of kidney transplantation. In the future, along with a robust evaluation by non-inferiority trials, continuous (prospective) verification of long-term results using high-quality research designs, such as randomized trials, will be essential.

6. Conclusions

This study first explored the relationship between UHC and medical innovations. The results suggested that expansion of the real economy and public investment is necessary for the progress of the medical system. Next, the method of explaining the medical and socioeconomic value of lifesaving was explained using HD research reports as examples. Based on the findings of previous studies, we highlighted case studies on the cost-effectiveness of renal replacement therapy and clarified that the performance of KT was generally better than that of other therapies. Finally, research on the medical economics of marginal donors against the backdrop of considering measures to promote KT was introduced. In the future, it will be important to select an appropriate therapy to further increase its clinical value for patients with ESRD.

Acknowledgements

We gratefully acknowledge the work of the past and present members of our study. This manuscript received significant help from Dr. Yoshiko Yamamoto. Section 5 of this chapter was funded by the Japan Agency for Medical Research and Development (research project title: Investigating new evidence to understand the safety of kidney transplantation from marginal donors).

Conflict of interest

The authors declare no conflict of interest.

Other declarations

It was ensured that articles in other languages cited in this paper were acceptable secondary publications.

Author details

Tomoyuki Takura[1*], Naotsugu Ichimaru[2] and Atushi Aikawa[3]

1 Department of Healthcare Economics and Health Policy, Graduate School of Medicine, The University of Tokyo, Tokyo, Japan

2 Department of Urology, Kinki Central Hospital, Hyogo, Japan

3 Department of Nephrology, Toho University School of Medicine, Tokyo, Japan

*Address all correspondence to: ttakura@m.u-tokyo.ac.jp

References

[1] GBD Chronic Kidney Disease Collaboration. Global, regional, and national burden of chronic kidney disease, 1990-2017: A systematic analysis for the global burden of disease study 2017. Lancet. 2020;**395**(10225):709-733. DOI: 10.1016/S0140-6736(20)30045-3

[2] Takura T. Values and Prices of Medical Care - Towards the Era of Choice and Decision. Tokyo: Igaku-Shoin; 2021. pp. 0-276. (Japanese)

[3] Takura T. Clinical economic value explanation in neurology. Clinical Neurology. 2011;**50**(50):1055-1057 (Japanese)

[4] Takura T. Advanced medicine as an industrial policy. El Hospital. 2014;**73**(7):528-533 (Japanese)

[5] Takura T, Miura H. Socioeconomic determinants of universal health coverage in the Asian region. International Journal of Environmental Research and Public Health. 2022;**19**(4):2376. DOI: 10.3390/ijerph19042376

[6] Eastin RV, Arbogast GL. Demand and Supply Analysis: Introduction (READING 13). Charlottesville: CFA Institute; 2011. pp. 0-54. [Internet]. Available from: https://www.cfainstitute.org/-/media/documents/support/programs/cfa/prerequisite-economics-material-demand-and-supply-analysis-intro.ashx [Accessed: 2023-03-20]

[7] Takura T. Socio-economic considerations of universal health coverage: Focus on the concept of health care value and medical treatment Price. In: Tavares AI, editor. Health Insurance. London: IntechOpen; 2022. pp. 1-34. DOI: 10.5772/intechopen.104798

[8] Takura T. An evaluation of clinical economics and cases of cost-effectiveness. Internal Medicine. 2018;**57**(9):1191-1200. DOI: 10.2169/internalmedicine.9835-17

[9] Takura T, Hiramatsu M, Nakamoto H, et al. Health economic evaluation of peritoneal dialysis based on cost-effectiveness in Japan: A preliminary study. ClinicoEconomics and Outcomes Research. 2019;**25**(11):579-590. DOI: 10.2147/CEOR.S212911

[10] Takura T, Nakanishi T, Kawanishi H, el. Cost-effectiveness of maintenance Hemodialysis in Japan. Therapeutic Apheresis and Dialysis. 2015;**19**(5):441-449. DOI: 10.1111/1744-9987.12314

[11] Dor A et al. End-stage renal disease and economic incentives: the International Study of Health Care Organization and Financing (ISHCOF). Review International Journal of Health Care Finance and Economics. 2007;7(2-3):73-111

[12] Health at a Glance 2009: OECD Indicators. OECD; 2009

[13] Robinson BM et al. World, mortality risk is high soon after initiation of hemodialysis. Kidney International. 2014;**85**(1):158-65. / End-stage renal disease and economic incentives: ISHCOF

[14] Howell M, Walker RC, Howard K. Cost effectiveness of dialysis modalities: A systematic review of economic evaluations. Applied Health Economics and Health Policy. 2019;**17**(3):315-330. DOI: 10.1007/s40258-018-00455-2

[15] Busink E, Kendzia D, Kircelli F, et al. A systematic review of the cost-effectiveness of renal replacement

therapies, and consequences for decision-making in the end-stage renal disease treatment pathway. European Journal of Health Economics. 2022;**24**(3):377-392. DOI: 10.1007/s10198-022-01478-2

[16] Taha A, Iman Y, Hingwala J, et al. Patient navigators for CKD and kidney failure: A systematic review. Kidney Medicine. 2022;**4**(10):100540. DOI: 10.1016/j.xkme.2022.100540

[17] Takura T. Evaluation of the medical economic value of kidney transplantation. Journal of the Japanese Society of Clinical Kidney. Transplantation. 2017;**5**(2):113-121 (Japanese)

[18] Takura T, Kawanishi H, Minakuchi J, et al. Cost-effective analysis of online hemodiafiltration in Japan. Blood Purification. 2013;**35**(Suppl. 1):85-89

[19] Takura T, Ichimaru N. Health economic evaluation of marginal donors in kidney transplantation. Journal of the Japanese Society of Clinical Kidney. Transplantation. 2021;**9**(2):157-163 (Japanese)